Enhanced Recovery in the ICU after Cardiac Surgery & New Developments in Cardiopulmonary Resuscitation

Editors

DANIEL T. ENGELMAN
CLIFTON W. CALLAWAY

CRITICAL CARE CLINICS

www.criticalcare.theclinics.com

Consulting Editor
JOHN A. KELLUM

October 2020 • Volume 36 • Number 4

ELSEVIER

1600 John F. Kennedy Boulevard • Suite 1800 • Philadelphia, Pennsylvania, 19103-2899

http://www.theclinics.com

CRITICAL CARE CLINICS Volume 36, Number 4
October 2020 ISSN 0749-0704, ISBN-13: 978-0-323-72276-6

Editor: Kerry Holland
Developmental Editor: Casey Potter

Critical Care Clinics (ISSN: 0749-0704) is published quarterly by Elsevier Inc., 360 Park Avenue South, New York, NY 10010-1710. Months of issue are January, April, July, and October. Business and Editorial Offices: 1600 John F. Kennedy Blvd., Suite 1800, Philadelphia, PA 19103-2899. Customer Service Office: 6277 Sea Harbor Drive, Orlando, FL 32887-4800. Periodicals postage paid at New York, NY and additional mailing offices. Subscription prices are $250.00 per year for US individuals, $683.00 per year for US institutions, $100.00 per year for US students and residents, $285.00 per year for Canadian individuals, $856.00 per year for Canadian institutions, $318.00 per year for international individuals, $856.00 per year for international institutions, $100.00 per year for Canadian students/residents, and $150.00 per year for foreign students/residents. To receive student/resident rate, orders must be accompanied by name of affiliated institution, date of term, and the signature of program/residency coordinator on institution letterhead. Orders will be billed at individual rate until proof of status is received. Foreign air speed delivery is included in all *Clinics* subscription prices. All prices are subject to change without notice. POSTMASTER: Send address changes to *Critical Care Clinics*, Elsevier Periodicals Customer Service, 11830 Westline Industrial Drive, St. Louis, MO 63146. **Customer Service: 1-800-654-2452 (US). From outside of the US, call 1-314-447-8871. Fax: 1-314-447-8029. E-mail: journalscustomerservice-usa@elsevier.com (for print support) or journalsonlinesupport-usa@elsevier.com (for online support).**

Reprints. For copies of 100 or more of articles in this publication, please contact the Commercial Reprints Department, Elsevier Inc., 360 Park Avenue South, New York, NY 10010-1710. Tel.: 212-633-3874; Fax: 212-633-3820; E-mail: reprints@elsevier.com.

Critical Care Clinics is also published in Spanish by Editorial Inter-Medica, Junin 917, 1er A, 1113, Buenos Aires, Argentina.

Critical Care Clinics is covered in *MEDLINE/PubMed (Index Medicus)*, *EMBASE/Excerpta Medica*, *Current Concepts/Clinical Medicine*, *ISI/BIOMED*, and *Chemical Abstracts*.

Contributors

CONSULTING EDITOR

JOHN A. KELLUM, MD, MCCM
Professor, Critical Care Medicine, Medicine, Bioengineering and Clinical and Translational Science, Director, Center for Critical Care Nephrology, The Clinical Research Investigation and Systems Modeling of Acute Illness (CRISMA) Center, Vice Chair for Research, Department of Critical Care Medicine, University of Pittsburgh School of Medicine, Pittsburgh, Pennsylvania, USA

EDITORS

DANIEL T. ENGELMAN, MD
Associate Professor of Surgery, Heart and Vascular Program, Baystate Health and University of Massachusetts Medical School–Baystate, Springfield, Massachusetts, USA

CLIFTON W. CALLAWAY, MD, PhD
Professor and Vice-Chair of Emergency Medicine, University of Pittsburgh School of Medicine, Pittsburgh, Pennsylvania, USA

AUTHORS

KEITH B. ALLEN, MD
Department of Cardiothoracic Surgery, Saint Luke's Mid America Heart Institute, University of Missouri-Kansas City School of Medicine, Kansas City, Missouri, USA

JESSICA ERIN ALLENDER, PharmD
Cardiovascular and Thoracic Surgery, WakeMed Health and Hospitals, Raleigh, North Carolina, USA

RAKESH C. ARORA, MD, PhD
Cardiac Sciences Program, St. Boniface Hospital, Department of Surgery, Max Rady College of Medicine, University of Manitoba, Winnipeg, Manitoba, Canada

LINDA F. BARR, MD
Assistant Professor of Medicine, Division of Pulmonary and Critical Care Medicine, Johns Hopkins School of Medicine, Baltimore, Maryland, USA

JASON A. BARTOS, MD, PhD
Associate Professor, Cardiovascular Division, University of Minnesota, Center for Resuscitation Medicine, Minneapolis, Minnesota, USA

MARK R. BONNELL, MD
Department of Cardiothoracic Surgery, University of Toledo, Toledo, Ohio, USA

MICHAEL J. BOSS, MD
Chief Cardiac Anesthesia, University of Maryland Saint Joseph Medical Center, Towson, Maryland, USA

WILLIAM T. BRADFORD, MD
Cardiovascular and Thoracic Surgery, WakeMed Health and Hospitals, Raleigh, North Carolina, USA

BARRY BURSTEIN, MD
Division of Pulmonary and Critical Care Medicine, Department of Internal Medicine, Mayo Clinic, Rochester, Minnesota, USA

JESTIN N. CARLSON, MD, MS
Department of Emergency Medicine, Saint Vincent Hospital, Allegheny Health Network, Erie, Pennsylvania, USA

SUBHASIS CHATTERJEE, MD
Assistant Professor of Surgery, Michael E. DeBakey Department of Surgery, Baylor College of Medicine, Director Thoracic Surgical ICU and ECMO Program, Texas Heart Institute at CHI Baylor St. Luke's Medical Center, Division of Cardiovascular Surgery, Houston, Texas, USA

DAVID J. COHEN, MD
Department of Cardiology, Saint Luke's Mid America Heart Institute, University of Missouri-Kansas City School of Medicine, Kansas City, Missouri, USA

CAMERON DEZFULIAN, MD, FAHA
Associate Professor, Critical Care Medicine, Associate Professor, Clinical and Translational Sciences, University of Pittsburgh School of Medicine, Pittsburgh, Pennsylvania, USA

JILL ENGEL, NP
Division of Cardiovascular and Thoracic Surgery, Department of Surgery, Duke University Medical Center, Durham, North Carolina, USA

DANIEL T. ENGELMAN, MD
Associate Professor of Surgery, Heart and Vascular Program, Baystate Health and University of Massachusetts Medical School–Baystate, Springfield, Massachusetts, USA

RICHARD M. ENGELMAN, MD
Clinical Professor Emeritus of Surgery at Tufts University School of Medicine, Heart and Vascular Program, Baystate Health and University of Massachusetts Medical School–Baystate, Springfield, Massachusetts, USA

NICK FLETCHER, MBBS, FRCA, FFICM
Consultant Cardiac Anaesthetist, St George's University Hospitals, Chair of the Institute of Anaesthesia and Critical Care, Cleveland Clinic, London, United Kingdom

MARC W. GERDISCH, MD
Department of Cardiothoracic Surgery, Franciscan Health Heart Center, Indianapolis, Indiana, USA

JOHN GREHAN, MD, PhD
Department of Cardiothoracic Surgery, Allina Health, Saint Paul, Minnesota, USA

KENDRA J. GRUBB, MD
Department of Cardiothoracic Surgery, Emory University, Atlanta, Georgia, USA

T. SLOANE GUY, MD
Department of Surgery, Division of Cardiac Surgery, Sidney Kimmel Medical College, Thomas Jefferson University, Philadelphia, Pennsylvania, USA

AILEEN HILL, MD
Department of Intensive Care Medicine, 3CARE—Cardiovascular Critical Care and Anesthesia Evaluation and Research, University Hospital RWTH Aachen, Aachen, Germany

GUILLAUME L. HOAREAU, PhD
Assistant Professor, Division of Emergency Medicine, University of Utah School of Medicine, Salt Lake City, Utah, USA

ALICE HUTIN, MD, PhD
Assistant Professor, SAMU de Paris, Necker Hospital, Paris, France

MARJAN JAHANGIRI, MBBS, MS, FRCS (CTh)
Professor of Cardiac Surgery, Department of Cardiothoracic Surgery, St George's Hospital, London, United Kingdom

OLIVER K. JAWITZ, MD
Division of Cardiovascular and Thoracic Surgery, Department of Surgery, Duke Clinical Research Institute, Duke University Medical Center, Durham, North Carolina, USA

SHRUTI JAYAKUMAR, MBBS
Cardiac Surgery Research Fellow, Department of Cardiothoracic Surgery, St George's Hospital, London, United Kingdom

JACOB C. JENTZER, MD, FACC, FAHA
Assistant Professor of Medicine, Division of Pulmonary and Critical Care Medicine, Departments of Internal Medicine and Cardiovascular Medicine, Mayo Clinic, Rochester, Minnesota, USA

MICHAEL AUSTIN JOHNSON, MD, PhD
Assistant Professor, Division of Emergency Medicine, University of Utah School of Medicine, Salt Lake City, Utah, USA

MIRA KÜLLMAR, MD
Department of Anesthesiology, Intensive Care and Pain Medicine, University of Münster, Münster, Germany

ALI KHOYNEZHAD, MD, PhD, FACS, FHRS
Professor of Surgery at UCLA, Director of Cardiovascular Surgery, MemorialCare Heart and Vascular Institute, MemorialCare Long Beach Medical Center, Long Beach, California, USA

LIONEL LAMHAUT, MD, PhD
Associate Professor, SAMU de Paris, Necker Hospital, Paris, France

KEVIN P. LANDOLFO, MD
Department of Cardiothoracic Surgery, Mayo Clinic, Jacksonville, Florida, USA

ERIC J. LAVONAS, MD, MS
Faculty Physician, Department of Emergency Medicine, Rocky Mountain Poison and Drug Safety, Denver Health, Denver, Colorado, USA; Professor, Department of Emergency Medicine, University of Colorado School of Medicine, Aurora, Colorado, USA

KEVIN W. LOBDELL, MD
Professor, Atrium Health-Sanger Heart and Vascular Institute Cardiac Surgery, Charlotte, North Carolina, USA

MICHAEL A. MAZZEFFI, MD, MPH, MSc
Associate Professor of Anesthesiology, University of Maryland School of Medicine, Baltimore, Maryland, USA

GINA McCONNELL, RN
Cardiovascular and Thoracic Surgery, WakeMed Health and Hospitals, Raleigh, North Carolina, USA

CIANA McCARTHY, MB, FCAI, JFICMI, EDIC, MEd
Critical Care Clinical Fellow, St Georges University Hospital, London, United Kingdom

LAURIE J. MORRISON, MD, MSc, FRCPC
Clinician Scientist, Rescu, Li Ka Shing Knowledge Institute, St Michael's Hospital, Professor, Division of Emergency Medicine, Department of Medicine, Faculty of Medicine, University of Toronto, Toronto, Ontario, Canada

YOSHIFUMI NAKA, MD, PhD
Division of Cardiothoracic Surgery, Department of Surgery, Columbia University Irving Medical Center, New York, New York, USA

NIRAV C. PATEL, MD
Department of Cardiothoracic Surgery, Lenox Hill Hospital, New York, New York, USA

RAWN SALENGER, MD
Assistant Professor of Surgery, University of Maryland School of Medicine, Baltimore, Maryland, USA

MICHAEL SANDER, MD
Professor, Department of Anesthesiology, Intensive Care Medicine and Pain Therapy, University Hospital Giessen, Justus-Liebig University Giessen, Giessen, Germany; Charity Medical University, Berlin, Germany

ROHAN SANJANWALA, MD, MPH
Cardiac Sciences Program, St. Boniface Hospital, Winnipeg, Manitoba, Canada

CHRISTIAN STOPPE, MD, FAHA
Department of Intensive Care Medicine, 3CARE—Cardiovascular Critical Care and Anesthesia Evaluation and Research, University Hospital RWTH Aachen, Aachen, Germany; Department of Anesthesiology, Intensive Care Medicine and Pain Therapy, University Hospital Würzburg, Würzburg, Germany

BRADLEY S. TAYLOR, MD
Associate Professor of Surgery, University of Maryland School of Medicine, Baltimore, Maryland, USA

VINOD H. THOURANI, MD
Department of Cardiovascular Surgery, Marcus Heart and Vascular Center, Piedmont Heart Institute, Atlanta, Georgia, USA

JOSEPH L. TONNA, MD
Assistant Professor, Division of Emergency Medicine, University of Utah School of Medicine, Division of Cardiothoracic Surgery, University of Utah, Salt Lake City, Utah, USA

NANA-MARIA WAGNER, MD
Department of Anesthesiology, Intensive Care and Pain Medicine, University of Münster, Münster, Germany

HENRY E. WANG, MD, MS
Department of Emergency Medicine, The University of Texas Health Science Center at Houston, Houston, Texas, USA

JUDSON B. WILLIAMS, MD, MHS
Division of Cardiovascular and Thoracic Surgery, Department of Surgery, Duke University Medical Center, Durham, North Carolina, USA; Cardiovascular and Thoracic Surgery, WakeMed Health and Hospitals, Raleigh, North Carolina, USA

SCOTT T. YOUNGQUIST, MD, MS
Associate Professor, Division of Emergency Medicine, University of Utah School of Medicine, Salt Lake City, Utah, USA

ALEXANDER ZARBOCK, MD
Department of Anesthesiology, Intensive Care and Pain Medicine, University of Münster, Münster, Germany

Contents

How to Start an Enhanced Recovery After Surgery Cardiac Program   571

Oliver K. Jawitz, William T. Bradford, Gina McConnell, Jill Engel, Jessica Erin Allender, and Judson B. Williams

In this review the authors introduce a practical approach to guide the initiation of an enhanced recovery after surgery (ERAS) cardiac surgery program. The first step in implementation is organizing a dedicated multidisciplinary ERAS cardiac team composed of representatives from nursing, surgery, anesthesiology, and other relevant allied health groups. Identifying a program coordinator or navigator who will have responsibilities for developing and implementing educational initiatives, troubleshooting, monitoring progress and setbacks, and data collection is also vital for success. An institution-specific protocol is then developed by leveraging national guidelines and local expertise.

Surgical Site Infections in Cardiac Surgery   581

Shruti Jayakumar, Ali Khoynezhad, and Marjan Jahangiri

Surgical site infection (SSI) can be a significant complication of cardiac surgery, delaying recovery and acting as a barrier to enhanced recovery after cardiac surgery. Several risk factors predisposing patients to SSI including smoking, excessive alcohol intake, hyperglycemia, hypoalbuminemia, hypo- or hyperthermia, and Staphylococcus aureus colonization are discussed. Various measures can be taken to abolish these factors and minimize the risk of SSI. Glycemic control should be optimized preoperatively, and hyperglycemia should be avoided perioperatively with the use of intravenous insulin infusions. All patients should receive topical intranasal Staphylococcus aureus decolonization and intravenous cephalosporin if not penicillin allergic.

Preoperative Treatment of Malnutrition and Sarcopenia in Cardiac Surgery: New Frontiers   593

Aileen Hill, Rakesh C. Arora, Daniel T. Engelman, and Christian Stoppe

Cardiac surgery is performed more often in a population with an increasing number of comorbidities. Although these surgeries can be lifesaving, they disturb homeostasis and may induce a temporary overall loss of physiologic function. The required postoperative intensive care unit and hospital stay often lead to a mid- to long-term decline of nutritional and physical status, mental health, and health-related quality of life. Prehabilitation before elective surgery might be an opportunity to optimize the state of the patient. This article discusses current evidence and potential effects of preoperative optimization of nutrition and physical status before cardiac surgery.

Marc W. Gerdisch, Keith B. Allen, Yoshifumi Naka, Mark R. Bonnell, Kevin P. Landolfo, John Grehan, Kendra J. Grubb, David J. Cohen, T. Sloane Guy, Nirav C. Patel, and Vinod H. Thourani

Enhanced recovery after surgery (ERAS) protocols recognize early postoperative mobilization as a driver of faster postoperative recovery, return to normal activities, and improved long-term patient outcomes. For patients undergoing open cardiac surgery, an opportunity for facilitating earlier mobilization and a return to normal activity lies in the use of improved techniques to stabilize the sternal osteotomy. By following the key orthopedic principles of approximation, compression, and rigid fixation, a more nuanced approach to sternal precaution protocols is possible, which may enable earlier patient mobilization, physical rehabilitation, and recovery.

Linda F. Barr, Michael J. Boss, Michael A. Mazzeffi, Bradley S. Taylor, and Rawn Salenger

Multimodal pain management of cardiac surgical patients is a paradigm shift in postoperative care. This promising approach features complementary medications and techniques that spare opioids and improves symptomatic and functional recovery. Although the specific elements remain to be defined, the collaboration of the health care team and patient and continuous iterative programmatic improvements are important pillars of this approach.

Kevin W. Lobdell, Subhasis Chatterjee, and Michael Sander

Goal-directed therapy couples therapeutic interventions with physiologic and metabolic targets to mitigate a patient's modifiable risks for death and complications. Goal-directed therapy attempts to improve quality-of-care metrics, including length of stay, rate of readmission, and cost per case. Debate persists around specific parameters and goals, the risk profiles that may benefit, and associated therapeutic strategies. Goal-directed therapy has demonstrated reduced complication rates and lengths of stay in noncardiac surgery studies. Establishing goal-directed therapy's early promise and role in cardiac surgery—namely, producing fewer complications and deaths—will require larger studies, including those with greater focus on high-risk patients.

Ciana McCarthy and Nick Fletcher

Prolonged intubation and mechanical ventilation following cardiac surgery have been associated with increased hospital and intensive care unit length of stays; higher health care costs; and morbidity resulting from atelectasis, intrapulmonary shunting, and pneumonia. Early extubation was developed as a strategy in the 1990s to reduce the high-dose opiate regimes and long ventilator times. Early extubation is a key component of the enhanced recovery pathway following cardiac surgery and enables early mobilization and early return to a normal diet. The plan to extubate should start as soon as the patient is scheduled for cardiac surgery and continue throughout the perioperative period.

This review provides an overview for health care teams involved in the perioperative care of cardiac surgery patients. The intention is to summarize key determinants of delirium, its impact on short- and long-term outcomes as well as to discuss effective management strategies. The first component of this review examines the prevalence and the factors associated with an increased risk of postoperative delirium. A multitude of predisposing (eg, baseline vulnerability and comorbidities) and precipitating (eg, type of cardiac surgery and postoperative care) factors that contribute to the occurrence of delirium are discussed.

Cardiac surgery–associated acute kidney injury (CSA-AKI) is a common complication after cardiac surgery and associated with a worse outcome. The pathogenesis of CSA-AKI is complex and multifactorial. Therapeutic options for severe CSA-AKI are limited to renal replacement therapy constituting a supportive measure. Therefore, risk identification, prevention, and early diagnosis are of utmost importance to improve patient outcomes. This review aims to provide an overview of the diagnosis, pathophysiologic mechanisms, and risk factors of CSA-AKI and delineates the strategies for AKI prevention available to improve patient outcomes after cardiac surgery.

Airway management during cardiac arrest has undergone several advancements. Endotracheal intubation (ETI) often is considered the gold standard for airway management in cardiac arrest; however, other options exist. Recent prospective randomized trials have compared outcomes in bag-valve mask ventilation and supraglottic airways to ETI in out-of-hospital cardiac arrest. ETI, if performed early in resuscitation, is associated with worse patient outcomes and has been de-emphasized so as

recurrent opioid effects. Patients with opioid overdose may be admitted to the intensive care unit for naloxone infusions, treatment of noncardiogenic pulmonary edema, autonomic instability, or sequelae of hypoxia-ischemia or cardiac arrest. Primary and secondary prevention are important to reduce the number of people with life-threatening opioid overdose.

Comprehensive Cardiac Care After Cardiac Arrest

Barry Burstein and Jacob C. Jentzer

Cardiac arrest (CA) results in multiorgan ischemia until return of spontaneous circulation and often is followed by a low-flow shock state. Upon restoration of circulation and organ perfusion, resuscitative teams must act quickly to achieve clinical stability while simultaneously addressing the underlying etiology of the initial event. Optimal cardiovascular care demands focused management of the post–cardiac arrest syndrome and associated shock. Acute coronary syndrome should be considered and managed in a timely manner, because early revascularization improves patient outcomes and may suppress refractory arrhythmias. This review outlines the diagnostic and therapeutic considerations that define optimal cardiovascular care after CA.

CRITICAL CARE CLINICS

THE CLINICS ARE AVAILABLE ONLINE!
Access your subscription at:
www.theclinics.com

Section 1: Enhanced Recovery in the ICU After Cardiac Surgery

Preface

The Journey from Fast Tracking to Enhanced Recovery

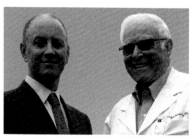

Daniel T. Engelman, MD, *Editor*, and Richard M. Engelman, MD

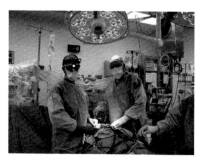

Daniel T. Engelman, MD and Richard M. Engelman, MD

My life's work in cardiac surgery began in 1968 at New York University, when I was a resident with Drs Frank Spencer and George Green. At that time, coronary bypass grafting (CABG) was just emerging as a therapeutic option for selected patients with symptomatic coronary artery disease. Dr Green had introduced internal mammary artery utilization, but saphenous veins were still our routine conduit of choice. Anesthesia was a combination of high-dose opioids, benzodiazepines, and long-acting inhalational agents. Patients remained intubated until at least the day after surgery and were on mandatory bedrest in the intensive care unit (ICU) for a minimum of 48 hours. Cardiac rehabilitation didn't begin before 72 hours and allowed only for very limited ambulation. Discharge was routinely 1 to 2 weeks after surgery, and patients were encouraged to remain sedentary for the next 4 to 6 weeks. These practices remained the standard for cardiac surgical perioperative care for decades, and morbidity following surgery was not inconsequential.

About 10 years later, I moved to Baystate Medical Center in Springfield, Massachusetts, where I founded the first cardiac surgical program in the western half of the state. In the early 1990s, I read an article by Bernard Krohn and colleagues in the *Journal of Thoracic and Cardiovascular Surgery* describing early discharge from The Hospital of the Good Samaritan in Los Angeles, and the excellent long-term results they achieved by paying close attention to perioperative care.[1] With this in mind, in 1992 we began a collaboration with colleagues at Hartford Hospital in Connecticut to develop what we called a "Fast-Track" approach to care for CABG patients. Our process to care included the following:

Crit Care Clin 36 (2020) xv–xviii
https://doi.org/10.1016/j.ccc.2020.07.010
0749-0704/20/© 2020 Published by Elsevier Inc.

1. Recruitment of a Fast-Track Coordinator to oversee patient care
2. Development of an evidence-based Care Pathway
3. Documentation of compliance and an appreciation of Care Pathway variance with attention paid to deviation from the Pathway
4. Involvement of a multidisciplinary team, including anesthesiology and critical care

The results of our efforts were documented in a presentation at the American College of Surgeons Surgical Forum[2] in 1993 and a 1994 publication in the *Annals of Thoracic Surgery*.[3] A review of consecutive patients undergoing CABG surgery 6 months before (N = 282) and 6 months after (N = 280) program implementation found that 48% of Fast-Track patients could be discharged early (3 to 5 days after surgery), nearly double the rate prior to Fast-Track implementation, with no increases in morbidity or mortality. Extubation times, ICU stay, and overall hospital stay were also dramatically reduced. The critical components were early extubation (<8 hours), limitation of intravenous fluids, control of atrial arrhythmias, normalization of gut function, and early ambulation. The discharge procedure incorporated the patient's family in the recovery process and utilized a Clinical Coordinator, Case Manager, Fast-Track Coordinator, and an outpatient Nurse Practitioner. As soon as it became apparent how effective this process was for CABG patients, we incorporated the same approach for all cardiac surgical procedures.

In 1993, the Baystate Cardiac Surgical program, together with Toronto General Hospital and Oxford Heart Centre, organized a live, international, multidisciplinary teleconference to describe and promote the Fast-Track approach, with attendees representing 40 cardiac surgical institutions. Since our first publication in 1994, there have been more than 700 peer-reviewed articles written about Fast-Track recovery in all surgical subspecialties. I am gratified that tens of thousands of patients have benefited from shorter lengths of stay and improved outcomes following all types of surgery, based on these guiding principles.

—Richard M. Engelman, MD

In 1999, I followed in my father's footsteps, becoming a board-certified cardiothoracic surgeon after graduating from Brigham and Women's Hospital in Boston, Massachusetts. As my career progressed, I noticed waning interest in the Fast-Track protocols popularized by my father in the 1990s, coincident with increasing provider concern about patient-reported outcomes and the costs associated with care.[4] Unfortunately, the potential risks of readmissions secondary to an early discharge, or poor HCAHPS (Hospital Consumer Assessment of Healthcare Providers and Systems) survey scores from patients with perceived excessive pain,[5] threatened to outweigh the benefits of these Fast-Track protocols.

Changes in cardiac surgical training and practice patterns also played roles. As percutaneous interventional techniques improved, they replaced some of the open cardiac surgical volume and changed workflows. There was an increased emphasis on reducing any and all delays between patient evaluation and surgical procedures. Preoperative optimization was at odds with this new urgency.

Furthermore, national and international cardiac surgical conferences mainly focused on technique while devoting far less time and didactic material to evidence-based best practices in perioperative care. Cardiac surgical training programs were shortened, and the emphasis on preoperative and postoperative care was reduced. Finally, postoperative patient care has increasingly become the responsibility of critical care specialists, as surgeons spent a greater proportion of their time in the operating room performing longer and more complex procedures.

In 2017, after reading multiple articles about the success of the Enhanced Recovery After Surgery (ERAS) Programs in most surgical specialties, I and a group of like-minded cardiac surgeons, decided to explore opportunities for introducing these same principles to cardiac surgery. The national and international interest was tremendous. A few early studies were simultaneously being conducted outlining enhanced recovery protocols demonstrating improved outcomes within our specialty.[6] What was old was now new again.

That same year, we formed the nonprofit ERAS Cardiac Society with the mission to improve surgical care and recovery through research, education, audit, and implementation of evidence-based best practices. The society's membership was distributed evenly among anesthesiologists, intensivists, and cardiac surgeons specializing in perioperative care. After a formal collaboration with the international ERAS Society,[7] our first guidelines were published in 2019 in *JAMA Surgery*.[8] The international interest in this topic has been extraordinary. This report has been downloaded over 140,000 times and was the most viewed article, in the highest-impact surgical journal in 2019.[9]

In this issue of *Critical Care Clinics*, we summarize 9 major topics in Enhanced Recovery After Cardiac Surgery. The articles begin with preoperative optimization and follow the patient through the intraoperative and, finally, postoperative phases of recovery.

Advances in cardiac surgical operative techniques and myocardial protection have dramatically improved outcomes. An unfortunate and unintended consequence is that 80% of the preventable morbidity and mortality following cardiac surgery is now occurring outside of the operating room.[10] Our hope is that a renewed emphasis on evidence-based best practices and standardized perioperative care will reduce overall morbidity and mortality and improve patient-centric care.

The Fast-Track recovery protocols that began under my father's leadership in 1992 will continue to evolve as more data are published from around the world. What was initially designed to speed up discharge has now evolved to emphasize improvement in each patient's perceptions of their ability to return to their presurgical state with the least discomfort, the fewest complications, and a minimal interruption in their daily lives.

This issue of *Critical Care Clinics* would never have been possible without the extraordinary contributions of the true "father" of Enhanced Recovery After Cardiac Surgery, Dr Richard Engelman. It is therefore dedicated to all of those patients who have already benefited and who will benefit in the future from special attention to standardizing evidence-based best practices in perioperative care. I would like to personally thank my father for starting us on this long but worthwhile journey.

—Daniel T. Engelman, MD

Daniel T. Engelman, MD
Richard M. Engelman, MD
Heart and Vascular Program
Baystate Health and University of Massachusetts Medical School–Baystate
759 Chestnut Street
Springfield, MA 01199, USA

E-mail address:
daniel.engelman@baystatehealth.org

REFERENCES

1. Krohn BG, Kay JH, Mendez MA, et al. Rapid sustained recovery after cardiac operations. J Thorac Cardiovasc Surg 1990;100(2):194–7.
2. Deaton DW, Engelman RM, Rousou J, et al. Fast track recovery of the cardiac surgical patient. Surg Forum 1993;44:223–5.
3. Engelman RM, Rousou JA, Flack JE 3rd, et al. Fast-track recovery of the coronary bypass patient. Ann Thorac Surg 1994;58(6):1742–6.
4. Shahian DM, Jacobs JP, Badhwar V, et al. Risk aversion and public reporting. part 1: observations from cardiac surgery and interventional cardiology. Ann Thorac Surg 2017;104(6):2093–101.
5. Available at: https://www.cms.gov/Medicare/Quality-Initiatives-Patient-Assessment-Instruments/HospitalQualityInits/HospitalHCAHPS. Accessed August 4, 2020.
6. Williams JB, McConnell G, Allender JE, et al. One-year results from the first US-based enhanced recovery after cardiac surgery (ERAS Cardiac) program. J Thorac Cardiovasc Surg 2019;157(5):1881–8.
7. Available at: https://www.businesswire.com/news/home/20180619006294/en/ERAS-Cardiac-Surgery-Officially-Joins-ERAS-Society. Accessed August 4, 2020.
8. Engelman DT, Ben Ali W, Williams JB, et al. Guidelines for perioperative care in cardiac surgery: enhanced recovery after surgery society recommendations. JAMA Surg 2019;154(8):755–66.
9. Kibbe MR. JAMA Surgery—The Year in Review, 2019. JAMA Surgery 2020;155:377–8.
10. Shannon FL, Fazzalari FL, Theurer PF, et al. A method to evaluate cardiac surgery mortality: phase of care mortality analysis. Ann Thorac Surg 2012;93(1):36–43.

How to Start an Enhanced Recovery After Surgery Cardiac Program

Oliver K. Jawitz, MD[a,b], William T. Bradford, MD[c],
Gina McConnell, RN[c], Jill Engel, NP[d], Jessica Erin Allender, PharmD[c],
Judson B. Williams, MD, MHS[a,c],*

KEYWORDS

- ERAS • Enhanced recovery • Cardiac surgery • Perioperative care

KEY POINTS

- Organizing a multidisciplinary enhanced recovery after surgery (ERAS) cardiac team with a dedicated program coordinator is key to launching a successful cardiac enhanced recovery initiative.
- The most important component of a successful ERAS cardiac program is an institution-specific protocol that is standardized and agreed on by all relevant stakeholders.
- After ERAS initiation, regular monitoring should be performed to identify protocol deviations, search for adverse events, and achieve the continuous quality improvement that is central to an ERAS cardiac program.

BACKGROUND

Since first introduced in Denmark in the 1990s, enhanced recovery after surgery (ERAS) programs have now become increasingly prevalent among surgical centers in North America, Western Europe, and indeed worldwide.[1] Although initially targeting patients undergoing major abdominal operations, ERAS protocols have since been developed and expanded to address inflammation, endocrine function, metabolism, pain, as well as surgical and anesthetic complications in patients undergoing many specialty procedures including orthopedic, gynecologic, urologic, head and neck, thoracic, and now cardiac.[2,3] General surgery ERAS programs have consisted of

[a] Division of Cardiovascular and Thoracic Surgery, Department of Surgery, Duke University Medical Center, Box 3443, Durham, NC 27710, USA; [b] Duke Clinical Research Institute, Duke University Medical Center, Box 3443, Durham, NC 27710, USA; [c] Cardiovascular and Thoracic Surgery, WakeMed Health and Hospitals, 3000 New Bern Avenue, Suite 1100, Raleigh, NC 27610, USA; [d] Division of Cardiovascular and Thoracic Surgery, Department of Surgery, Duke University Medical Center, DUMC 3442, 2301 Erwin Road, Durham, NC 27710, USA
* Corresponding author. Cardiovascular and Thoracic Surgery, WakeMed Health and Hospitals, 3000 New Bern Avenue, Suite 1100, Raleigh, NC 27610.
E-mail address: judson.williams@duke.edu
Twitter: @ojawitzMD (O.K.J.); @JudsonBWilliams (J.B.W.)

Crit Care Clin 36 (2020) 571–579
https://doi.org/10.1016/j.ccc.2020.07.001
0749-0704/20/© 2020 Elsevier Inc. All rights reserved.
criticalcare.theclinics.com

efforts to optimize medications and patient education, minimize invasiveness, promote multimodal opioid-sparing analgesia, mitigate complications, and encourage early mobilization.[4] Such programs have resulted in a substantial improvement in hospital length of stay, as well as reductions in complications, readmissions, and overall health care costs.[4–6] Procedure-specific protocols for nongeneral surgery specialties have since been developed in recent years with supporting scientific evidence.[7]

Although cardiac surgery has been a relatively late adopter of an officially labeled "ERAS" pathway, outcomes-based quality improvement efforts have been widespread for decades. In the 1990s, the cardiac surgery "fast-track" movement was initiated by Dr Richard Engelman and others, with an aim to limit intensive care unit (ICU) length of stay through a balanced anesthetic technique with reduced opioid dependency, patient education, early extubation, and mobilization.[8] This approach successfully reduced ICU and hospital lengths of stay by 20%, as well as ventilator times by 30% without any adverse increase in morbidity or mortality.[9,10]

Other examples of highly impactful patient care improvement efforts include the design of multiple risk stratification models, the building of large cardiac surgery databases, and the development of multidisciplinary practice guidelines.[11–17] In 2019, the ERAS cardiac expert consensus statement was published, marking the culmination of a diverse, multidisciplinary effort to systematically evaluate the evidence supporting clinical practices in perioperative cardiac surgery.[18] Here, the authors introduce a practical approach to guide the initiation of an ERAS cardiac surgery program with the aim of implementing similar evidence-based best practices.

ORGANIZING A DEDICATED ENHANCED RECOVERY AFTER SURGERY CARDIAC TEAM

The first step in implementing a successful ERAS cardiac program is organizing a dedicated ERAS cardiac team. This team must be multidisciplinary in nature, with representation from all key stakeholders including nursing, surgery, anesthesiology, and other relevant allied health groups. The team will meet frequently and be tasked with developing their own center-specific ERAS cardiac protocol, ensuring all interested parties have an opportunity to provide input, develop, and rollout education initiatives for program dissemination and finally perform continuous process monitoring, evaluation, and improvement.

Identification of a Program Coordinator

One of the most important members of the ERAS cardiac team is the program coordinator or navigator, who is often a nurse champion who will oversee all aspects of the ERAS program design and development. Specifically, the coordinator will have responsibilities for developing and implementing educational initiatives, troubleshooting, monitoring progress and setbacks, and data collection. Engaging nursing staff in peer-to-peer education is particularly important, as many ERAS cardiac interventions are nursing based and will not be successful without broad buy-in from these essential frontline team members.

Identification of Specialty Champions

Specialty champions must be identified from both cardiac surgery and anesthesiology. These individuals will serve the important role of helping develop and implement a center-specific ERAS protocol that will be acceptable to their clinician colleagues. Historically, surgeons and anesthesiologists have often used varied approaches to patient care, making the process of standardization quite challenging.

These physician preferences are often based on personal experience, training, and culture, rather than based on evidence or guidelines validated in the literature. Successful implementation of an ERAS program, however, requires all caregivers to adopt a standardized evidence-based approach without deviation. As such, these specialty champions are essential and should be empowered to represent their respective groups or partners. Many institutions will also require a critical care unit physician champion depending on the role of a designated ICU team in the postoperative care. Intensivists are in a unique position to oversee all aspects of ERAS protocol implementation in the immediate postoperative period. Indeed, what will be learned in support of a cardiac surgical program will be beneficial for support of perioperative and posttrauma patients in general.

Identification of Key Allied Health Representatives

The perioperative management of cardiac surgery patients is complex, often requiring knowledgeable pharmacists, intensivists, perfusionists, cardiologists, physical therapists, advance practice providers, and others. Successful ERAS cardiac teams include champions from these areas, based on local surgical models of care. We have found that pharmacy champions are essential in determining potential medication interactions under ERAS protocols, particularly among immunosuppressed patient populations and those with other complex medical conditions. A pharmacy champion also brings knowledge of best-value pharmacologic multimodal analgesia alternatives and changes in local purchasing prices for pharmacologic components of the pathway. Champions from the perfusion team can spearhead efforts surrounding goal-directed perfusion, a burgeoning area of growth with roll-out of advanced perfusion monitoring linked with the electronic medical record.

DESIGNING AN ENHANCED RECOVERY AFTER SURGERY CARDIAC PROTOCOL

After organizing a dedicated ERAS cardiac team, the first major task is to design a mutually agreed on setting-specific ERAS protocol. Although many ERAS cardiac principals are key to all programs, such as multimodal analgesia and early extubation, a one-size-fits-all approach is not likely to be successful. Institutional differences may influence pathway components, such as the presence or absence of 24-hour skilled cardiothoracic critical care coverage, which may influence the type of invasive and noninvasive monitoring used. Local expertise should be used and local barriers acknowledged, to achieve a nuanced individualized evidence-based pathway for care.

Standardization is the Key Driver of Success

Although designing an ERAS protocol for the management of all aspects of perioperative cardiac surgical care is a noble endeavor, the most important aspect of a successful ERAS cardiac surgical program is standardization. It is important to recognize that cardiac surgery patients are a unique population, and unlike many other surgical specialties with ERAS interventions, the patients incorporate cardiopulmonary bypass, hypothermia, extracorporeal support, and hemodynamic manipulations. The complexity of perioperative care in these patients mandates a multidisciplinary approach with multiple involved stakeholders. As such, if consensus is unachievable for particular interventions, leaving those out of the current iteration of the protocol is preferable, rather than derailing the entire enhanced recovery effort. Furthermore, the protocol should only include agreed-upon interventions, mitigating the need for practitioners to "opt out" of interventions that did not achieve consensus. Visual education tools also provide an important means of furthering consensus and standardization of the key goals and maintain the focus on patient-centered care (**Fig. 1**).

Leverage National Guidelines

Although ERAS programs in cardiac surgery are a relatively recent development, multiple national guidelines, society statements, and published protocols for program design have been published and should all be leveraged in the design of the setting-specific ERAS program.[19–22] This includes the recent 2019 systematic review and consensus statement by Engelman and colleagues,[18] which used the American College of Cardiology/American Heart Association "Classification of Recommendations and Level of Evidence" approach to review and grade aspects of ERAS cardiac protocols based on published meta-analyses, randomized controlled trials, large nonrandomized studies, and reviews.[23] The body of literature with existing evidence for perioperative cardiac interventions should be rigorously reviewed by the ERAS cardiac team, including the risks and benefits of each ERAS component, until consensus regarding a comprehensive set of perioperative practices can be achieved.

Leverage Local Expertise

In addition to using published guidelines in the creation of an ERAS program, ERAS cardiac teams should also carefully consider areas of local expertise. For example, a program with experience in parasternal nerve blocks may consider this intervention as part of the opioid-sparing measures in the protocol. Similarly, interventions by experts in patient-reported outcomes, ICU delirium, and biomarkers may be incorporated into a successful ERAS cardiac initiative. Leveraging local expertise not only has the potential to improve patient care in a standardized fashion but also promotes broad multidisciplinary buy-in for the program and provides additional avenues for data collection and other academic pursuits.

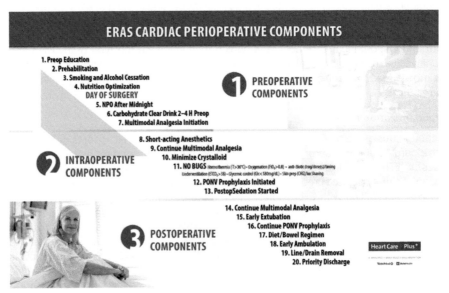

Fig. 1. A visual used in the ERAS cardiac program in Raleigh, NC, USA.

RECEIVING INPUT FROM ALL KEY STAKEHOLDERS

Successful ERAS cardiac programs are designed using input and feedback from key stakeholders, including patients. The importance of reaching out to all potentially affected care providers cannot be overstated.

Identify Barriers

Table 1 reviews barriers and interventions for successful development and roll-out of an ERAS cardiac pathway. Input from all key stakeholders enables the expedient identification of all potential barriers to the implementation of a working ERAS protocol. Tailoring the protocol to the specific health system and environment of care is vital to success. Because achieving buy-in from the entire team is often a central problem in implementing an ERAS protocol, each stakeholder must be individually engaged. Ensuring that each clinician and discipline that would be affected by the standardization of care processes feels valued and contributory is of utmost importance in addressing barriers and facilitating adoption. Although this process is indeed time consuming and potentially resource intensive, this effort will substantially increase the likelihood of success after the protocol is initiated.

Identify Enablers

Just as important as identifying potential barriers to protocol implementation is identifying enablers. ERAS program enablers may include individuals from the nursing staff, physical therapy, the ICU, or even cardiology with a strong desire to improve patient care. These individuals should be approached early in the program design process to promote a successful rollout of the ERAS protocol. In addition, site-based grant funding for any component of the ERAS cardiac program should be thoroughly investigated. These funding sources have the potential to be extremely valuable, particularly because health systems increase their focus on readmission prevention, length-of-stay reduction, and opioid minimization.

IMPLEMENTING EFFECTIVE EDUCATIONAL INITIATIVES

A vital component of the development of an ERAS cardiac program is education. Although some members of the care team may be familiar with ERAS protocols in

Table 1		
Barriers and interventions used for successful implementation of an ERAS cardiac pathway		
Barrier	**Description**	**Intervention**
Lack of evidence for ERAS in cardiac surgery	Paucity of published data from similar institutions with ERAS cardiac experience	Literature review for each component; subject matter experts consulted
Physician preferences	Surgeon, anesthesiologist, and intensivist preferences	Champions empowered from each group; information technology standardization
Financial	No mechanism existed to pay for interventions	Meetings with health system administration regarding value-added
Engagement and education of staff	Hundreds of staff members from inpatient and outpatient care units required education and input	Education and unit-based meetings with ERAS cardiac champion

other surgical specialties, it is important to train all individuals on the new specific standardized ERAS cardiac pathway. This includes surgeons, anesthesiologists, nurse educators, ICU nurses, nurse anesthetists, advanced practice providers, step-down nurses, dieticians, pharmacists, administration/management, as well as outpatient, preoperative, intraoperative, and discharge staff. Education becomes a continuous process as new hires are a reality in each phase of care, from preoperative secretarial staff to intraoperative nursing and postoperative advance practice providers. In addition to providing formal education opportunities regarding the individual elements of the ERAS cardiac pathway, it is beneficial to frequently emphasize that the overall goal is to create a standardized approach for improved patient care.

IMPLEMENTATION TIMELINE

START
Core team identified

1–2 MO
- Literature, facility resources and provider preferences reviewed to develop pathway
- Metrics determined and baseline metrics before implementation recorded
- Obtain executive sponsorship and support

3–4 MO
- Education of providers along every component including changes to current treatment, new treatments, reasons for the change, and expectations of every provider

6 MO
- ERAS for Cardiac Surgery started practice wide
- Opportunities for feedback to the core team including barriers, compliance, successes, and areas to improve
- Core team remained in constant communication with one another with every barrier that arose and would quickly respond to the ones reporting the barrier and possibly reeducate providers if needed

9–12 MO
- Metrics analyzed often for changes that have occurred both positive and negative with a response to negative changes if needed in pathway
- After initial implementation and metric analysis, further possible changes to pathway explored and implemented for following phases

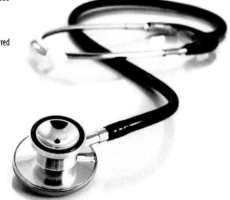

Fig. 2. Sample timeline for the development and implementation of an ERAS cardiac program.

PURSUING CONTINUOUS PROCESS IMPROVEMENT

Before ERAS implementation, audit allows ERAS cardiac teams to establish baseline guideline compliance, length of ICU and hospital stay, and track complications, to set a benchmark for postprotocol initiation improvements. After the beginning of the ERAS pathway, regular monitoring is performed for identifying protocol deviations, searching for adverse events, and achieving the continuous quality improvement that is central to the ERAS cardiac program. Efforts should be focused on areas where compliance is low, iterating toward improved outcomes.[24] In most situations, the nurse or advance practice provider champion on the ERAS cardiac team assumes primary responsibility for investigating deviations in protocol, concerns or potential adverse events, and facilitating process improvements. This individual also serves as the communication link between team members and the multidisciplinary members involved in patient care. At regularly scheduled ERAS cardiac meetings, the nurse champion is able to convey to the rest of the team how effective the program has been, address concerns, and consider modifications as warranted. Suggestions and changes may come from stakeholders across the health system or may be the result of new evidence in the scientific literature. Over time, ensuring successful implementation of the ERAS program will become less burdensome; however, the nurse or advanced practice provider champion will continue to play a major role in facilitating process improvements and monitoring patient outcomes. The team's clinical pharmacist can lead audits and monitor opioid use, whereas data analysts can collect program outcomes, including total opioid use, length of stay, readmissions, and costs of care.

Optimize the Use of the Electronic Medical Record

The electronic medical record (EMR) can be an invaluable tool for ensuring ERAS protocol adherence, rolling out updates to the ERAS care pathway, and identifying patients who may require additional perioperative optimization. Local EMR programming experts should be engaged for building automated preoperative and postoperative order sets, promoting standardization and improving efficiency. Furthermore, the EMR should be used to alert the clinical team about medication interactions as well as highlight important preoperative testing and laboratory results, which may trigger action for preoperative medical optimization.

SUMMARY: BUILDING A TIMELINE FOR SUCCESS

The ERAS cardiac pathway is an example of value-based care applied to cardiac surgery patients, with primary goals of early recovery, opioid minimization, and cost reduction. Protocol standardization and achieving broad multidisciplinary buy-in for all of the pathway interventions is critical to ensuring a successful ERAS rollout. This requires a motivated ERAS cardiac coordinator, as well as a team of engaged champions from each phase of care and discipline. Continuous quality improvement with assimilation of new evidence and close monitoring of clinical outcomes will make an ERAS cardiac program nimble and sustainable. A sample timeline is provided (**Fig. 2**), which outlines the development and implementation of an ERAS cardiac program in a period of 9 to 12 months.

DISCLOSURE

The authors have nothing to disclose.

REFERENCES

1. Kehlet H, Dahl JB. Anaesthesia, surgery, and challenges in postoperative recovery. Lancet 2003;362(9399):1921–8.
2. Carmichael JC, Keller DS, Baldini G, et al. Clinical practice guideline for enhanced recovery after colon and rectal surgery from the American Society of Colon and Rectal Surgeons (ASCRS) and Society of American Gastrointestinal and Endoscopic Surgeons (SAGES). Surg Endosc 2017;31(9):3412–36.
3. ERAS Society. History of the ERAS Society. 2019. Available at: http://erassociety.org/about/history/. Accessed July 1, 2019.
4. Greco M, Capretti G, Beretta L, et al. Enhanced recovery program in colorectal surgery: a meta-analysis of randomized controlled trials. World J Surg 2014; 38(6):1531–41.
5. Gustafsson UO, Oppelstrup H, Thorell A, et al. Adherence to the ERAS protocol is associated with 5-year survival after colorectal cancer surgery: a retrospective cohort study. World J Surg 2016;40(7):1741–7.
6. Feldheiser A, Aziz O, Baldini G, et al. Enhanced Recovery after Surgery (ERAS) for gastrointestinal surgery, part 2: consensus statement for anaesthesia practice. Acta Anaesthesiol Scand 2016;60(3):289–334.
7. Ljungqvist O, Scott M, Fearon KC. Enhanced recovery after surgery: a review. JAMA Surg 2017;152(3):292–8.
8. Engelman RM, Rousou JA, Flack JE 3rd, et al. Fast-track recovery of the coronary bypass patient. Ann Thorac Surg 1994;58(6):1742–6.
9. Myles PS, Daly DJ, Djaiani G, et al. A systematic review of the safety and effectiveness of fast-track cardiac anesthesia. Anesthesiology 2003;99(4):982–7.
10. Wong WT, Lai VK, Chee YE, et al. Fast-track cardiac care for adult cardiac surgical patients. Cochrane Database Syst Rev 2016;(9):CD003587.
11. Shahian DM, O'Brien SM, Filardo G, et al. The Society of Thoracic Surgeons 2008 cardiac surgery risk models: part 1–coronary artery bypass grafting surgery. Ann Thorac Surg 2009;88(1 Suppl):S2–22.
12. O'Brien SM, Shahian DM, Filardo G, et al. The Society of Thoracic Surgeons 2008 cardiac surgery risk models: part 2–isolated valve surgery. Ann Thorac Surg 2009;88(1 Suppl):S23–42.
13. Shahian DM, O'Brien SM, Filardo G, et al. The Society of Thoracic Surgeons 2008 cardiac surgery risk models: part 3–valve plus coronary artery bypass grafting surgery. Ann Thorac Surg 2009;88(1 Suppl):S43–62.
14. Nashef SA, Roques F, Sharples LD, et al. EuroSCORE II. Eur J Cardiothorac Surg 2012;41(4):734–44 [discussion: 744–5].
15. Hagan PG, Nienaber CA, Isselbacher EM, et al. The International Registry of Acute Aortic Dissection (IRAD): new insights into an old disease. JAMA 2000; 283(7):897–903.
16. Edwards FH, Engelman RM, Houck P, et al. The Society of Thoracic Surgeons practice guideline series: antibiotic prophylaxis in cardiac surgery, part i: duration. Ann Thorac Surg 2006;81(1):397–404.
17. Engelman R, Baker RA, Likosky DS, et al. The Society of Thoracic Surgeons, The Society of Cardiovascular Anesthesiologists, and The American Society of Extra-Corporeal Technology: clinical practice guidelines for cardiopulmonary bypass–temperature management during cardiopulmonary bypass. Ann Thorac Surg 2015;100(2):748–57.

18. Engelman DT, Ben Ali W, Williams JB, et al. Guidelines for perioperative care in cardiac surgery: enhanced recovery after surgery society recommendations. JAMA Surg 2019;154(8):755–66.
19. McConnell G, Woltz P, Bradford WT, et al. Enhanced recovery after cardiac surgery program to improve patient outcomes. Nursing 2018;48(11):24–31.
20. Williams JB, McConnell G, Allender JE, et al. One-year results from the first US-based enhanced recovery after cardiac surgery (ERAS Cardiac) program. J Thorac Cardiovasc Surg 2019;157(5):1881–8.
21. Fleming IO, Garratt C, Guha R, et al. Aggregation of marginal gains in cardiac surgery: feasibility of a perioperative care bundle for enhanced recovery in cardiac surgical patients. J Cardiothorac Vasc Anesth 2016;30(3):665–70.
22. Krzych L, Kucewicz-Czech E. It is time for enhanced recovery after surgery in cardiac surgery. Kardiol Pol 2017;75(5):415–20.
23. Jacobs AK, Anderson JL, Halperin JL, et al. The evolution and future of ACC/AHA clinical practice guidelines: a 30-year journey: a report of the American College of Cardiology/American Heart Association Task Force on practice guidelines. Circulation 2014;130(14):1208–17.
24. Nelson G, Dowdy SC, Lasala J, et al. Enhanced recovery after surgery (ERAS(R)) in gynecologic oncology - practical considerations for program development. Gynecol Oncol 2017;147(3):617–20.

Surgical Site Infections in Cardiac Surgery

Shruti Jayakumar, MBBS[a], Ali Khoynezhad, MD, PhD, FHRS[b],
Marjan Jahangiri, MBBS, MS, FRCS (CTh)[a,*]

KEYWORDS

- Surgical site infection • Sternal wound infections • Mediastinitis • Cardiac surgery

KEY POINTS

- Patients scheduled to undergo cardiac surgery should have preoperative hemoglobin A_{1c} testing. The glycemic state should be optimized with a combination of conservative and medical therapies.
- Hyperglycemia should be avoided both in the perioperative and postoperative periods. Intravenous insulin infusions are recommended if hyperglycemia is present.
- As part of a surgical site infection prevention bundle, all patients should receive topical intranasal *Staphylococcus aureus* decolonization before surgery and an intravenous cephalosporin within 60 minutes before skin incision. An additional dose of intravenous vancomycin can be given 60 to 120 minutes before skin incision in patients known to have methicillin-resistant *Staphylococcus aureus* colonization.
- Clipping should be used immediately before surgery instead of shaving.
- Normothermia should be maintained and hypoxia should be avoided.

INTRODUCTION

Surgical site infection (SSI) can be significantly detrimental to a patient's recovery. A SSI may result in sepsis, increased postoperative pain, impede early mobilization and increase hospital stay and mortality. It is also associated with a substantial financial burden,[1] especially in cases of deep sternal infection. Minimizing the risk of SSI is imperative to an enhanced recovery after surgery program.

There are several known risk factors for the development of SSIs. The main predisposing factors are diabetes, smoking, obesity, and poor nutrition, which are all known to impair wound healing. Risk factors related to the operation include prolonged procedures, blood transfusion, and inadequate surgical scrub or skin preparation. In addition, physiologic states of hyperglycemia, hypo- or hyperthermia, and hypoxia both intra- and postoperatively are associated with an increased risk of SSI due to its negative effects on wound healing.[2]

[a] Department of Cardiothoracic Surgery, St. George's Hospital, Blackshaw Road, London SW17 0QT, UK; [b] MemorialCare Heart and Vascular Institute, MemorialCare Long Beach Medical Center, 2801 Atlantic Avenue, Long Beach, CA 90806, USA
* Corresponding author.
E-mail address: marjan.jahangiri@stgeorges.nhs.uk

Crit Care Clin 36 (2020) 581–592
https://doi.org/10.1016/j.ccc.2020.06.006
0749-0704/20/Crown Copyright © 2020 Published by Elsevier Inc. All rights reserved.
criticalcare.theclinics.com

Rigorous SSI prevention is particularly important in cardiac surgery. Infection risk is increased by use of chest drains, cardiopulmonary bypass, and an additional number of secondary surgical sites after conduit harvesting. In addition, internal mammary artery harvesting can increase the risk of both superficial and deep sternal wound infection particularly with bilateral harvests, due to a reduction in blood supply to the sternum. This risk is significantly greater in patients with diabetes.[3] Cardiac surgical care should include bundles to minimize SSI. These should be aimed not only at enforcing sterile patient preparation and wound closure but also at optimizing patients preoperatively to minimize SSI risk (**Fig. 1**, **Table 1**).

DEFINITIONS

An SSI is defined as any infection arising from a site of surgery and can be classed into superficial and deep, generally referring to the incision site, although more serious SSIs may involve organs or implanted material.[4]

Superficial Sternal Wound Infections

Superficial sternal wound infections involve only the skin, subcutaneous tissue, and pectoralis fascia without any bony or hardware involvement, presenting with clinical features of discharge, erythema, and low-grade fevers.[5] They occur in up to 8% of patients undergoing cardiac surgery and are associated with hospital readmission and increased costs.[6] Superficial sternal wound infections are typically treated with intravenous antibiotics and wound care as needed, although improperly treated infections may progress to involve the bone.

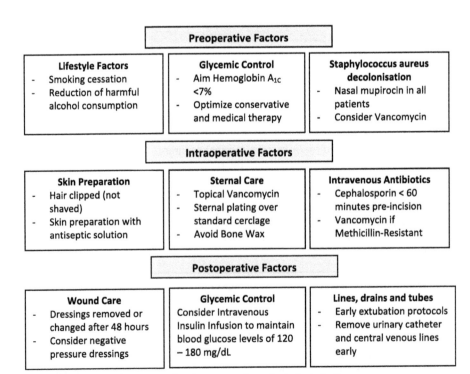

Fig. 1. Factors contributing to development of surgical site infections.

Table 1
Summary of evidence

Modifiable Factors	Recommendations	Level of Evidence
Smoking	Smoking cessation at least 4 wk preoperatively	I C-LD
Harmful or excessive alcohol intake	Minimize or abstain from alcohol for at least 3 wk and ideally 8 wk	I C-LD
Staphylococcus aureus colonization	Topical intranasal mupirocin preoperatively for decolonization	I A
Hair over surgical site	Hair should be clipped not shaved immediately before surgery	I C
Hyperglycemia	Glycosylated hemoglobin (HbA1c) screening in all patients with appropriate glycemic control measures	I B-R
	Peri- and postoperative hyperglycemia should be avoided with intravenous insulin infusions if needed	IIa B-NR
Nutritional deficiencies	Correction of nutritional deficiencies in patients with hypoalbuminemia preoperatively	IIa C-LD
Perioperative antibiotics	Weight-adjusted dose of intravenous cephalosporins should be administered within 60 min before skin incision	I A
	If the operation is >4 h or cardiopulmonary bypass time is >120 min, this should be redosed	I A
	Intravenous vancomycin should be administered if MRSA positive	I B-R
Hyperthermia	Hyperthermia should be avoided during rewarming with cardiopulmonary bypass	III (Harm)
Topical antibiotics	Topical vancomycin paste may be used on cut sternal edges	I B-R
Sternal plating	Rigid sternal fixation should be used to improve sternal healing, particularly in high-risk patients	IIa B-R
Bone wax	Bone wax should be avoided to minimize nonunion	III (Harm)
Wound care	Dressings should be removed or changed after 48 h	I A
Hypoxia	Hypoxia should be avoided	IIa B-NR
Hypothermia	Persistent hypothermia should be avoided postoperatively and in critical care	IB

Abbreviations: LD, limited data; MRSA, methicillin-resistant *Staphylococcus aureus*; NR, non-randomized studies; R, randomized studies.

Deep Sternal Wound Infections

Deep sternal wound infections are characterized by sternal dehiscence and instability and represent a smaller proportion of cardiac SSIs (reported incidence of 0.75%–1.8%).[6–8] Clinical features include purulent discharge and sternal instability. Mediastinitis is a potentially life-threatening complication representing a more widespread and serious type of deep sternal wound infection. Treatment of deep sternal wound infection involves intravenous antibiotics, and patients are readmitted to the hospital for intensive treatment until clinically improved. In addition, patients will usually require surgical debridement and wound management with vacuum drainage and occasional flap reconstruction if undergoing a sternectomy.

Harvest Site Infections

Coronary artery bypass graft surgery (CABG) has the added risk of harvest site infections at conduit surgical sites, which involve the leg for long saphenous vein harvests or the forearm for radial artery harvests. Leg wounds are the most common site of infection in CABG patients with infection rates of up to 15.4%.[9] Open saphenous vein harvesting is associated with an increased risk of harvest site infections compared with endoscopic harvesting.[10]

PREOPERATIVE INTERVENTIONS: BEFORE ADMISSION
Glycemic Control

Optimal glycemic control is one of the most important factors in minimizing risk of SSIs.[11] All patients who undergo elective cardiac surgery should be screened for diabetes preoperatively. Glycemic control should be optimized in advance of surgery, with both conservative interventions and optimization of medical therapy to achieve a hemoglobin A_{1c} (HbA$_{1c}$) of less than 7%, although this should ideally be less than 6.5%.[12] Patients should also be educated regarding exercise, diet, smoking cessation, and alcohol intake, which are important measures for optimizing glycemic control.[12–14] In hyperglycemic patients undergoing urgent or emergency surgery, the use of intravenous insulin infusions should be considered, particularly if blood glucose levels remain elevated (higher than 180 mg/dL). If used, the rate of insulin infusion should be titrated to maintain blood glucose levels of 120 to 180 mg/dL.[13,14] In addition to reducing wound complications, improving glycemic control significantly reduces postoperative morbidity and mortality.

Nutritional Status

Poor nutritional status is associated with negative effects on wound healing, which is a complex process composed of the clotting cascade, neutrophil and macrophage infiltration followed by angiogenesis, granulation tissue formation, and epithelialization. These physiologic processes require significant energy consumption and adequate stores of carbohydrate, protein, amino acids, vitamins (particularly vitamin C), and minerals.[15] Malnutrition and poor metabolic states have been shown to result in decreased wound tensile strength and collagen synthesis and reduced neutrophil and macrophage activity, which leads to both impaired wound healing and poor defense against potential wound infections,[16] leading to increased SSIs. Correction of nutritional deficiencies preoperatively may therefore reduce the risk of SSIs.

Albumin is most commonly used as a clinical marker of nutritional status, and patients with serum albumin levels less than 3.5 g/dL are at higher risk of developing postoperative wound complications.[17] In patients undergoing cardiac surgery, serum prealbumin levels of less than 20 mg/dL were associated with increased risk of postoperative infections.[18] Although no clear evidence or guidelines for preoperative supplementation in cardiac surgery exists, oral nutritional supplementation 5 to 7 days preoperatively in malnourished patients undergoing colorectal surgery reduced the risk of postoperative infections.[19] There is also some evidence to suggest that oral nutritional supplements for 5 days before cardiac surgery can enhance the immune response, thus reducing the incidence of SSIs.[20]

Lifestyle Factors

Smoking, in particular, is strongly associated with delayed wound healing as well as increased susceptibility to infections, thereby increasing the risk of SSIs. Although few studies exist on the effect of smoking on cardiac surgery outcomes, this can be extrapolated from other studies. Preoperative smoking cessation for a period of at least 3 to 4 weeks preoperatively has been shown to improve inflammatory cellular functions and reduce the incidence of SSI.[21–23] Excessive alcohol intake is also an important risk factor for the development of wound complications including SSIs due to suppression of the immune response; this improves 2 weeks after abstinence and normalizes after 8 weeks.[23]

Smoking cessation and minimization of alcohol consumption are low-cost measures that may be easily implemented. All patients should therefore be screened for cigarette smoking and alcohol consumption preoperatively using validated screening tools. Current smokers should be offered nicotine replacement therapies or referred to a smoking cessation service. Patients with alcohol intake exceeding recommended guidelines should be encouraged to abstain for at least 8 weeks preoperatively or referred to a specialist unit if at risk for withdrawal seizures requiring detoxification.[23]

PREOPERATIVE INTERVENTIONS ON ADMISSION

Staphylococcus aureus is a leading cause of postprocedural infections including both superficial and deep SSI.[24,25] In one study, methicillin-sensitive *S aureus* accounted for 28.3% of SSIs, whereas methicillin-resistant *S aureus* was isolated in 14.6% of SSIs, together accounting for almost 50% of SSIs following CABG.[26] Moreover, *S aureus* is a major cause of mediastinitis and is the culprit organism in 20% to 36% of cases.[27,28]

Up to 20% to 45% of patients may be carriers for *S aureus*, which most commonly colonizes the anterior nares. Although this maybe harmless when patients are healthy, colonized patients face up to a 6-fold increase in risk of staphylococcal infections following both medical and surgical procedures, including bacteremia. Nasal *S aureus* colonization has been strongly correlated with postoperative SSI. The risk of SSI following cardiac surgery in colonized patients is up to 9 times the risk of noncolonized patients, and this is augmented in patients with diabetes.[29]

Intranasal mupirocin for nasal decolonization is an effective and low-cost method to significantly reduce the incidence of sternal wound infection in both diabetic and nondiabetic patients.[30] SSI prevention bundles should also include a dose of a cephalosporin antibiotic administered immediately before surgery. In addition, patients who are colonized with methicillin-resistant *S aureus* should also receive a dose of a glycopeptide antibiotic, such as vancomycin, in addition to the standard prophylaxis regime.[31] Universal decolonization, where all patients are treated prophylactically, is more cost-effective and provides greater increase in quality-of-life adjusted years than targeted decolonization provided only to patients who are culture positive.[32] Skin decontamination with a chlorhexidine gluconate shower the day before surgery can reduce bacterial counts but is not associated with a reduction in SSI rate.[33] Previous studies have investigated the use of a vaccine against *S aureus* in patients undergoing cardiac surgery but found no benefit, rather demonstrating increased rates of mortality in patients who developed *S aureus* infections despite vaccinations, suggesting the development of resistant or more aggressive strains.[34]

INTRAOPERATIVE INTERVENTIONS
Perioperative Antibiotics

All patients should receive intravenous prophylactic antibiotics less than 60 minutes before skin incision[35,36] in the form of a weight-adjusted dose of cephalosporin such as cefuroxime or cefazolin. In patients considered at risk of having methicillin-resistant *S aureus* an additional dose of vancomycin should be given 60 to 120 minutes before the skin incision. A further dose of cephalosporin should be given in procedures lasting greater than 4 hours or if cardiopulmonary bypass time exceeds 2 hours.[37,38] In cases of type I hypersensitivity reactions (eg, anaphylaxis) to beta-lactam antibiotics, vancomycin may be given instead, although additional gram-negative coverage should be considered. This is usually an aminoglycoside such as gentamicin. However, this must be used with caution when given in conjunction with vancomycin, due to its ototoxic and nephrotoxic effects, which may be amplified following cardiopulmonary bypass due to reduced renal clearance. Cephalosporins may be administered for up to 48 hours following cardiac surgery but should not be routinely continued beyond this period.[37,39,40] Although Center for Disease Control has recommended discontinuation of antibiotics beyond the intraoperative period,[41] the evidence supporting single-dose antibiotics in cardiac surgery is limited.[42]

Patient Preparation and Sterile Fields

Hair should be clipped around surgical sites using electric clippers before surgery. Shaving may be associated with an increased risk of SSI and should not be undertaken.[43] Skin preparation at the time of surgery should be with a povidone iodine or chlorhexidine solution. In addition, when grafts are harvested from secondary surgical sites during CABG, a dedicated set of sterile instruments should be used for each different harvest site, and these should be kept separate from instruments used in the chest. Separate sterile fields should be used to minimize the risk of cross-contamination. Sterile surgical gloves and gowns should also be changed when moving from secondary surgical sites to the chest. In addition, some evidence suggests changing sterile surgical gloves immediately before wound closure.[44]

Glycemic Control

Surgery activates a physiologic stress response, resulting in release of cortisol, which subsequently leads to hyperglycemia. In addition, in cardiac surgery, increased oxidative stress and the proinflammatory response following cardiopulmonary bypass augment this response. This dysregulation of glucose control is often more severe in patients with preexisting diabetes. As previously discussed, hyperglycemia is significantly associated with development of SSI. Intensive perioperative glycemic control has been shown to improve postoperative outcomes and reduce the incidence of SSI in a wide range of patients including diabetic and nondiabetic populations.[45,46] Insulin infusions may be started to maintain tight blood glucose control, particularly in patients with serum glucose levels persistently greater than 160 mg/dL to 180 mg/dL postoperatively. A blood glucose range of 120 to 180 mg/dL should be targeted perioperatively, and multiple studies have demonstrated a significant reduction in sternal wound infection by maintaining blood glucose levels of less than 180 mg/dL.[11,13] More intensive regimes also exist, although this may be associated with hypoglycemia, which should be avoided in the postoperative period, as it is associated with an increased incidence of cardiorespiratory complications, stroke, and mortality.[47–49]

Operative Techniques and Sternal Closure

Wire cerclage is a well-established technique for sternotomy closure and is used to realign the cut ends of the sternum. Stainless steel wires are either passed through the entire thickness of bone on either side (transsternal) or around the sternum (parasternal) and tightened to adjoin both halves of the sternum. Although it continues to be widely used, it does not prevent sternal movement, particularly from side to side, which causes extended postoperative pain, and may impair bone and wound healing.

Sternal movement, particularly longitudinal movements, may be reduced by using figure of 8 cable wires and is associated with a reduction in wound infections.[50,51]

Sternal fixation with rigid plating provides significantly better sternal healing and union with a reduction in wound complications and SSIs including mediastinitis, as well as reduction in pain and improved quality of life.[52,53] In addition, a recent study found sternal plating to not be associated with increased costs compared with standard wire cerclage.[54] Sternal plating should be considered in all patients but particularly in patients who are at higher risk of sternal complications and SSIs.

Bone wax was previously used to reduce sternal bleeding but is not recommended, as it prevents bone union and acts as a foreign body, resulting in sternal dehiscence and wound infections.[55] Topical vancomycin paste may be applied to the cut sternal edges after sternotomy and just before closure and has been shown to significantly reduce the incidence of sternal wound infection in both diabetic and nondiabetic patient cohorts.[56,57]

The use of triclosan-coated sutures has been suggested, but there is little established benefit from their use and evidence is mixed. No reduction in SSI was demonstrated in multiple randomized trials in patients undergoing colorectal and orthopedic surgery.[58,59] The use of triclosan-coated sutures reported a reduction in SSIs following great saphenous vein harvesting,[60] but this benefit was not seen in another similar trial.[61]

POSTOPERATIVE INTERVENTIONS
Wound Care

Dressings should be changed 48 hours postoperatively. Negative pressure dressings may be used in patients at higher risk of SSI. In patients with sternal drainage but without clinical evidence of wound infection, prophylactic negative pressure dressings or wound therapy may be used to promote wound healing and minimize the risk of SSI.

Maintenance of Metabolic Homeostasis

Maintenance of adequate oxygenation is important to promote wound healing, as well as minimize the risk of pneumonia and other infections. In addition, maintenance of normothermia is vital in the postoperative period to prevent coagulopathies, improve the immune response, and aid wound healing.[62] Persistent hypothermia lasting 2 to 5 hours following cardiac surgery is associated with increased bleeding and coagulopathies necessitating transfusions and results in increased infections.[63] Extended hypothermia should be avoided by using forced-air warming blankets.[64] Minimal evidence exists for the prophylactic use of warmed irrigation or fluids to prevent hypothermia, but if hypothermia remains a persistent problem lasting greater than 5 hours following intensive care admission, patients should be treated with warmed irrigation or intravenous fluids.[65]

Hyperthermia can occur with rewarming following cardiopulmonary bypass and is a risk factor for mediastinitis, particularly in diabetic patients.[66] Therefore, hyperthermia should be avoided during rewarming and in the immediate postoperative period. This includes the hyperthermic return of blood from the cardiopulmonary bypass machine, which would be necessary if the patient is to be warmed up to 37°C (98.6°F).[67,68] Given the temperature gradient necessary to warm the patient, the recommendation is to warm arterial blood up to 36°C (96.8°F) and continue to normothermia with forced-air warming systems.

As previously mentioned, glycemic control is very important in the postoperative period and should be maintained with intravenous insulin infusion when needed.

However, hypoglycemia should be strictly avoided, as this is associated with an increase in morbidity and mortality. This risk is considerably increased when hypoglycemia follows periods of hyperglycemia.[47]

Lines, Drains, and Tubes

Postoperative cardiac surgical patients are intubated, catheterized, and usually have multiple forms of invasive monitoring including a central venous catheter and an arterial line, as well as peripheral cannulas. All these lines and tubes can serve as potential sources of infection postoperatively. Although not directly in the surgical site, the presence of infection elsewhere can increase the risk of SSI through cross-contamination and via the blood stream. Device-associated infection is one of the leading causes of sepsis, accounting for up to 25.6% of all health care–associated infections.[69] Of this group, catheter-associated urinary tract infections and central-catheter–associated blood stream infection account for 5.5% and 2.4%, respectively of health care–associated infections, whereas most of the device-associated infections (7.7% of health care–associated infections) are ventilator-associated pneumonitis.

Early extubation strategies may be used to facilitate extubation within 6 hours postoperatively. These targeted protocols typically involve low-dose opioid anesthesia, which reduce the rates of pneumonia and sepsis that have been associated with increased ICU readmission, reintubation, and length of stay. All of these are detrimental in themselves but also serve as risk factors for development of SSIs.[70]

The use of postoperative chest drains are important to prevent build-up of blood or fluid, which may cause tamponade or hemothorax. However, chest drains, as any other invasive device or foreign body, serves as a potential source for infection and may be safely removed when drainage becomes serous in appearance rather than waiting for cessation of drainage.[71]

SUMMARY

Reducing the magnitude of risk factors for SSIs can minimize the morbidity, mortality, and length of stay following cardiac surgery. Preoperative optimization of lifestyle factors including smoking cessation, minimization of alcohol intake, and improvement of diet as well as glycemic control are vital to improving wound healing and SSI reduction. Variable rate insulin infusions should be commenced perioperatively in the event of hyperglycemia. Staphylococcus decolonization, adequate skin preparation with clipping of hair over surgical sites, and topical vancomycin paste over sternal edges can reduce the risk of SSIs. Normothermia and normoxia should be maintained in the peri- and postoperative periods to preserve metabolic homeostasis, prevent coagulopathy, and enable wound healing. Postoperative strategies should include early removal of lines, drains, and tubes, as well as early extubation, reducing potential sources of infection. These evidence-based, targeted measures are key to ensuring optimal outcomes for patients following cardiac surgery.

DISCLOSURE

The authors have no conflicts of interest to disclose.

REFERENCES

1. Loop FD, Lytle BW, Cosgrove DM, et al. J. Maxwell Chamberlain Memorial Paper. Sternal wound complications after isolated coronary artery bypass grafting: early

and late mortality, morbidity, and cost of care. Ann Thorac Surg 1990;49(2): 179–86 [discussion: 186–7].

2. Cheadle WG. Risk factors for surgical site infection. Surg Infect (Larchmt) 2006; 7(s1):s7–11.

3. Grossi EA, Esposito R, Harris LJ, et al. Sternal wound infections and use of internal mammary artery grafts. J Thorac Cardiovasc Surg 1991;102(3):342–6 [discussion: 346–7].

4. Anderson DJ, Podgorny K, Berríos-Torres SI, et al. Strategies to prevent surgical site infections in acute care hospitals: 2014 update. Infect Control Hosp Epidemiol 2014;35(6):605–27.

5. Lazar HL, Salm TV, Engelman R, et al. Prevention and management of sternal wound infections. J Thorac Cardiovasc Surg 2016;152:962–72.

6. Ridderstolpe L, Gill H, Granfeldt H, et al. Superficial and deep sternal wound complications: incidence, risk factors and mortality. Eur J Cardiothorac Surg 2001;20(6):1168–75.

7. Filsoufi F, Castillo JG, Rahmanian PB, et al. Epidemiology of deep sternal wound infection in cardiac surgery. J Cardiothorac Vasc Anesth 2009;23(4):488–94.

8. Borger MA, Rao V, Weisel RD, et al. Deep sternal wound infection: risk factors and outcomes. Ann Thorac Surg 1998;65(4):1050–6.

9. Vuorisalo S, Haukipuro K, Pokela R, et al. Risk features for surgical-site infections in coronary artery bypass surgery. Infect Control Hosp Epidemiol 1998;19(4):240–7.

10. Gulack BC, Kirkwood KA, Shi W, et al. Secondary surgical-site infection after coronary artery bypass grafting: a multi-institutional prospective cohort study. J Thorac Cardiovasc Surg 2018;155(4):1555–62.e1.

11. Zerr, MBA KJ, Furnary MDAP, et al. Glucose control lowers the risk of wound infection in diabetics after open heart operations. Ann Thorac Surg 1997;63(2): 356–61.

12. Wong J, Zoungas S, Wright C, et al. Evidence-based guidelines for perioperative management of diabetes in cardiac and vascular surgery. World J Surg 2010; 34(3):500–13.

13. Lazar HL, Chipkin SR, Fitzgerald CA, et al. Tight glycemic control in diabetic coronary artery bypass graft patients improves perioperative outcomes and decreases recurrent ischemic events. Circulation 2004;109(12):1497–502.

14. Lazar HL, McDonnell MM, Chipkin S, et al. Effects of aggressive versus moderate glycemic control on clinical outcomes in diabetic coronary artery bypass graft patients. Ann Surg 2011;254(3):458–64.

15. Arnold M, Barbul A. Nutrition and wound healing. Plast Reconstr Surg 2006; 117(SUPPLEMENT):42S–58S.

16. Casey J, Flinn WR, Yao JS, et al. Correlation of immune and nutritional status with wound complications in patients undergoing vascular operations. Surgery 1983; 93(6):822–7.

17. Gu A, Malahias M-A, Strigelli V, et al. Preoperative malnutrition negatively correlates with postoperative wound complications and infection after total joint arthroplasty: a systematic review and meta-analysis. J Arthroplasty 2019;34(5): 1013–24.

18. Yu P-J, Cassiere HA, Dellis SL, et al. Impact of preoperative prealbumin on outcomes after cardiac surgery. J Parenter Enteral Nutr 2015;39(7):870–4.

19. Waitzberg DL, Saito H, Plank LD, et al. Postsurgical infections are reduced with specialized nutrition support. World J Surg 2006;30(8):1592–604.

20. Tepaske R, te Velthuis H, Oudemans-van Straaten HM, et al. Effect of preoperative oral immune-enhancing nutritional supplement on patients at high risk of

infection after cardiac surgery: a randomised placebo-controlled trial. Lancet 2001;358(9283):696–701.

21. Sørensen LT. Wound healing and infection in surgery. The clinical impact of smoking and smoking cessation: a systematic review and meta-analysis. Arch Surg 2012;147(4):373–83.

22. Sørensen LT. Wound Healing and Infection in Surgery: the pathophysiological impact of smoking, smoking cessation, and nicotine replacement therapy: a systematic review. Ann Surg 2012;255(6):1069–79.

23. Tønnesen H, Nielsen PR, Lauritzen JB, et al. Smoking and alcohol intervention before surgery: evidence for best practice. Br J Anaesth 2009;102(3):297–306.

24. Paling FP, Olsen K, Ohneberg K, et al. Risk prediction for Staphylococcus aureus surgical site infection following cardiothoracic surgery; A secondary analysis of the V710-P003 trial. PLoS One 2018;13(3):e0193445.

25. Bode LGM, Kluytmans JAJW, Wertheim HFL, et al. Preventing Surgical-Site Infections in Nasal Carriers of Staphylococcus Aureus. N Engl J Med 2010; 362(1):9–17.

26. Si D, Rajmokan M, Lakhan P, et al. Surgical site infections following coronary artery bypass graft procedures: 10 years of surveillance data. BMC Infect Dis 2014;14:318.

27. Lemaignen A, Birgand G, Ghodhbane W, et al. Sternal wound infection after cardiac surgery: incidence and risk factors according to clinical presentation. Clin Microbiol Infect 2015;21(7). 674.e11-e18.

28. Ma J-G, An J-X. Deep sternal wound infection after cardiac surgery: a comparison of three different wound infection types and an analysis of antibiotic resistance. J Thorac Dis 2018;10(1):377–87.

29. Kluytmans JAJW, Mouton JW, Ijzerman EPF, et al. Nasal carriage of staphylococcus aureus as a major risk factor for wound infections after cardiac surgery. J Infect Dis 1995;171(1):216–9.

30. Cimochowski GE, Harostock MD, Brown R, et al. Intranasal mupirocin reduces sternal wound infection after open heart surgery in diabetics and nondiabetics. Ann Thorac Surg 2001;71(5):1572–9.

31. Schweizer M, Perencevich E, McDanel J, et al. Effectiveness of a bundled intervention of decolonization and prophylaxis to decrease Gram positive surgical site infections after cardiac or orthopedic surgery: systematic review and meta-analysis. BMJ 2013;346:f2743.

32. Hong JC, Saraswat MK, Ellison TA, et al. Staphylococcus aureus prevention strategies in cardiac surgery: a cost-effectiveness analysis. Ann Thorac Surg 2018; 105(1):47–53.

33. Kuhme T, Isaksson B, Dahlin L-G. Wound contamination in cardiac surgery. A systematic quantitative and qualitative study of bacterial growth in sternal wounds in cardiac surgery patients. J Pathol Microbiol Immunol 2007;115(9):1001–7.

34. Fowler VG, Allen KB, Moreira ED, et al. Effect of an investigational vaccine for preventing Staphylococcus aureus infections after cardiothoracic surgery. JAMA 2013;309(13):1368.

35. Ban KA, Minei JP, Laronga C, et al. American College of Surgeons and Surgical Infection Society: surgical site infection guidelines, 2016 update. J Am Coll Surg 2017;224(1):59–74.

36. Leaper D, Burman-Roy S, Palanca A, et al. Prevention and treatment of surgical site infection: summary of NICE guidance. BMJ 2008;337:a1924.

37. Edwards FH, Engelman RM, Houck P, et al, Society of Thoracic Surgeons. The Society of Thoracic Surgeons practice guideline series: antibiotic prophylaxis in cardiac surgery, part i: duration. Ann Thorac Surg 2006;81(1):397–404.

38. Engelman R, Shahian D, Shemin R, et al. The Society of Thoracic Surgeons prac-tice guideline series: antibiotic prophylaxis in cardiac surgery, part II: antibiotic choice. Ann Thorac Surg 2007;83(4):1569–76.
39. Harbarth S, Samore MH, Lichtenberg D, et al. Prolonged antibiotic prophylaxis after cardiovascular surgery and its effect on surgical site infections and antimi-crobial resistance. Circulation 2000;101(25):2916–21.
40. Trent Magruder J, Grimm JC, Dungan SP, et al. Continuous intraoperative cefazolin infusion may reduce surgical site infections during cardiac surgical procedures: a propensity-matched analysis. J Cardiothorac Vasc Anesth 2015;29(6):1582–7.
41. Berríos-Torres SI, Umscheid CA, Bratzler DW, et al. Centers for Disease Control and Prevention guideline for the prevention of surgical site infection, 2017. JAMA Surg 2017;152(8):784.
42. Tamayo E, Gualis J, Flórez S, et al. Comparative study of single-dose and 24-hour multiple-dose antibiotic prophylaxis for cardiac surgery. J Thorac Cardiovasc Surg 2008;136(6):1522–7.
43. Tanner J, Norrie P, Melen K. Preoperative hair removal to reduce surgical site infection. Cochrane Database Syst Rev 2011;(11):CD004122.
44. Vij SC, Kartha G, Krishnamurthi V, et al. Simple operating room bundle reduces super-ficial surgical site infections after major urologic surgery. Urology 2018;112:66–8.
45. Fish LH, Weaver TW, Moore AL, et al. Value of postoperative blood glucose in predicting complications and length of stay after coronary artery bypass grafting. Am J Cardiol 2003;92(1):74–6.
46. Doenst T, Wijeysundera D, Karkouti K, et al. Hyperglycemia during cardiopulmo-nary bypass is an independent risk factor for mortality in patients undergoing car-diac surgery. J Thorac Cardiovasc Surg 2005;130(4):1144.
47. Johnston LE, Kirby JL, Downs EA, et al. Postoperative hypoglycemia is associ-ated with worse outcomes after cardiac operations. Ann Thorac Surg 2017; 103(2):526–32.
48. D'Ancona G, Bertuzzi F, Sacchi L, et al. Iatrogenic hypoglycemia secondary to tight glucose control is an independent determinant for mortality and cardiac morbidity. Eur J Cardiothorac Surg 2011;40(2):360–6.
49. Gandhi GY, Nuttall GA, Abel MD, et al. Intensive intraoperative insulin therapy versus conventional glucose management during cardiac surgery. Ann Intern Med 2007;146(4):233.
50. Almdahl SM, Halvorsen P, Veel T, et al. Avoidance of noninfectious sternal dehis-cence: figure-of-8 wiring is superior to straight wire closure. Scand Cardiovasc J 2013;47(4):247–50.
51. Bottio T, Rizzoli G, Vida V, et al. Double crisscross sternal wiring and chest wound infections: a prospective randomized study. J Thorac Cardiovasc Surg 2003; 126(5):1352–6.
52. Allen KB, Thourani VH, Naka Y, et al. Randomized, multicenter trial comparing sternotomy closure with rigid plate fixation to wire cerclage. J Thorac Cardiovasc Surg 2017;153(4):888–96.e1.
53. Raman J, Lehmann S, Zehr K, et al. Sternal closure with rigid plate fixation versus wire closure: a randomized controlled multicenter trial. Ann Thorac Surg 2012; 94(6):1854–61.
54. Allen KB, Thourani VH, Naka Y, et al. Rigid plate fixation versus wire cerclage: patient-reported and economic outcomes from a randomized trial. Ann Thorac Surg 2018;105(5):1344–50.

55. Steingrímsson S, Gustafsson R, Gudbjartsson T, et al. Sternocutaneous fistulas after cardiac surgery: incidence and late outcome during a ten-year follow-up. Ann Thorac Surg 2009;88(6):1910–5.

56. Vander Salm TJ, Okike ON, Pasque MK, et al. Reduction of sternal infection by application of topical vancomycin. J Thorac Cardiovasc Surg 1989;98(4):618–22.

57. Lazar HL, Ketchedjian A, Haime M, et al. Topical vancomycin in combination with perioperative antibiotics and tight glycemic control helps to eliminate sternal wound infections. J Thorac Cardiovasc Surg 2014;148(3):1035–8, 1038–40.

58. Sandini M, Mattavelli I, Nespoli L, et al. Systematic review and meta-analysis of sutures coated with triclosan for the prevention of surgical site infection after elective colorectal surgery according to the PRISMA statement. Medicine (Baltimore) 2016;95(35):e4057.

59. Sprowson AP, Jensen C, Parsons N, et al. The effect of triclosan-coated sutures on the rate of surgical site infection after hip and knee arthroplasty: a double-blind randomized controlled trial of 2546 patients. Bone Joint J 2018;100-B(3):296–302.

60. Thimour-Bergström L, Roman-Emanuel C, Scherstén H, et al. Triclosan-coated sutures reduce surgical site infection after open vein harvesting in coronary artery bypass grafting patients: a randomized controlled trial. Eur J Cardiothorac Surg 2013;44(5):931–8.

61. Seim BE, Tønnessen T, Woldbaek PR. Triclosan-coated sutures do not reduce leg wound infections after coronary artery bypass grafting. Interact Cardiovasc Thorac Surg 2012;15(3):411–5.

62. Leslie K, Sessler DI. The implications of hypothermia for early tracheal extubation following cardiac surgery. J Cardiothorac Vasc Anesth 1998;12(6 Suppl 2):30–4 [discussion: 41–4].

63. Sessler DI. Perioperative thermoregulation and heat balance. Lancet 2016; 387(10038):2655–64.

64. Engelen S, Himpe D, Borms S, et al. An evaluation of underbody forced-air and resistive heating during hypothermic, on-pump cardiac surgery. Anaesthesia 2011;66(2):104–10.

65. Campbell G, Alderson P, Smith AF, et al. Warming of intravenous and irrigation fluids for preventing inadvertent perioperative hypothermia. Cochrane Database Syst Rev 2015;(4):CD009891.

66. Groom RC, Rassias AJ, Cormack JE, et al. Highest core temperature during cardiopulmonary bypass and rate of mediastinitis. Perfusion 2004;19(2):119–25.

67. Grocott HP, Mackensen GB, Grigore AM, et al. Postoperative hyperthermia is associated with cognitive dysfunction after coronary artery bypass graft surgery. Stroke 2002;33(2):537–41.

68. Nussmeier NA. Management of temperature during and after cardiac surgery. Tex Heart Inst J 2005;32(4):472–6. Available at: http://www.ncbi.nlm.nih.gov/pubmed/16429889. Accessed August 19, 2019.

69. Magill SS, Edwards JR, Bamberg W, et al. Multistate point-prevalence survey of health care–associated infections. N Engl J Med 2014;370(13):1198–208.

70. Camp SL, Stamou SC, Stiegel RM, et al. Quality improvement program increases early tracheal extubation rate and decreases pulmonary complications and resource utilization after cardiac surgery. J Card Surg 2009;24(4):414–23.

71. Gercekoglu H, Aydin NB, Dagdeviren B, et al. Effect of timing of chest tube removal on development of pericardial effusion following cardiac surgery. J Card Surg 2003;18(3):217–24.

Preoperative Treatment of Malnutrition and Sarcopenia in Cardiac Surgery: New Frontiers

Aileen Hill, MD[a],*, Rakesh C. Arora, MD, PhD[b,c],
Daniel T. Engelman, MD[d], Christian Stoppe, MD[a,e]

KEYWORDS

- Prehabilitation • Critical care • Cardiac surgery • Malnutrition • Sarcopenia
- Nutrition therapy • Exercise

KEY POINTS

- Malnutrition and sarcopenia are frequent comorbidities in cardiac surgery patients and negatively affect the patient's short- and long-term outcomes.
- The preoperative period may represent an attractive time window to diagnose malnutrition and sarcopenia and initiate therapy to optimize the patient's nutritional status and physical function before surgery.
- It is hoped that prehabilitation through a combination of enhanced nutrition and exercise may permit the deconditioned and malnourished patient to withstand the stresses of surgery and shorten the recovery phase.

INTRODUCTION

Hundreds of thousands of cardiac surgeries are performed worldwide each year.[1–3] More complex cardiac surgery is performed on an increasingly older population with frequent comorbidities and higher perioperative risk profiles including malnutrition and frailty.[2,4,5]

Although cardiac surgery can be vital for the patient's survival, it is associated with a systemic inflammatory syndrome and disturbs homeostasis, which complicates the postoperative course of these patients.[6] In the past, several strategies have been developed to modulate and decrease the inflammatory response, such as less

[a] Department of Intensive Care Medicine, 3CARE—Cardiovascular Critical Care & Anesthesia Evaluation and Research, University Hospital RWTH Aachen, Pauwelsstraße 30, Aachen D-52074, Germany; [b] Cardiac Sciences Program, St. Boniface Hospital, CR3015-369 Tache Avenue, Winnipeg, Manitoba R2H 2A6, Canada; [c] Department of Surgery, Max Rady College of Medicine, University of Manitoba, Winnipeg, Manitoba, Canada; [d] Heart and Vascular Program, Baystate Health and University of Massachusetts Medical School–Baystate, 759 Chestnut Street, Springfield, MA 01199, USA; [e] Department of Anesthesiology, Intensive Care Medicine and Pain Therapy, University Hospital Würzburg, Würzburg, Germany
* Corresponding author.
E-mail address: ahill@ukaachen.de

Crit Care Clin 36 (2020) 593–616
https://doi.org/10.1016/j.ccc.2020.06.002
0749-0704/20/© 2020 Elsevier Inc. All rights reserved.

invasive transcatheter procedures, less blood product use, and the use of leukocyte filters during cardiopulmonary bypass.[1,7] These improvements have led to shorter times to extubation, but other outcomes such as operative morbidity and mortality, rates of new onset of atrial fibrillation, stroke, renal failure, prolonged ventilation, deep sternal wound infection, and readmissions have remained essentially unchanged.[1] Acute and persistent organ dysfunction still occurs frequently after cardiac surgery and consequently affects the patient's outcome and health-related quality of life.[8,9]

The complications may in some cases outweigh the benefits of the operation. Postoperative complications are a major determinant of morbidity, mortality, length of hospital stay, hospital costs, and quality of life after heart surgery.[10] Major infections, stroke, and continued inotrope requirement within the first 3 months have a detrimental effect on subsequent survival.[11–21] This combination of more complex cardiac surgery procedures being undertaken in an increasingly comorbid population, leads to a growing incidence of prolonged recovery both in the intensive care and hospital environment. New strategies to improve the long-term outcome and health-related quality of life for these patients are urgently needed.[22]

Preoperative factors, such as age, comorbidities, nutritional status, and muscle mass have a major impact on the physical functioning of patients postoperatively in the intensive care unit (ICU) and for years after discharge.[23–25] Two of the most frequent comorbidities of patients undergoing cardiac surgery are malnutrition and sarcopenia. Both entities lead to muscle and body wasting and contribute to poor mobility and function.[26] The impact of body wasting on the outcome of cardiac surgery patients is summarized in **Fig. 1**.

Preoperative optimization of these factors (prehabilitation) before elective cardiac surgery is an attractive option with promising effects. Data from adequately designed randomized controlled trials and meta-analyses are rare in the field of cardiac surgery. This review discusses the impact of malnutrition and sarcopenia on the outcome and current evidence regarding the preoperative treatment of these entities.

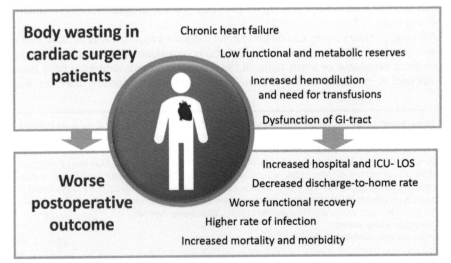

Fig. 1. Impact of body wasting in cardiac surgery patients on patient outcome. GI, gastrointestinal tract; ICU, intensive care unit; LOS, length of stay.

OPTIMIZATION OF NUTRITIONAL STATUS
Impact of Malnutrition and Cachexia

Malnutrition is defined as a subacute or chronic state of disordered nutrition that leads to altered body composition (decreased fat free mass) and body cell mass leading to diminished physical and mental function and impaired clinical outcome from disease.[27] Malnutrition affects up to 46% of cardiac surgery patients[28] and up to 50% of patients with heart failure.[29] Cardiac cachexia is defined as an involuntary loss of more than 5% of nonedematous body weight associated with an advanced stage of heart failure. In special subpopulations, such as patients before left ventricular assist device implantation, the incidence of cardiac cachexia is up to 33%[29–32] (**Box 1**).

Malnutrition and cardiac cachexia have a large influence on mortality after cardiac surgery and remain independent predictors of death, associated with a mortality rate of 20% to 40% per year.[23] They are associated with a greater loss of function, higher rates of infection, an increased inflammatory response, a higher risk for pneumonia and pulmonary dysfunction, increased hospital and ICU length of stay, decreased discharge to home rate, and thus higher morbidity and mortality.[23]

Not only chronic malnutrition, but iatrogenic malnutrition owing to decreased oral intake during any preoperative hospital stay and acute perioperative starvation, which occurs frequently in this clinical setting, contribute to malnutrition in these patients.[32] Postoperative malnutrition during the ICU stay further aggravates a patient's suboptimal nutritional state and negatively influences the postoperative systemic inflammation reaction and ultimately patients' outcomes.[32] Rahman and colleagues[33] recently demonstrated in an international nutrition survey in critically ill cardiac surgery patients that both energy and protein supplementation is inadequate. Additionally, patients undergoing cardiovascular surgery are at a higher risk for iatrogenic malnutrition owing to the withholding of nutritional support during the early postoperative course. In this analysis, the mean time from ICU admission to initiation of enteral nutrition was 2.3 ± 1.8 days and 40% of patients received no nutrition therapy at all.[33,34] A significant lack of macronutrients and micronutrients has been observed in several small observational studies, which impedes a patient's metabolism, leads to increased postoperative complications, and prolongs wound healing leading to overall worse outcomes.[23]

Box 1
Pathogenesis of malnutrition and cachexia

- Alterations in appetite and food intake
- Increased resting energy expenditure
- Excretion of proinflammatory cytokines
- Neuroendocrine abnormalities
  - Activation of the sympathetic nervous system
  - Activation of the renin-angiotensin-aldosterone axis
  - Activation of natriuretic peptide
  - Increase in cortisol
  - Greater growth hormone resistance
  - Insulin resistance

Data from Adam Rahman, Syed Jafry, Khursheed Jeejeebhoy, A Dave Nagpal, Barbara Pisani, and Ravi Agarwala. Malnutrition and cachexia in heart failure. *JPEN. Journal of parenteral and enteral nutrition*, 40:475–486, May 2016. And Stephan von Haehling, Nicole Ebner, Marcelo R Dos Santos, Jochen Springer, and Stefan D Anker. Muscle wasting and cachexia in heart failure: mechanisms and therapies. *Nature reviews. Cardiology*, 14:323–341, June 2017.

These conditions are major contributors to postoperative complications (eg, infections) and the development of organ dysfunction in the ICU (eg, lung and kidney)[33–42] and ultimately lead to weakness and an inability to ambulate, and significantly influence the patients' long-term outcomes. Despite the growing evidence demonstrating the detrimental effects on chronic and acute malnutrition on high-risk cardiac surgery patients, routine nutritional screening has rarely been implemented in every day clinical practice and no specific nutritional guidelines exist for this patient population.[43] When using only traditional methods, such as body mass index and weight loss, one-half of the patients with low fat-free mass index are falsely classified as well-nourished.[44] Therefore, an adequate nutritional risk assessment is crucial to identify and treat patients who are cachectic or malnourished. In this context, recent evidence indicates that the combined use of EUROScore, cardiopulmonary bypass time, and nutrition risk screening tools, such as the Nutrition Risk Screening 2002 and the Mini Nutritional Assessment, are useful for prediction of prolonged ICU length of stay in cardiac surgery patients.[45] If confirmed in prospectively adequately powered studies, this model may help to preoperatively identify patients with potential prolonged ICU stay who may benefit from early initiated nutrition therapy.

Nutrition Interventions Before Cardiac Surgery

Chronically malnourished patients or patients at risk for acute malnutrition (patients with high surgical risk and anticipated prolonged ICU stays) may be the cohort that benefits most from an intense perioperative medical nutrition therapy.[45] In the postoperative setting, mechanical ventilation, the effects of sedatives, nausea and anorexia, and the overall proinflammatory and catabolic status of the patient, may present obstacles for effective nutrition therapy. However, most of these factors are not present preoperatively. Therefore, in patients undergoing elective cardiac surgery, the preoperative phase may represent an attractive time window for optimized nutrition therapy. This therapy may include special/targeted nutritional counseling and nutrition optimization strategies to improve the nutrition status, physical function, and mental health (eg, depression) and potentially also optimize glycemic and lipid profiles.[46]

One possibility to further improve nutrition preoperatively is the additional administration of oral nutrition supplements. The goals of oral nutrition supplements is to optimize daily nutrition intake by providing a high-caloric and high-protein diet to avoid fluid and salt overload and to replenish vitamins and trace elements, which ideally attenuates the systemic inflammatory and metabolic response to surgery.[47–50] Different contents of macronutrients and micronutrients and volumes per unit are commercially available as sip feeds, pudding, or powder to cater to the needs of the individual patient. Oral nutrition supplements are safe and cost effective for all patients regardless of their baseline nutritional state[51–54]; however, the effects are more pronounced in high-risk and malnourished patients.[55–57] Preoperative oral nutrition supplements have demonstrated beneficial effects in patients through decreased weight loss, decreased rate of complications, decreased hospital LOS and lower rates of malnutrition-associated complications.[58–63]

The European Society of Parenteral and Enteral Nutrition recommends medical nutrition therapy for a period of 7 to 14 days preoperatively for severely malnourished patients undergoing elective surgery, even if the surgery has to be delayed.[64] The management strategies will not be suitable for those patients who require more urgent cardiac surgery procedures. This circumstance highlights the need to determine alternative effective strategies for these patients with a shorter time window for optimization. This is currently being tested in the PROPER-LVAD study (approved by the ethics committee of Medical Faculty RWTH Aachen, EK313/19, registration on clinicaltrials. gov: NCT04205760).

Preoperatively administered immunomodulating adjuvant supplements containing arginine, omega-3 fatty acids, and nucleotides have been shown to improve the postoperative immune response, gut oxygenation, and intestinal microperfusion to decrease the overall infection rate, hospital length of stay and postoperative complications in smaller studies.[51,63] This finding has led some to recommend an oral nutrition supplement, which includes arginine, omega-3 fatty acids, and nucleotides if feasible.[64] There are only a few rather small studies on preoperative oral nutrition supplement for patients with heart failure and cardiac cachexia (**Table 1**), which have demonstrated feasibility and safety, as well as good patient compliance. The potential benefits have stimulated an increased interest to further study these strategies in high-risk patient populations.

OPTIMIZATION OF MUSCLE MASS AND PHYSICAL FUNCTION
Impact of Sarcopenia

Sarcopenia, frailty, and diminished functional status are predictors of unfavorable outcomes. Frailty is a multidimensional syndrome that leads to increased vulnerability in the patient with the inability to cope with stressor events, such as surgery.[69] Sarcopenia (a component of the frailty phenotype) is defined as low muscle strength, low muscle quantity or quality, and low physical performance.[70] Sarcopenia and frailty are commonly (although not exclusively) associated with aging and immobility. Chronic illness, such as heart disease, can exacerbate this process. A screening tool for sarcopenia or frailty has yet to be validated in patients undergoing cardiac surgery or in patients with heart failure, but most rely on the assessment of muscle mass, muscle strength, or physical function. The SARC-F questionnaire, a low handgrip strength, a low gait speed, a short walking distance in the 6-minute walk test, and quadriceps strength are possibilities to assess muscle function.[47,71] Psoas muscle area[72,73] and quadriceps ultrasound[74,75] have proven to be useful for the assessment of muscle mass, if dual-energy x-ray absorptiometry or lumbar cross-sections of computed tomography scans or MRI are not available.[70]

Sarcopenia occurs in 5% to 13% of people between 60 and 70 years of age and in 27% of patients undergoing cardiac surgery,[76] leading to impaired functional capacity.[77] Sarcopenia and frailty are predictors of longer ICU and hospital lengths of stay, higher postdischarge mortality, a lower quality of life, and a lesser likelihood of discharge to home.[24,76–84] Sarcopenia is an independent predictor for decreased survival in patients undergoing cardiac surgery in patients older than 70 years.[85] A recent meta-analysis concluded that frail cardiac surgery patients have a greater likelihood of dying, higher morbidity and functional decline, and more major adverse cardiac and cerebrovascular events, regardless of the definition of frailty.[86]

Body wasting can be detected preoperatively, especially in older adults patients before elective surgery.[87,88] During the preoperative "waiting period," many changes in physiology owing to decreased mobility have been observed, specifically decreased muscle strength, respiratory muscle strength, and cardiac function. This process is mediated through atrophy of the heart muscle, which clinically occurs as decreased stroke volume, increased resting heart rate, and an increase in orthostatic intolerance.[89] The process of a declining functional state during a hospital stay has been called "hospitalization-associated disability," and affects one-third of patients.[87,88,90–92] A major cause of iatrogenic disability is a lack of mobilization owing to excessive bedrest and lack of physical therapy after surgery.[93]

Table 1
Selected studies addressing preoperative ONS in cardiac surgery and chronic heart failure

Author and Year	Number and Type of Patients	Nutrition Intervention	Results
Paccagnella et al,[65] 1994	6 patients with mitral valve disease and heart failure	20–30 kcal/kg/d, 2 wk before and 3 wk after surgery	Nutrition is safe in severe heart failure, improvement in clinical status
Tepaske et al,[66] 2001	50 preoperative cardiac surgery patients	Immune enhancing ONS, 5–10 L during 5–10 d	No adverse effects Improvement in preoperative host defense, decreased number of postoperative infections, better renal function, decreased requirement for inotropes Trend toward reduction in hospital LOS
Aquilani et al,[67] 2008	38 stable patients with chronic heart failure, muscle-depleted normal weight	Supplementation of essential amino acids for 8 wk	Weight gain Trend toward improved insulin resistance Decreased lactate and pyruvate levels Improved exercise output Improved peak oxygen consumption Increased walking capacity
Rozentryt et al,[68] 2010	29 patients with chronic heart failure	ONS: 600 kcal, 20 g of protein for 6 wk	Increase in body weight Significant improvement in QOL Systemic reduction in TNF-α levels

Abbreviations: LOS, length of stay; ONS, oral nutrition supplement; QOL, quality of life; TNF-α, tumor necrosis factor.
Data from Refs.[65–68]

If a preoperative physical impairment is paired with the expected postoperative decline of function, the overall functional level might drop into a critical zone, where the patient needs a prolonged period to recover.[50,88] The ability to walk can be limited after cardiac surgery[5,94] and ICU-acquired weakness is observed in many ICU patients in the absence of formal mobilization protocols, resulting from increased protein degradation rates.[95,96] Although the published data for ICU-acquired weakness in cardiac surgery are limited, the reported incidence of ICU-acquired weakness ranges from 25% to 100% in critically ill patients. Up to 30% of muscle mass is lost within the first 10 days of ICU admission,[74,78,82,97–100] leading to substantial functional limitations in the activities of daily living, which may persist for years after discharge.[94,101–104] The possibility that sarcopenia and frailty can predict the occurrence of ICU-acquired weakness has not been studied extensively. However, there has been a shift in research and clinical practice from the use of sedation and bedrest toward early exercise in the ICU to counteract the phenomenon of immobilization-induced loss of muscle mass and function.[105–111] In combination with an intensive nutritional therapy protocol, preoperative optimization of physical function and muscle mass might be more effective than solely using postoperative rehabilitation. Postoperatively, sedation, edema, and drug effects are greater and opportunities for exercise are more restricted owing to pain, drains, catheters, or movement restriction applied after surgery. Therefore, prehabilitation programs have gained increasing interest in the past few years.

Effects of Preoperative Physical Exercise

Preoperative physical exercise is known to be safe and beneficial in cardiac surgery and other surgical patients[5,17,64,81,112–123] and has been especially used in older adult patients. Preoperative exercise decreases sympathetic overactivity, improves insulin sensitivity, and increases the ratio of lean body mass to body fat.[124] There are 3 possible approaches to preoperative physical therapy, which may be combined and tailored to the individual patient:

- Aerobic exercise to strengthen the cardiovascular system,
- Respiratory exercise to strengthen the respiratory system, and
- Strength exercises to increase muscle strength.

Two Cochrane reviews and several systematic reviews regarding preoperative physical therapy and preoperative inspiratory muscle training for elective cardiac surgery patients concluded that these treatments resulted in[5,125–127]:

- Fewer postoperative pulmonary complications,
- Decreased hospital length of stay,
- Improved physical function, and
- Improved quality of life.

Although several studies have proven the effectiveness and safety of exercise in patients before elective cardiac surgery, most studies focused on patients classified as an intermediate grade of heart failure (New York Heart Association grades II and III) and only a few studies have investigated the effects of preoperative aerobic exercise training (**Table 2**). In-bed cycling is a physiotherapeutic approach gaining popularity during the last few years and several studies are currently being conducted. The technique can be used preoperatively or postoperatively, actively or passively, and has proven to be safe, well-tolerated, and feasible in critically ill patients.[115,128–134] In-bed cycling focuses on the lower limb muscles, which are especially affected by immobilization and are critical to ambulation and functional independence.[135,136] Several studies also demonstrated benefits from passive exercise.[137,138]

Solution to Both: Combined Interventions?

The recent Enhanced Recovery After Surgery Cardiac Society's guideline state "prehabilitation enables patients to withstand the stress of surgery by augmenting functional capacity. It improves physical and psychological readiness for surgery,

Table 2
Selected studies of exercise in patients with heart failure, preoperative cardiosurgical patients and ICU patients

Author and Year	Number and Type of Patients	Description of Exercise Intervention	Results
Arthur et al,[139] 2000	249 low-risk CABG	Supervised exercise + education 90 min twice/week for 8 wk Intensity: 40%–70% of functional capacity	Reduced hospital, ICU, and postoperative LOS Improved QOL More patients participate in postoperative physical therapy
Herdy et al,[114] 2008	56 waiting CABG	Exercise program > 5 d	Shorter time to extubation reduction in postoperative pulmonary complications shorter hospital length of stay
Rosenfeldt et al,[140] 2011	Cardiac surgery	Aerobic exercise and mental training 2×60 min/week for > 2 wk Intensity: 60% of maximum heart rate	No significant changes
Tung et al,[141] 2012	35 elective cardiac surgeries, NYHA I- III	Individualized exercise using a treadmill 40–60 min, 1–2/week, >3 times Intensity: 50%–60% pVO_2	Out of bed earlier, improvement in QOL
Sawatzky et al,[142] 2014	17 elective CABG	Exercise and education classes for 60 min/d, twice a week for at least 4 wk	Increased walking distance in 6MWD, improved gait speed, higher enrollment in cardiac rehabilitation

Abbreviations: 6MWD, 6-minute walking test; CABG, coronary artery bypass grafting; EF, ejection fraction; HRR, heart rate reserve; LOS, length-of stay; NYHA, New York Heart Association grade; ONS, oral nutritional supplement; pVO_2, peak oxygen consumption; QOL, quality of life.
   Data from Refs.[114,139–142]

reduces postoperative complications and the length of stay, and improves the transition from the hospital to the community. A cardiac prehabilitation program should include education, nutritional optimization, exercise training, social support, and anxiety reduction, although current existing evidence is limited."[124]

Given the multifactorial etiologies of cardiac disease and the intertwined pathogenetic pathways of cardiac cachexia and sarcopenia (**Fig. 2**), a combined intervention treating all aspects seems promising and desirable.[50]

Very often, sarcopenia and cardiac cachexia occur together and lead to multifocal complications in patients with advanced heart failure as well as in survivors of complex surgical procedures. Disturbances include loss of muscle mass and weight (body wasting), hospital- and ICU-acquired weakness, increased mortality, functional and cognitive impairment, anxiety, and decreased health-related quality of life (as shown

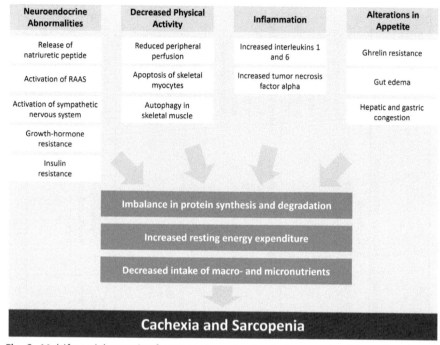

Fig. 2. Multifactorial genesis of sarcopenia and cachexia in patients with cardiac disease. RAAS, renin–angiotensin–aldosterone system.

in **Fig. 1**). Therefore, a sensible therapeutic approach would be a treatment of both sarcopenia and cachexia through a combination of nutritional therapy and exercise.[78,100,143–149] Because postoperative inflammation induces catabolism, this phenomenon can potentially aggravate a preexisting malnourished state. Therefore, a preoperative intervention seems promising to improve the nutritional and functional condition of these patients. Patients scheduled for elective cardiac surgery should be screened early for malnutrition and functional abilities with interventions directed toward improving nutritional status.[23,43] Postoperatively, protocols from the Enhanced Recovery After Surgery Society suggest a bundle of perioperative care elements to promote the rapid recovery of surgical patients.[124,150,151]

Available evidence demonstrates that neither pure exercise[152–154] nor sole adequacy of energy–protein intake alone[67,74,78,143,153,155–161] are sufficient to improve nutritional and functional status and induce anabolism. Additionally, in view of the background of sarcopenic obesity, neither pure weight gain nor gain of fat mass without the building up of muscle mass should be the main target of therapy.[162,163] To build up or prevent the loss of muscle mass as well as to improve physical function and health-related quality of life, adequate nutritional intake and physical exercise are both necessary.[47,59,164–167] In this context, small randomized and controlled studies have addressed combined nutrition and exercise interventions that have demonstrated the greatest benefits (**Table 3**). To our knowledge, there are no completed studies regarding the preoperative optimization of nutrition and physical exercise in patients scheduled for elective cardiac surgery.

In addition to the strategies previously discussed, several concepts have already been proposed to treat sarcopenia and cardiac cachexia, as summarized in **Fig. 3**.

Table 3
Review of some studies of combined nutrition and exercise interventions

Author and Year	Number and Type of Patients	Trial Duration	Nutrition Intervention	Exercise Intervention	Results
Fiatarone et al,[168] 1993, Fiatarone et al,[156] 1994	100 frail nursing home residents	10 wk	Multinutrient supplement 360 kcal/d	3 days/week Lower extremity resistance training (hip and knee extensors)	High-intensity resistance exercise is feasible and effective, while nutrient supplementation without exercise does not reduce frailty
Bonnefoy et al,[152] 2003	57 frail elderly volunteers	9 mo	2 × 200 mL ONS (200 kcal and 15 g of protein each)	60 min 3 times/wk (strength, balance and flexibility exercises)	Muscle power and BMI increased in patients with dietary supplements Exercise improved functional tests
Kim et al,[130] 2012	155 women aged 75 and older	3 mo	3 g of leucine-rich essential amino acid mixture twice a day	60-min training program 2 d/wk	Increased walking speed in exercise groups Increase of muscle mass and knee extension strength in exercise and nutrition group
Jones et al,[169] 2015	93 critically ill patients	3 mo	Essential amino acid supplement drink twice daily for 3 mo	Enhanced physiotherapy and structured exercise for 6 wk	Patients receiving both interventions had the greatest improvement of function and reduction in rates of anxiety

Study	Population	Duration	Nutritional intervention	Exercise intervention	Outcome
Molnar et al,[170] 2016	34 elderly patients at a long care facility	3 mo	ONS (20 g protein, 10 g amino acids, 9 g carbohydrates, 3 g fat)	Regular, standard length physiotherapy sessions, mostly strengthening exercise 30 min 2 times a wk	Physical exercise alone: no significant improvement in skeletal muscle mass or strength. Combined intervention: significantly increased muscle strength
Sandmael et al,[171] 2017	41 patients with head and neck cancer	During RT: 6 wk, or after RT: 3 wk	ONS, at least 1 each weekday with 350 kcal	Progressive resistance training, including aerobic warm up and strength exercises	Different interventions between the groups, mitigation of loss of muscle mass in both groups
Solheim et al,[172] 2017	46 cachectic patients with lung and pancreatic cancer	6 wk	Two ONS with 2 g EPA/d, nutritional counseling	Home-based Aerobic component: 30 min, 2 times weekly Resistance exercise: of 6 individualized exercises 3 times weekly for 20 min	Compliance at home: 60% for exercise, and 48% for nutritional supplements, no significant effect on physical activity or muscle mass. No adverse events Similar survival between the groups
Minnella et al,[173] 2018	51 patients before esophagogastric resection for cancer	Median of 36 d	Food-based dietary advice, whey protein supplement, protein target: 1.2–1.5 g/kg/d	Individualized, home-based exercise training program, aerobic exercise 3 d/wk, strength exercise 1 d/wk, each min	Significant change in walking distance both preoperatively and postoperatively, no changes in complications, LOS, mortality or readmission

(continued on next page)

Table 3
(continued)

Author and Year	Number and Type of Patients	Trial Duration	Nutrition Intervention	Exercise Intervention	Results
Francois et al,[174] 2018	53 adult patients with type II diabetes	12 wk	Postexercise milk, milk protein, or placebo supplementation 3 times a week (intervention group)	Cardio and resistance-based HIIT (4–10 × 1 min at 90% maximal heart rate) 3 times a week (both groups)	Improved femoral artery intima media thickness, carotid-femoral pulse wave velocity heart rate in both groups, no differences between nutrition groups for all outcomes
Invernizzi et al,[175] 2019	32 patients 3 mo after hip fracture	2 mo	Dietetic counseling and 4 g/d of essential amino acids (interventional group only)	Physical exercise rehabilitative program (5sessions of 40 min/wk for 2 wk, followed by a home-based exercise protocol) (both groups)	Amino acid supplementation did not show greater improvements in primary outcome measures compared with nutritional counseling alone, but a combined intervention showed significant improvement in sarcopenic patients

Abbreviations: BMI, body mass index; EPA, eicosapentaenoic acid; HIIT, high-intensity interval training; LOS, length of stay; ONS, oral nutrition supplement; RT, radiotherapy.

Data from Refs.[130,152,156,168–175]

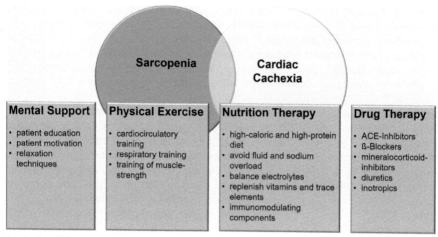

Fig. 3. Possible treatment options for cardiac cachexia and sarcopenia. ACE, angiotensin-converting enzyme.

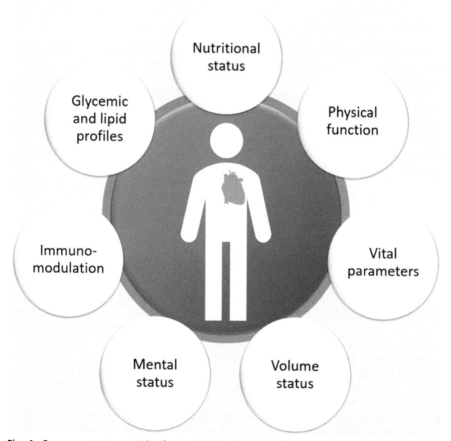

Fig. 4. Components to consider for prehabilitation in cardiac surgery.

Regarding the optimization of drug therapy, administering the maximum dosage of angiotensin-converting enzyme inhibitors, β-blockers, and mineralocorticoid receptor antagonists have been described.[47] Although many other drugs could possibly be beneficial in the treatment of muscle wasting in patients with heart failure, none of the potential treatments, such as appetite stimulants, anti-inflammatory substances, or anabolic agents in combination with nutritional supplements have proven beneficial.[29,47]

Different preoperative combinations of treatments, such as nutrition and exercise therapy, respiratory and cardiocirculatory training, psychological interventions and optimization of drug therapy have been summarized by the term "prehabilitation" and shown efficacy in improving patient outcomes. Some of these components are summarized in **Fig. 4**. Prehabilitation improved postoperative pain and physical function, decreased postoperative complication rates and length of stay, and improved quality of life, as well as functional capacity in different groups of patients.[64,87,88,111,121,176–178] Frail and sarcopenic patients may benefit most from prehabilitation.[47,64,179–181]

Given the currently available evidence, and a recent multidisciplinary consensus statement of international experts[43] a combined preoperative nutritional and exercise intervention may improve functional status, reduce complication and infection rates and improve quality of life.

SUMMARY

Malnutrition, cardiac cachexia, sarcopenia, and frailty have a strong impact on long-term outcomes in patients undergoing cardiac surgery. Despite many patients staying only a limited time in the ICU, they may experience a postoperative decline of physical function that affects their quality of life for months or even years. In the setting of an increasingly older adult population with a greater incidence of comorbidities, new strategies are urgently needed to improve outcomes. Although rehabilitation after surgery has been established worldwide for years, the interdisciplinary preoperative optimization of patients called "prehabilitation" has only recently gained interest. It is hoped that prehabilitation may permit the deconditioned and malnourished patient to withstand the stresses of surgery and shorten the recovery phase. As part of this process, the optimization of nutritional and physical status may represent promising strategies in malnourished and sarcopenic patients. However, the lack of reliable studies for screening and interventions to reverse the malnutrition and sarcopenia in these patients undergoing cardiac surgery strongly advocates further research in this area.

DISCLOSURE

C. Stoppe has received lecture fees and travel expenses by Fresenius Kabi and consulting fees from Fresenius Kabi and Biosyn. C. Stoppe received a co-funding grant from Baxter Healthcare Corporation for a study of postoperative protein supplementation. C. Stoppe has received a grant from B. Braun to conduct a study of exercise and nutrition in critically ill patients. A. Hill and C. Stoppe have received a grant by Fresenius Kabi to perform a trial of prehabilitation. A. Hill was supported by the "clinician scientist program" of the Faculty of Medicine of the RWTH Aachen University. D.T. Engelman is a consultant for Edwards Lifesciences. All authors declare no further conflict of interest that may be perceived as inappropriately influencing the representation or interpretation of reported research results. Disclosures for R.C. Arora have not been made but will be given subsequently.

REFERENCES

1. D'Agostino RS, Jacobs JP, Badhwar V, et al. The society of thoracic surgeons adult cardiac surgery database: 2019 update on outcomes and quality. Ann Thorac Surg 2019;107:24–32.
2. Beckmann A, Meyer R, Lewandowski J, et al. German heart surgery report 2018: the annual updated registry of the German society for thoracic and cardiovascular surgery. Thorac Cardiovasc Surg 2019;67:331–44.
3. Peter Z, Yacoub M, Zühlke L, et al. Global unmet needs in cardiac surgery. Glob Heart 2018;13:293–303.
4. Grover A, Gorman K, Dall TM, et al. Shortage of cardiothoracic surgeons is likely by 2020. Circulation 2009;120:488–94.
5. Reed H, Malone D. Effectiveness of preoperative physical therapy for elective cardiac surgery. Phys Ther 2015;95:160–6.
6. Hall R. Identification of inflammatory mediators and their modulation by strategies for the management of the systemic inflammatory response during cardiac surgery. J Cardiothorac Vasc Anesth 2013;27:983–1033.
7. Landis RC, Brown JR, Fitzgerald D, et al. Attenuating the systemic inflammatory response to adult cardiopulmonary bypass: a critical review of the evidence base. J Extra Corpor Technol 2014;46:197–211.
8. Stoppe C, McDonald B, Benstoem C, et al. Evaluation of persistent organ dysfunction plus death as a novel composite outcome in cardiac surgical patients. J Cardiothorac Vasc Anesth 2016;30:30–8.
9. Hill A, Wendt S, Benstoem C, et al. Vitamin c to improve organ dysfunction in cardiac surgery patients-review and pragmatic approach. Nutrients 2018; 10:974.
10. Hoogeboom TJ, Dronkers JJ, Erik HJ, et al. Merits of exercise therapy before and after major surgery. Curr Opin Anaesthesiol 2014;27:161–6.
11. Benjamin EJ, Blaha MJ, Chiuve SE, et al. Paul Muntner, American heart association Statistics committee, and stroke Statistics Subcommittee. Heart disease and stroke statistics-2017 update: a report from the American Heart Association. Circulation 2017;135:e146–603.
12. A Diegeler. Externe stationaere qualitaetssicherung herz- und lungentransplantation herzunterstuetzungssysteme/kunstherzen. 8. Qualitaetssicherungskonferenz des Gemeinsamen Bundesausschusses Berlin, 29. September 2016, 2016.
13. Kirklin JK, Pagani FD, Kormos RL, et al. Eighth annual INTERMACS report: special focus on framing the impact of adverse events. J Heart Lung Transplant 2017;36:1080–6.
14. Lampropulos JF, Kim N, Wang Y, et al. Trends in left ventricular assist device use and outcomes among Medicare beneficiaries, 2004-2011. Open heart 2014;1: e000109.
15. Prinzing A, Herold Ulf, Anna B, et al. Left ventricular assist devices-current state and perspectives. J Thorac Dis 2016;8:E660–6.
16. Bouza E, Hortal J, Munoz P, et al, European Study Group on Nosocomial Infections, and European Workgroup of Cardiothoracic Intensivists. Postoperative infections after major heart surgery and prevention of ventilator-associated pneumonia: a one-day European prevalence study (esgni-008). J Hosp Infect 2006;64:224–30.
17. Garcia-Delgado M, Navarrete-Sanchez I, Colmenero M. Preventing and managing perioperative pulmonary complications following cardiac surgery. Curr Opin Anaesthesiol 2014;27:146–52.

18. He S, Chen B, Li W, et al. Ventilator-associated pneumonia after cardiac surgery: a meta-analysis and systematic review. J Thorac Cardiovasc Surg 2014;148: 3148–55.e1–5.

19. Hortal J, Munoz P, Cuerpo G, et al. European Study Group on Nosocomial Infections, and European Workgroup of Cardiothoracic Intensivists. Ventilator-associated pneumonia in patients undergoing major heart surgery: an incidence study in Europe. Crit Care 2009;13:R80.

20. Ibanez J, Riera M, Amezaga R, et al. Long-term mortality after pneumonia in cardiac surgery patients: a propensity-matched analysis. J Intensive Care Med 2016;31:34–40.

21. Sheng W, Xing Q-S, Hou W-M, et al. Independent risk factors for ventilator-associated pneumonia after cardiac surgery. J Invest Surg 2014;27:256–61.

22. Herman CR, Buth KJ, Jean-Francois L, et al. Development of a predictive model for major adverse cardiac events in a coronary artery bypass and valve population. J Cardiothorac Surg 2013;8:177.

23. Hill A, Nesterova E, Lomivorotov V, et al. Current evidence about nutrition support in cardiac surgery patients-what do we know? Nutrients 2018;10:597.

24. Parry SM, Huang M, Needham DM. Evaluating physical functioning in critical care: considerations for clinical practice and research. Crit Care 2017;21:249.

25. Silberman S, Bitran D, Fink D, et al. Very prolonged stay in the intensive care unit after cardiac operations: early results and late survival. Ann Thorac Surg 2013; 96:15–21 [discussion: 21–2].

26. Ebner N, D Anker S, von Haehling S. Recent developments in the field of cachexia, sarcopenia, and muscle wasting: highlights from the 11th cachexia conference. J Cachexia Sarcopenia Muscle 2019;10:218–25.

27. Cederholm T, Bosaeus I, Barazzoni R, et al. Diagnostic criteria for malnutrition - an ESPEN consensus statement. Clin Nutr 2015;34:335–40.

28. Ringaitiené D, Gineitytė D, Vicka V, et al. Preoperative risk factors of malnutrition for cardiac surgery patients. Acta Med Litu 2016;23:99–109.

29. Adam R, Syed J, Jeejeebhoy K, et al. Malnutrition and cachexia in heart failure. JPEN J Parenter Enteral Nutr 2016;40:475–86.

30. Pichette M, Liszkowski M, Ducharme A. Preoperative optimization of the heart failure patient undergoing cardiac surgery. Can J Cardiol 2017;33:72–9.

31. Sundararajan S, Kiernan MS, DeNofrio D, et al. Cachexia is common in ventricular assist device recipients but not predictive of mortality. J Card Fail 2016;22: S57–8.

32. von Haehling S, Markus SA, D Anker S. Prevalence and clinical impact of cachexia in chronic illness in Europe, USA, and Japan: facts and numbers update 2016. J Cachexia Sarcopenia Muscle 2016;7:507–9.

33. Rahman A, Hasan RM, Agarwala R, et al. Identifying critically-ill patients who will benefit most from nutritional therapy: further validation of the "modified nutric" nutritional risk assessment tool. Clin Nutr 2016;35:158–62.

34. Stoppe C, Whitlock R, Arora RC, et al. Nutrition support in cardiac surgery patients: be calm and feed on! J Thorac Cardiovasc Surg 2019;158:1103–8.

35. Bendavid I, Singer P, Theilla M, et al. Nutrition day ICU: a 7 year worldwide prevalence study of nutrition practice in intensive care. Clin Nutr 2017;36(4):1122–9.

36. Drover JW, Cahill NE, Kutsogiannis J, et al. Nutrition therapy for the critically ill surgical patient: we need to do better! JPEN J Parenter enteral Nutr 2010;34: 644–52.

37. Cahill NE, Dhaliwal R, Day AG, et al. Nutrition therapy in the critical care setting: what is "best achievable" practice? an international multicenter observational study. Crit Care Med 2010;38:395–401.
38. Goldhill DR, Whelpton R, Winyard JA, et al. Gastric emptying in patients the day after cardiac surgery. Anaesthesia 1995;50:122–5.
39. Ohri SK, Velissaris T. Gastrointestinal dysfunction following cardiac surgery. Perfusion 2006;21:215–23.
40. Adam R, Wu T, Ryan B, et al. Malnutrition matters in Canadian hospitalized patients: malnutrition risk in hospitalized patients in a tertiary care center using the malnutrition universal screening tool. Nutr Clin Pract 2015;30:709–13.
41. Rossi M, Sganga G, Mazzone M, et al. Cardiopulmonary bypass in man: role of the intestine in a self-limiting inflammatory response with demonstrable bacterial translocation. Ann Thorac Surg 2004;77:612–8.
42. Wei X, Day AG, Ouellette-Kuntz H, et al. The association between nutritional adequacy and long-term outcomes in critically ill patients requiring prolonged mechanical ventilation: a multicenter cohort study. Crit Care Med 2015;43:1569–79.
43. Stoppe C, Goetzenich A, Whitman G, et al. Role of nutrition support in adult cardiac surgery: a consensus statement from an international multidisciplinary expert group on nutrition in cardiac surgery. Crit Care 2017;21:131.
44. van Venrooij LMW, de Vos R, Zijlstra E, et al. The impact of low preoperative fat-free body mass on infections and length of stay after cardiac surgery: a prospective cohort study. J Thorac Cardiovasc Surg 2011;142:1263–9.
45. Stoppe C, Ney J, Vladimir V, et al. Prediction of prolonged ICU stay in cardiac surgery patients as a useful method to identify nutrition risk in cardiac surgery patients: a post hoc analysis of a prospective observational study. JPEN J Parenter enteral Nutr 2018;43(6):768–79.
46. George S, Zafirova Z. Ten years experiences with preoperative evaluation clinic for day admission cardiac and major vascular surgical patients: model for "perioperative anesthesia and surgical home. Semin Cardiothorac Vasc Anesth 2016;20:120–32.
47. von Haehling S, Ebner N, Dos Santos MR, et al. Muscle wasting and cachexia in heart failure: mechanisms and therapies. Nat Rev Cardiol 2017;14:323–41.
48. Weijs PJM, Cynober L, DeLegge M, et al. Proteins and amino acids are fundamental to optimal nutrition support in critically ill patients. Crit Care 2014;18:591.
49. Weijs PJM, Stapel SN, de Groot SDW, et al. Optimal protein and energy nutrition decreases mortality in mechanically ventilated, critically ill patients: a prospective observational cohort study. JPEN J Parenter enteral Nutr 2012;36:60–8.
50. Gillis C, Wischmeyer PE. Pre-operative nutrition and the elective surgical patient: why, how and what? Anaesthesia 2019;74(Suppl 1):27–35.
51. Bharadwaj S, Trivax B, Tandon P, et al. Should perioperative immunonutrition for elective surgery be the current standard of care? Gastroenterol Rep 2016;4: 87–95.
52. Braga M. Perioperative immunonutrition and gut function. Curr Opin Clin Nutr Metab Care 2012;15:485–8.
53. Braga M, Gianotti L. Preoperative immunonutrition: cost-benefit analysis. JPEN J Parenter enteral Nutr 2005;29:S57–61.
54. Muscaritoli M, Krznaric Z, Singer P, et al. Effectiveness and efficacy of nutritional therapy: a systematic review following Cochrane methodology. Clin Nutr 2017; 36(4):939–57.
55. Braga M, Wischmeyer PE, Drover J, et al. Clinical evidence for pharmaconutrition in major elective surgery. JPEN J Parenter Enteral Nutr 2013;37:66S–72S.

56. Compher C, Chittams J, Sammarco T, et al. Greater protein and energy intake may be associated with improved mortality in higher risk critically ill patients: a multicenter, multinational observational study. Crit Care Med 2017;45:156–63.

57. Parsons EL, Stratton RJ, Cawood AL, et al. Oral nutritional supplements in a randomised trial are more effective than dietary advice at improving quality of life in malnourished care home residents. Clin Nutr 2017;36(1):134–42.

58. Brown PP, Kugelmass AD, Cohen DJ, et al. The frequency and cost of complications associated with coronary artery bypass grafting surgery: results from the United States Medicare program. Ann Thorac Surg 2008;85:1980–6.

59. Evans DC, Martindale RG, Kiraly LN, et al. Nutrition optimization prior to surgery. Nutr Clin Pract 2014;29:10–21.

60. Drover JW, Dhaliwal R, Weitzel L, et al. Perioperative use of arginine-supplemented diets: a systematic review of the evidence. J Am Coll Surg 2011;212:385–99, 399.e1.

61. National Collaborating Centre for Acute Care. Nutrition support in adults Oral nutrition support, enteral tube feeding and parenteral nutrition. London: National Collaborating Centre for Acute Care; 2006. Available at: www.rcseng.ac.uk.

62. Smedley F, Bowling T, James M, et al. Randomized clinical trial of the effects of preoperative and postoperative oral nutritional supplements on clinical course and cost of care. Br J Surg 2004;91:983–90.

63. Waitzberg DL, Saito H, D Plank L, et al. Postsurgical infections are reduced with specialized nutrition support. World J Surg 2006;30:1592–604.

64. Weimann A, Braga M, Franco C, et al. ESPEN guideline: clinical nutrition in surgery. Clin Nutr 2017;36(3):623–50.

65. Paccagnella A, Calò MA, Caenaro G, et al. Cardiac cachexia: preoperative and postoperative nutrition management. JPEN J Parenter Enteral Nutr 1994;18(5):409–16.

66. Tepaske R, Velthuis H, Oudemans-van Straaten HM, et al. Effect of preoperative oral immune-enhancing nutritional supplement on patients at high risk of infection after cardiac surgery: a randomised placebo-controlled trial. Lancet 2001; 358:696–701.

67. Aquilani R, Opasich C, Gualco A, et al. Adequate energy-protein intake is not enough to improve nutritional and metabolic status in muscle-depleted patients with chronic heart failure. Eur J Heart Fail 2008;10:1127–35.

68. Rozentryt P, von Haehling S, Lainscak M, et al. The effects of a high-caloric protein-rich oral nutritional supplement in patients with chronic heart failure and cachexia on quality of life, body composition, and inflammation markers: a randomized, double-blind pilot study. J Cachexia Sarcopenia Muscle 2010;1:35–42.

69. Clegg A, Young J, Iliffe S, et al. Frailty in elderly people. Lancet 2013;381: 752–62.

70. Cruz-Jentoft AJ, Bahat G, Bauer JÃ, et al. Writing group for the European Working group on sarcopenia in older people 2 (EWGSOP2), and the Extended group for EWGSOP2. Sarcopenia: revised European consensus on definition and diagnosis. Age Ageing 2019;48:16–31.

71. Malmstrom TK, Miller DK, Simonsick EM, et al. SARC-F: a symptom score to predict persons with sarcopenia at risk for poor functional outcomes. J Cachexia Sarcopenia Muscle 2016;7:28–36.

72. Hawkins RB, Mehaffey JH, Charles EJ, et al. Psoas muscle size predicts risk-adjusted outcomes after surgical aortic valve replacement. Ann Thorac Surg 2018;106:39–45.

73. Balsam LB. Psoas muscle area: a new standard for frailty assessment in cardiac surgery? J Thorac Dis 2018;10:S3846–9.

74. Puthucheary ZA, Rawal J, McPhail M, et al. Acute skeletal muscle wasting in critical illness. JAMA 2013;310:1591–600.

75. Mourtzakis M, Parry S, Connolly B, et al. Skeletal muscle ultrasound in critical care: a tool in need of translation. Ann Am Thorac Soc 2017;14:1495–503.

76. Teng C-H, Chen S-Y, Wei Y-C, et al. Effects of sarcopenia on functional improvement over the first year after cardiac surgery: a cohort study. Eur J Cardiovasc Nurs 2019;18:309–17.

77. Saitoh M, Ishida J, Doehner W, et al. Anker, and Jochen Springer. Sarcopenia, cachexia, and muscle performance in heart failure: review update 2016. Int J Cardiol 2017;238:5–11.

78. Bear DE, Wandrag L, Merriweather JL, et al, Grocott, and Enhanced Recovery After Critical Illness Programme Group (ERACIP) investigators. The role of nutritional support in the physical and functional recovery of critically ill patients: a narrative review. Crit Care 2017;21:226.

79. Cooper LB, Hammill BG, Allen LA, et al. Assessing frailty in patients undergoing destination therapy left ventricular assist device: observations from interagency registry for mechanically assisted circulatory support. ASAIO J 2017;64(1): 16–23.

80. Dronkers JJ, Chorus AMJ, U van Meeteren NL, et al. The association of preoperative physical fitness and physical activity with outcome after scheduled major abdominal surgery. Anaesthesia 2013;68:67–73.

81. Friedman J, Lussiez A, Sullivan J, et al. Implications of sarcopenia in major surgery. Nutr Clin Pract 2015;30:175–9.

82. Jolley SE, Bunnell AE, Hough CL. ICU-acquired weakness. Chest 2016;150: 1129–40.

83. Moran J, Wilson F, Guinan E, et al. Role of cardiopulmonary exercise testing as a risk-assessment method in patients undergoing intra-abdominal surgery: a systematic review. Br J Anaesth]2016;116:177–91.

84. Springer J, Anker MS, Stefan DA. Advances in cachexia and sarcopenia research in the heart failure context: call for action. J Cardiovasc Med (Hagerstown) 2016;17:860–2.

85. Okamura H, Kimura N, Tanno K, et al. The impact of preoperative sarcopenia, defined based on psoas muscle area, on long-term outcomes of heart valve surgery. J Thorac Cardiovasc Surg 2018. https://doi.org/10.1016/j.jtcvs.2018. 06.098.

86. Sepehri A, Beggs T, Hassan A, et al. The impact of frailty on outcomes after cardiac surgery: a systematic review. J Thorac Cardiovasc Surg 2014;148:3110–7.

87. Covinsky KE, Palmer RM, Fortinsky RH, et al. Loss of independence in activities of daily living in older adults hospitalized with medical illnesses: increased vulnerability with age. J Am Geriatr Soc 2003;51:451–8.

88. Punt IM, van der Most R, Bongers BC, et al. [improving pre- and perioperative hospital care: major elective surgery]. Bundesgesundheitsblatt Gesundheitsforschung Gesundheitsschutz 2017;60:410–8.

89. Hulzebos EHJ, U van Meeteren NL. Making the elderly fit for surgery. Br J Surg 2016;103:e12–5.

90. Covinsky KE, Pierluissi E, Johnston CB. Hospitalization-associated disability: "she was probably able to ambulate, but I'm not sure. JAMA 2011;306:1782–93.

91. Palleschi L, Luca Fimognari F, Pierantozzi A, et al. Acute functional decline before hospitalization in older patients. Geriatr Gerontol Int 2014;14:769–77.

92. Wischmeyer PE, Puthucheary Z, San Millan I, et al. Muscle mass and physical recovery in ICU: innovations for targeting of nutrition and exercise. Curr Opin Crit Care]2017;23:269–78.

93. Sourdet S, Lafont C, Rolland Y, et al. Preventable iatrogenic disability in elderly patients during hospitalization. J Am Med Directors Assoc 2015;16:674–81.

94. van der Schaaf M, Dettling DS, Beelen A, et al. Poor functional status immediately after discharge from an intensive care unit. Disabil Rehabil 2008;30: 1812–8.

95. Klaude M, Mori M, Tjaeder I, et al. Protein metabolism and gene expression in skeletal muscle of critically ill patients with sepsis. Clin Sci 2012;122:133–42.

96. Rooyackers O, Jan W. Imaging opens possibilities both to target and to evaluate nutrition in critical illness. Crit Care 2014;18(144).

97. De Jonghe B, Sharshar T, Lefaucheur J-P, et al. Paresis acquired in the intensive care unit: a prospective multicenter study. JAMA 2002;288(22):2859–67.

98. Kress JP, Hall JB. ICU-acquired weakness and recovery from critical illness. N Engl J Med 2014;370:1626–35.

99. Paddon-Jones D, Sheffield-Moore M, Cree MG, et al. Atrophy and impaired muscle protein synthesis during prolonged inactivity and stress. J Clin Endocrinol Metab 2006;91:4836–41.

100. Zorowitz RD. ICU-acquired weakness: a rehabilitation perspective of diagnosis, treatment, and functional management. Chest 2016;150:966–71.

101. Ali NA, O'Brien JM Jr, Hoffmann P, et al. Acquired weakness, handgrip strength, and mortality in critically ill patients. Am J Respir Crit Care Med 2008;178(3): 261–8.

102. Cheung AM, Tansey CM, George T, et al. Two-year outcomes, health care use, and costs of survivors of acute respiratory distress syndrome. Am J Respir Crit Care Med 2006;174(5):538–44.

103. Herridge MS, Cheung AM, Tansey CM, et al. One-year outcomes in survivors of the acute respiratory distress syndrome. N Engl J Med 2003;348(8):683–93.

104. Herridge MS, Catherine MT, Matté A, et al. Functional disability 5 years after acute respiratory distress syndrome. N Engl J Med 2011;364(14):1293–304.

105. Bailey P, Thomsen GE, Spuhler VJ, et al. Early activity is feasible and safe in respiratory failure patients. Crit Care Med 2007;35(1):139–45.

106. Denehy L, Skinner EH, Lara E, et al. Exercise rehabilitation for patients with critical illness: a randomized controlled trial with 12 months of follow-up. Crit Care 2013;17(4):R156.

107. Morris PE, Goad A, Thompson C, et al. Early intensive care unit mobility therapy in the treatment of acute respiratory failure. Crit Care Med 2008;36(8):2238–43.

108. Needham DM, Korupolu R, Zanni JM, et al. Early physical medicine and rehabilitation for patients with acute respiratory failure: a quality improvement project. Arch Phys Med Rehabil 2010;91(4):536–42.

109. Schaller SJ, Anstey M, Blobner M, et al, International Early SOMS guided Mobilization Research Initiative. Early, goal-directed mobilisation in the surgical intensive care unit: a randomised controlled trial. Lancet 2016;388:1377–88.

110. Schweickert WiD, Pohlman MC, Pohlman AS, et al. Early physical and occupational therapy in mechanically ventilated, critically ill patients: a randomised controlled trial. Lancet 2009;373(9678):1874–82.

111. Sricharoenchai T, Parker AM, Zanni JM, et al. Safety of physical therapy interventions in critically ill patients: a single-center prospective evaluation of 1110 intensive care unit admissions. J Crit Care 2014;29(3):395–400.

112. Dunne DFJ, Jack S, Jones RP, et al. Randomized clinical trial of prehabilitation before planned liver resection. Br J Surg 2016;103:504–12.
113. Gomes Neto M, Martinez BP, Fc Reis H, et al. Pre- and postoperative inspiratory muscle training in patients undergoing cardiac surgery: systematic review and meta-analysis. Clin Rehabil 2017;31:454–64.
114. Herdy AH, Marcchi PLB, Vila A, et al. Pre- and postoperative cardiopulmonary rehabilitation in hospitalized patients undergoing coronary artery bypass surgery: a randomized controlled trial. Am J Phys Med Rehabil 2008;87:714–9.
115. Hirschhorn AD, Richards DAB, Mungovan SF, et al. Does the mode of exercise influence recovery of functional capacity in the early postoperative period after coronary artery bypass graft surgery? a randomized controlled trial. Interactive Cardiovasc Thorac Surg 2012;15:995–1003.
116. Hulzebos EHJ, van Meeteren NLU, van den Buijs BJWM, et al. Feasibility of preoperative inspiratory muscle training in patients undergoing coronary artery bypass surgery with a high risk of postoperative pulmonary complications: a randomized controlled pilot study. Clin Rehabil 2006;20:949–59.
117. Hulzebos EHJ, Helders PJM, Favie NJ, et al. Preoperative intensive inspiratory muscle training to prevent postoperative pulmonary complications in high-risk patients undergoing CABG surgery: a randomized clinical trial. JAMA 2006; 296:1851–7.
118. Pouwels S, Stokmans RA, Willigendael EM, et al. Preoperative exercise therapy for elective major abdominal surgery: a systematic review. Int J Surg 2014;12(2): 134–40.
119. Snowdon D, Haines TP, Skinner EH. Preoperative intervention reduces postoperative pulmonary complications but not length of stay in cardiac surgical patients: a systematic review. J Physiother 2014;60:66–77.
120. Timmerman H, de Groot JF, Hulzebos HJ, et al. Feasibility and preliminary effectiveness of preoperative therapeutic exercise in patients with cancer: a pragmatic study. Physiother Theory Pract 2011;27:117–24.
121. Valkenet K, de Heer F, Backx FJG, et al. Effect of inspiratory muscle training before cardiac surgery in routine care. Phys Ther 2013;93:611–9.
122. Valkenet K, van de Port IGL, Dronkers JJ, et al. The effects of preoperative exercise therapy on postoperative outcome: a systematic review. Clin Rehabil 2011;25:99–111.
123. Weston M, Weston KL, Prentis JM, et al. High-intensity interval training (hit) for effective and time-efficient pre-surgical exercise interventions. Perioper Med (Lond) 2016;5:2.
124. Engelman DT, Ben Ali W, Williams JB, et al. Guidelines for perioperative care in cardiac surgery: Enhanced Recovery After Surgery Society recommendations. JAMA Surg 2019;154(8):755–66.
125. Hulzebos EHJ, Smit Y, Helders PPJM, et al. Preoperative physical therapy for elective cardiac surgery patients. Cochrane Database Syst Rev 2012;(11):CD010118.
126. Katsura M, Kuriyama A, Takeshima T, et al. Preoperative inspiratory muscle training for postoperative pulmonary complications in adults undergoing cardiac and major abdominal surgery. Cochrane Database Syst Rev 2015;(10):CD010356.
127. Mans CM, Reeve JC, Elkins MR. Postoperative outcomes following preoperative inspiratory muscle training in patients undergoing cardiothoracic or upper abdominal surgery: a systematic review and meta analysis. Clin Rehabil 2015; 29:426–38.

128. Burtin C, Clerckx B, Robbeets C, et al. Early exercise in critically ill patients enhances short-term functional recovery. Crit Care Med 2009;37:2499–505.

129. Kho ME, Molloy AJ, Clarke FJ, et al, Canadian Critical Care Trials Group. Trycycle: a prospective study of the safety and feasibility of early in-bed cycling in mechanically ventilated patients. PloS one 2016;11:e0167561.

130. Kim HK, Suzuki T, Saito K, et al. Effects of exercise and amino acid supplementation on body composition and physical function in community-dwelling elderly Japanese sarcopenic women: a randomized controlled trial. J Am Geriatr Soc 2012;60:16–23.

131. Kimawi I, Lamberjack B, Nelliot A, et al. Safety and feasibility of a protocolized approach to in-bed cycling exercise in the intensive care unit: quality improvement project. Phys Ther 2017;97:593–602.

132. Kayambu G, Boots R, Paratz J. Physical therapy for the critically ill in the ICU: a systematic review and meta-analysis. Crit Care Med 2013;41(6):1543–54.

133. Pires-Neto RC, Fogaça Kawaguchi YM, Hirota AS, et al. Very early passive cycling exercise in mechanically ventilated critically ill patients: physiological and safety aspects-a case series. PloS one 2013;8(9):e74182.

134. Rahimi RA, Skrzat J, Reddy DRS, et al. Physical rehabilitation of patients in the intensive care unit requiring extracorporeal membrane oxygenation: a small case series. Phys Ther 2013;93(2):248–55.

135. Guralnik JM, Ferrucci L, Simonsick EM, et al. Lower-extremity function in persons over the age of 70 years as a predictor of subsequent disability. N Engl J Med 1995;332(9):556–62.

136. LeBlanc AD, Schneider VS, Evans HJ, et al. Regional changes in muscle mass following 17 weeks of bed rest. J Appl Physiol 1992;73(5):2172–8.

137. Griffiths RD, Palmer TE, Helliwell T, et al. Effect of passive stretching on the wasting of muscle in the critically ill. Nutrition 1995;11(5):428â€–432.

138. Preiser J, Prato C, Harvengt A, et al. Passive cycling limits myofibrillar protein catabolism in unconscious patients: a pilot study. J Nov Physiother 2014;4:225.

139. Arthur HM, Daniels C, McKelvie R, et al. Effect of a preoperative intervention on preoperative and postoperative outcomes in low-risk patients awaiting elective coronary artery bypass graft surgery. a randomized, controlled trial. Ann Intern Med 2000;133:253–62.

140. Rosenfeldt F, Braun L, Spitzer O, et al. Physical conditioning and mental stress reduction–a randomised trial in patients undergoing cardiac surgery. BMC Complement Altern Med 2011;11:20.

141. Tung H-H, Shen S-F, Shih C-C, et al. Effects of a preoperative individualized exercise program on selected recovery variables for cardiac surgery patients: a pilot study. J Saudi Heart Assoc 2012;24(3):153–61.

142. Sawatzky J-AV, D Scott K, Ready AE, et al. Prehabilitation program for elective coronary artery bypass graft surgery patients: a pilot randomized controlled study. Clin Rehabil 2014;28:648–57.

143. Arabi YM, Casaer MP, Chapman M, et al. The intensive care medicine research agenda in nutrition and metabolism. Intensive Care Med 2017;43(9):1239–56.

144. Botros D, Gabriel S, Neri D, et al. Interventions to address chronic disease and HIV: strategies to promote exercise and nutrition among HIV-infected individuals. Curr HIV/AIDS Rep 2012;9(4):351–63.

145. Arora RC, Brown CH, Sanjanwala RM, et al. "New" prehabilitation: a 3-way approach to improve postoperative survival and health-related quality of life in cardiac surgery patients. Can J Cardiol 2018;34:839–49.

146. English KL, Douglas P-J. Protecting muscle mass and function in older adults during bed rest. Curr Opin Clin Nutr Metab Care 2010;13(1):34.
147. Heyland DK, Stapleton RD, Mourtzakis M, et al. Combining nutrition and exercise to optimize survival and recovery from critical illness: conceptual and methodological issues. Clin Nutr 2016;35:1196–206.
148. Kim J-S, Wilson JM, Lee S-R. Dietary implications on mechanisms of sarcopenia: roles of protein, amino acids and antioxidants. J Nutr Biochem 2010;21:1–13.
149. Villareal DT, Suresh C, Parimi N, et al. Weight loss, exercise, or both and physical function in obese older adults. N Engl J Med 2011;364(13):1218–29.
150. Gustafsson UO, Scott MJ, Schwenk W, et al. Ljungqvist, for perioperative care Enhanced Recovery After Surgery (ERAS) Society, European Society for Clinical Nutrition, Metabolism (ESPEN), International Association for Surgical Metabolism, and Nutrition (IASMEN). Guidelines for perioperative care in elective colonic surgery: Enhanced Recovery After Surgery (ERAS(r)) Society recommendations. World J Surg 2013;37:259–84.
151. Ljungqvist Olle. ERAS–Enhanced Recovery After Surgery: moving evidence-based perioperative care to practice. JPEN J Parenter Enteral Nutr 2014;38:559–66.
152. Bonnefoy M, Cornu C, Normand S, et al. The effects of exercise and protein–energy supplements on body composition and muscle function in frail elderly individuals: a long-term controlled randomised study. Br J Nutr 2003;89(5):731–8.
153. Trappe TA, Burd NA, Louis ES, et al. Influence of concurrent exercise or nutrition countermeasures on thigh and calf muscle size and function during 60 days of bed rest in women. Acta Physiol 2007;191(2):147–59.
154. Tieland M, Dirks ML, van der Zwaluw N, et al. Protein supplementation increases muscle mass gain during prolonged resistance-type exercise training in frail elderly people: a randomized, double-blind, placebo-controlled trial. J Am Med Directors Assoc 2012;13(8):713–9.
155. Ferrie S, Allman-Farinelli M, Daley M, et al. Protein requirements in the critically ill: a randomized controlled trial using parenteral nutrition. JPEN J Parenter Enteral Nutr 2016;40:795–805.
156. Fiatarone MA, O'Neill EF, Ryan ND, et al. Exercise training and nutritional supplementation for physical frailty in very elderly people. N Engl J Med 1994;330(25):1769–75.
157. Galvan E, Arentson-Lantz E, Lamon S, et al. Protecting skeletal muscle with protein and amino acid during periods of disuse. Nutrients 2016;8(7):404.
158. Hermans G, Casaer MP, Clerckx B, et al. Effect of tolerating macronutrient deficit on the development of intensive-care unit acquired weakness: a subanalysis of the EPANIC trial. Lancet Respir Med 2013;1:621–9.
159. Rasmussen BB, Phillips SM. Contractile and nutritional regulation of human muscle growth. Exerc Sport Sci Rev 2003;31:127–31.
160. Symons TB, Sheffield-Moore M, Mamerow MM, et al. The anabolic response to resistance exercise and a protein-rich meal is not diminished by age. J Nutr Health Aging 2011;15(5):376–81.
161. Warnold I, Eden E, Lundholm K. The inefficiency of total parenteral nutrition to stimulate protein synthesis in moderately malnourished patients. Ann Surg 1988;208:143–9.
162. Fearon KCH. Cancer cachexia and fat-muscle physiology. N Engl J Med 2011;365:565–7.
163. Visser M, van Venrooij LMW, Vulperhorst L, et al. Sarcopenic obesity is associated with adverse clinical outcome after cardiac surgery. Nutr Metab Cardiovasc Dis 2013;23(6):511–8.

164. Cermak NM, de Groot LCPGM, Saris WHM, et al. Protein supplementation augments the adaptive response of skeletal muscle to resistance-type exercise training: a meta-analysis. Am J Clin Nutr 2012;96(6):1454–64.

165. Luo D, Zheng L, Li S, et al. Effect of nutritional supplement combined with exercise intervention on sarcopenia in the elderly: a meta-analysis. Int J Nurs Sci 2017;4(4):389–401.

166. Kim H, Kim M, Kojima N, et al. Exercise and nutritional supplementation on community-dwelling elderly Japanese women with sarcopenic obesity: a randomized controlled trial. J Am Med Directors Assoc 2016;17:1011–9.

167. Payne C, Larkin PJ, McIlfatrick S, et al. Exercise and nutrition interventions in advanced lung cancer: a systematic review. Curr Oncol 2013;20:e321–37.

168. Fiatarone MA, O'Neill EF, Doyle N, et al. The Boston FICSIT study: the effects of resistance training and nutritional supplementation on physical frailty in the oldest old. J Am Geriatr Soc 1993;41(3):333–7.

169. Jones C, Eddleston J, McCairn A, et al. Improving rehabilitation after critical illness through outpatient physiotherapy classes and essential amino acid supplement: a randomized controlled trial. J Crit Care 2015;30(5):901–7.

170. Molnár A, Jónásné Sztruhár I, Csontos ÁA, et al. Special nutrition intervention is required for muscle protective efficacy of physical exercise in elderly people at highest risk of sarcopenia. Physiol Int 2016;103:368–76.

171. Sandmael JA, Bye A, Solheim TS, et al. Feasibility and preliminary effects of resistance training and nutritional supplements during versus after radiotherapy in patients with head and neck cancer: a pilot randomized trial. Cancer 2017;123:4440–8.

172. Solheim TS, Laird BJA, Balstad TR, et al. A randomized phase ii feasibility trial of a multimodal intervention for the management of cachexia in lung and pancreatic cancer. J Cachexia Sarcopenia Muscle 2017;8:778–88.

173. Minnella EM, Awasthi R, Loiselle S-E, et al. Effect of exercise and nutrition prehabilitation on functional capacity in esophagogastric cancer surgery: a randomized clinical trial. JAMA Surg 2018;153:1081–9.

174. Francois ME, Pistawka KJ, Halperin FA, et al. Cardiovascular benefits of combined interval training and post-exercise nutrition in type 2 diabetes. J Diabetes Complications 2018;32:226–33.

175. Invernizzi M, de Sire A, D'Andrea F, et al. Effects of essential amino acid supplementation and rehabilitation on functioning in hip fracture patients: a pilot randomized controlled trial. Aging Clin Exp Res 2019;31:1517–24.

176. Gill F, Dumville JC, Miles JNV, et al. prehabilitation" prior to CABG surgery improves physical functioning and depression. Int J Cardiol 2009;132:51–8.

177. Anderson EA. Preoperative preparation for cardiac surgery facilitates recovery, reduces psychological distress, and reduces the incidence of acute postoperative hypertension. J Consult Clin Psychol 1987;55:513–20.

178. Mina DS, Clarke H, Ritvo P, et al. Effect of total-body prehabilitation on postoperative outcomes: a systematic review and meta-analysis. Physiotherapy 2014; 100:196–207.

179. Castillo R, Haas A. Chest physical therapy: comparative efficacy of preoperative and postoperative in the elderly. Arch Phys Med Rehabil 1985;66:376–9.

180. de Morton NA, Keating JL, Jeffs K. Exercise for acutely hospitalised older medical patients. Cochrane Database Syst Rev 2007;(1):CD005955.

181. Silver JK, Baima J. Cancer prehabilitation: an opportunity to decrease treatment-related morbidity, increase cancer treatment options, and improve physical and psychological health outcomes. Am J Phys Med Rehabil 2013; 92:715–27.

Orthopedic Principles to Facilitate Enhanced Recovery After Cardiac Surgery

Marc W. Gerdisch, MD[a],*, Keith B. Allen, MD[b], Yoshifumi Naka, MD, PhD[c], Mark R. Bonnell, MD[d], Kevin P. Landolfo, MD[e], John Grehan, MD, PhD[f], Kendra J. Grubb, MD[g], David J. Cohen, MD[h], T. Sloane Guy, MD[i], Nirav C. Patel, MD[j], Vinod H. Thourani, MD[k]

KEYWORDS

- Median sternotomy • Sternal closure • Sternal fixation • Rigid fixation
- Wire cerclage • Sternal wiring • Sternal plating • Sternal bands

KEY POINTS

- Early patient mobilization is a major driver of recovery after cardiac surgery with open sternotomy.
- Instability of the healing sternal osteotomy hinders postoperative patient movement, causes pain, and puts patients at risk of complications, necessitating restrictive sternal precaution protocols.
- Sternal closure with wire cerclage does not adequately satisfy the three fundamental principles of orthopedic healing: approximation, compression, and rigid fixation.
- Selection of sternal closure methods according to orthopedic principles promotes accelerated recovery and return to normal activities while reducing pain and requirements for opioid analgesics.

---

[a] Department of Cardiothoracic Surgery, Franciscan Health Heart Center, 5255 East Stop 11 Road, Suite 200, Indianapolis, IN 46237, USA; [b] Department of Cardiothoracic Surgery, Saint Luke's Mid America Heart Institute, University of Missouri-Kansas City School of Medicine, 4320 Wornall Road, Suite 50-II, Kansas City, MO 64111, USA; [c] Division of Cardiothoracic Surgery, Department of Surgery, Columbia University Medical Center, 630 W 168th St, New York, NY 10032, USA; [d] Department of Cardiothoracic Surgery, University of Toledo, 1735 W Rocket Dr, Toledo, OH 43607, USA; [e] Department of Cardiothoracic Surgery, Mayo Clinic, 4500 San Pablo Road - Davis 321N, Jacksonville, FL 32224, USA; [f] Department of Cardiothoracic Surgery, Allina Health, 225 Smith Ave N, Nasseff Specialty Center, Suite 400, St Paul, MN 55102, USA; [g] Department of Cardiothoracic Surgery, Emory University, 550 Peachtree St NE, Davis Fischer 4th Floor, Atlanta, GA 30308, USA; [h] Department of Cardiology, Saint Luke's Mid America Heart Institute, University of Missouri-Kansas City School of Medicine, 4320 Wornall Road, Suite 50-II, Kansas City, MO 64111, USA; [i] Department of Surgery, Division of Cardiac Surgery, Sidney Kimmel Medical College, Thomas Jefferson University, 1025 Walnut St, Suite 607, Philadelphia, PA 19107, USA; [j] Department of Cardiothoracic Surgery, Lenox Hill Hospital, 130 East 77th Street, 4th Floor, New York, NY 10075, USA; [k] Department of Cardiovascular Surgery, Marcus Heart and Vascular Center, Piedmont Heart Institute, 95 Collier Road, Suite 5015, Atlanta, GA 30309, USA
* Corresponding author.
E-mail address: mgerdisch@openheart.net

Crit Care Clin 36 (2020) 617–630
https://doi.org/10.1016/j.ccc.2020.07.003
0749-0704/20/© 2020 The Authors. Published by Elsevier Inc. This is an open access article under the CC BY-NC-ND license (http://creativecommons.org/licenses/by-nc-nd/4.0/).

THE EVOLUTION FROM "FAST-TRACK" TO "ENHANCED RECOVERY" AFTER CARDIAC SURGERY

Around the world, clinical and economic analyses increasingly show that evidence-based initiatives to improve and shorten the course of in-hospital recovery positively affect quality of care, patient outcomes, and cost-effectiveness of care.[1-4] In Europe, the Enhanced Recovery After Surgery (ERAS) Society has formalized the movement to promote improvements in postsurgical recovery of patients by releasing a series of guidelines for multimodal, transdisciplinary care improvement.[1] Early successes improving recovery times and clinical outcomes after colorectal surgery have served as a model for the development of similar initiatives in gynecologic, bariatric, gastrointestinal, liver, and head and neck surgery.[1]

The general principles that have been formalized in current ERAS guidelines have been informally used in cardiac surgery for at least 3 decades. As early as 1990, Krohn and colleagues[5] verified that proactive prevention and prompt correction of noncardiac complications after surgery shortened hospital length of stay (LOS) and resulted in fewer readmissions. In 1994, Engelman and colleagues[6] found that a fast-track recovery protocol aimed at reducing complications and accelerating discharge was associated with statistically significant and clinically meaningful decreases in time to extubation, peak weight gain, intensive care unit (ICU) LOS, and overall hospital LOS without increases in morbidity or mortality.

Subsequent studies in both Europe and the United States built on these successes by gradually adding more ERAS principles to the perioperative process.[7] Zaouter and colleagues[8] (France) examined extubation outcomes and postoperative complications in 38 patients undergoing robotic, totally endoscopic coronary artery bypass grafting (CABG), managed according to an ERAS-guided protocol, compared with a matched cohort undergoing conventional CABG with traditional perioperative management. They found that patients in the robotic surgery/ERAS group could be safely extubated in the operating room, experienced lower transfusion rates, experienced shorter ICU stays (mean reduction of 24 hours), and experienced overall hospital stays (mean reduction of 4 days) compared with patients managed with standard care (P<.05). A notable variable in these procedures was the use of minimally invasive, sternum-sparing approaches in the robotic surgery group; the critical role of a stable sternum in the healing process is central to the present discussion.

In 2016, Fleming and colleagues[9] from the United Kingdom published the results of a prospective, observational study comparing outcomes in 105 consecutive adult patients undergoing any scheduled, elective cardiac surgery, before and after implementation of a perioperative care bundle based on ERAS principles. The aim was to evaluate whether small practice improvements distributed throughout the course of perioperative management could accumulate to result in meaningful gains in clinical outcomes. Even in this small study, the group managed according to ERAS principles (n = 52) experienced less postoperative morbidity and mortality and reported improved postoperative pain scores compared with patients who underwent surgery before the care bundle was implemented.

A clinical trial carried out in China and published in 2018 by Li and colleagues[10] evaluated outcomes after randomization to either an ERAS protocol or standard of care in 226 patients undergoing elective cardiac value procedures, with or without cardiac ablation and/or CABG. The study found that patients in the ERAS group spent significantly less time on mechanical ventilation, had a shorter stay in the ICU, and were ready for discharge a day earlier. Overall cost of care was also significantly reduced in the ERAS patients.

In 2019, Grant and colleagues[11] published a retrospective analysis of prospectively collected data from 451 consecutive patients undergoing CABG, valvular, or combination procedures, as part of a stepwise implementation of an institutional early-recovery program for cardiac surgery at their hospital. After stratifying patients into low- and high-compliance groups (based on how many protocol measures were followed) and then propensity-matching patients between groups, they found that implementation of their program significantly improved early extubation rates and hospital LOS.

Most recently, Williams and colleagues[12] published the results of a large feasibility study of prospectively collected, retrospectively reviewed data comparing outcomes in 443 US patients managed according to an ERAS-based protocol, versus 489 managed according to traditional standard of care. Standardized processes included preoperative patient education, carbohydrate loading 2 hours before general anesthesia, multimodal opioid-sparing analgesia, goal-directed perioperative insulin infusion, a rigorous bowel regimen, and early mobilization.[13] One-year clinical data and survey results showed ERAS-based patient management was associated with reduced median overall LOS (6 vs 7 days; $P<.01$), reduced ICU time (28 vs 43 hours; $P<.01$), lower rate of gastrointestinal complications (3.6% vs 6.8%; $P<.05$), and an 8 mg morphine equivalent reduction in opioid use in the first 24 hours postoperatively ($P<.01$). Patient satisfaction was also higher in the ERAS-managed group.

Based on the growing body of evidence regarding the individual practices that benefit recovery and outcomes after cardiac surgery, the ERAS Cardiac Society was formed in 2017 to develop a set of recommendations for the field. The founding group of cardiac surgeons, anesthesiologists, and intensivists published its first, expert-consensus review of evidence-based practices for Enhanced Recovery After Cardiac Surgery in 2019, in partnership with the ERAS Society.[14]

MEDIAN STERNOTOMY AS AN OBSTACLE AND OPPORTUNITY FOR ERAS AFTER CARDIAC SURGERY

ERAS guidelines across all disciplines are typically organized into preoperative, intraoperative, and postoperative strategies, each ranked by strength of recommendation (based on expected benefits vs potential harms) and by the quality of evidence underlying each recommendation. The Enhanced Recovery After Cardiac Surgery Society (ERAS Cardiac) guidelines are evidence based and are similar to those of other disciplines.[14] Recommended preoperative measures include optimization of glycemic control, kidney function, and nutrition; patient education; and cessation of smoking and hazardous alcohol consumption. Intraoperatively, the guidelines recommend use of protocols to reduce surgical site infections, avoidance of hyperthermia during patient rewarming on cardiopulmonary bypass, use of tranexamic acid or epsilon aminocaproic acid for bleeding management during on-pump cardiac surgical procedures, and use of rigid-plate fixation (RPF) to provide maximal stability to the healing osteotomy and potentially reduce the incidence of major sternal complications. Postoperative recommendations include continued perioperative management of glycemic control and kidney function; maintenance of normothermia, chest tube patency, and thromboprophylaxis; multimodal, opioid-sparing pain management; goal-directed fluid therapy; systematic screening for delirium; and extubation within 6 hours of surgery.

The ERAS Cardiac guidelines differ from those for other disciplines. First, the ERAS Cardiac recommendations do not emphasize use of minimally invasive surgical (MIS) approaches. Although MIS parasternal and minithoracotomy approaches have been developed for single-valve operations and select, combined cardiac surgical procedures, median sternotomy remains the most common incision for open heart surgery.[15]

Although it is an invasive procedure, median sternotomy provides access to every part of the heart and the large blood vessels within the chest. It is, therefore, likely to remain a common surgical approach for the foreseeable future.[16]

Second, the ERAS Cardiac guidelines include no specific recommendations for early postoperative enteral feeding and mobilization, even though these measures are known to work together to stimulate resumption of gut function, preserve musculoskeletal function, and promote a faster and safer return to normal activities after surgery.[17–22] A sternotomy incision limits early mobilization and rehabilitation activities. Although the ERAS Cardiac guidelines do recommend that cardiac surgery programs develop multidisciplinary institutional guidelines to address early feeding and mobilization,[14] traditional sternal precautions prioritize the stability of the bony union over patient mobility, greatly limiting opportunities for return to normal activity and physical rehabilitation in the postoperative recovery period.[17,18,23] The authors propose that the limitations that sternal healing imposes on early mobilization and physical activity during recovery represent a potential target for further gains in the pace of recovery and improved outcomes after cardiac surgery.

ORTHOPEDIC PRINCIPLES: THE RECIPE FOR SUCCESSFUL HEALING AND EARLY MOBILIZATION AFTER STERNOTOMY

Healing of osseous fractures, whether traumatic or as a result of surgical osteotomy or osteochondrotomy, depends on a complex interaction between biological processes and biomechanical forces.[24–27] The biomechanical principles that promote successful healing include accurate reapproximation, alignment, and reduction of the osteotomy gap to foster restoration of blood flow and cellular communication; compression that is adequate to encourage osteosynthesis but not so excessive as to impede blood flow; and rigid fixation of the union to stabilize it against movement and prevent recurring microfractures.[24–27]

Stability of the sternum promotes revascularization and bone formation. In contrast, instability in the presence of repetitive distractive tensile loads and shear forces allows bone-on-bone movement within the osteotomy. Such movement promotes the formation of a fibrocartilaginous callous that must later remodel into ossified bone, or it may inhibit the healing process altogether.[25,28]

Like all other bone fractures, the sternotomy is governed by these same orthopedic principles and biological processes. It is also subject to continuous forces from breathing, coughing, movements of the head, spine, and upper extremities, and ambulation. A critical role of the healthy sternum is to provide flexible support and central communication and distribution of the forces from these activities.[28] Sternal instability after closure is closely associated with poor sternal healing, deep sternal wound infection (DSWI), and sternal dehiscence or nonunion, as well as postoperative pain and increased requirement for analgesia.[29,30] These sternal complications represent major drivers of postsurgical morbidity and mortality after cardiac surgery, especially in high-risk patients. The incidence of sternal wound infection is as high as 5%, and mediastinitis has been reported to occur in 0.8% to 2.3% of patients.[31] DSWI in particular is associated with as much as a 4-fold increase in 1-year postoperative mortality, 3-fold increase in length of hospital stay, and 2.5-fold higher cost of care compared with patients without infection.[32]

Even though early postoperative mobilization and resumption of physical activities are known to be advantageous to healing of bone fractures and to functional recovery in general,[18,23,26] cardiothoracic surgeons face a dilemma in choosing methods for sternal closure, governed by the effort to balance 2 potential risks: one, that patient movements and consequent forces on an unstable sternal union will disrupt healing and invite infection; and two, that devices providing rigid fixation represent an obstacle to emergent sternal reentry.[33]

Newer techniques and devices for closure, coupled with higher-quality evidence regarding their relative ability to stabilize the sternum for optimal healing, suggest a path toward reducing the influence of sternal healing as a limiting factor on the ERAS principle of early mobilization and return to normal activity.

STERNAL-CLOSURE TECHNIQUES IN THE CONTEXT OF ORTHOPEDIC PRINCIPLES
Wire Cerclage

Traditional wire cerclage remains by far the most common technique for sternal closure after median sternotomy,[16] leaving cardiac surgeons as the only specialty that still relies on wire cerclage for postosteotomy fixation. In this technique, the cut edges of the sternal osteotomy are brought together at 5 to 8 levels with lengths of stainless-steel surgical wire, wrapped around or through the bone and tightened (**Fig. 1**). This technique is simple and inexpensive to implement, and in case of emergent need for sternal reentry, the wires can readily be cut for removal.

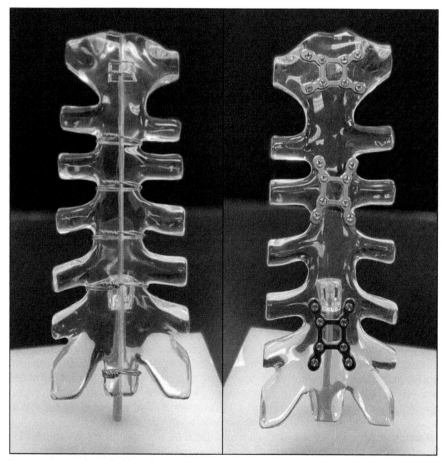

Fig. 1. Wire cerclage (*left*) and RPF (*right*). Photographs provided by Zimmer Biomet.

Wire cerclage provides for 2 of the 3 essential requirements for sternal union, namely, approximation and compression.[34] However, it has been shown that wire cerclage provides, at best, suboptimal fixation and stabilization of the healing bone.[28] It is also notable that the low ratio of surface-area contact between wire and bone concentrates the compressive forces along the wires, with the potential for notching or cutting of the bone and even complete transverse sternal fracture.[28] Although alternative techniques for single-wire cerclage, such as double-wire, figure-of-8, and Robicsek's weave, have been developed to improve the relative distribution of compressive forces,[16,35] they have not been shown to reduce rates of sternal dehiscence or DSWI compared with single wires.[36,37] Furthermore, despite providing a range of compressive forces, none of these approaches address the biomechanical problem of inadequate fixation.[35] Rigid Fixation is especially critical in patients who are considered to be high risk because of morbid obesity, chronic obstructive pulmonary disease, diabetes mellitus, or other comorbidities, because sternal dehiscence is associated with a markedly higher mortality in these patients.[30]

Steel Bands

Stainless-steel bands have been explored as a potential adjunct to wires, chiefly because their wider profile provides for improved contact surface area between the band and bone, thus potentially reducing wire pull-through and preventing transverse fractures as the mechanism for failure. Three studies have found that the use of steel bands in combination with standard wiring reduces the risk of sternal dehiscence compared with single steel wires used alone.[38–40] However, none of the studies found that steel bands reliably reduced the incidence of mediastinitis.

Criticisms of steel bands include that their structural rigidity prevents them from conforming to the patient-specific shape of the sternum. The bands also do not have a mechanism to lock them in place after tightening, and they may be difficult to remove in case of the need for sternal reentry.[16] Furthermore, although steel bands adequately satisfy the requirements for approximation and compression, the directional forces are similar to wires and do not provide rigid fixation.

Polymer Cable Ties

A newer alternative to steel wires or bands is cable ties made of polyether ether ketone (PEEK), a high-performance, biocompatible, nickel-free polymer that has been used since the 1990s to replace metal in a growing number of implanted medical devices.[41] The polymer cable ties work according to a principle similar to steel bands, but are more flexible and malleable.[41] The recommended use is to place 5 ties along the sternum (the first transsternally through the manubrial bone, 3 peristernal bands through the intercostal spaces, and the fifth transsternally through the xiphoid region). The free end of each tie is passed through the locking head at the other end, tightened by hand to ensure accurate sternal approximation, and then tensioned to a force of 200 N using a system-specific application device, which also cuts away excess tie material. As with steel bands, the cable ties are wider than surgical wire (4.2 mm vs 0.7 mm for US Pharmacopeia 5 steel wire) and thus provide increased area of contact between implant and bone, potentially reducing the risk of sternal damage. In support of this idea, PEEK-based cable ties have been shown, in engineering studies, to have equivalent or better static-loading strength, fatigue strength, and resistance to bone cut-through compared with stainless-steel surgical wire.[42,43]

A commercially available polymer sternal cable-tie system has been evaluated in several studies, with mixed results.[41,44–47] A retrospective comparison of 95 sternotomies closed with polymer cable ties versus 498 closed with transverse, interrupted figure-of-8 stainless-steel wires found no difference in superficial or DSWI between groups.[47] Another retrospective, nonrandomized comparison found that DSWI occurred in 2.6% (8/309) of patients who underwent sternal closure with surgical wires alone versus no occurrences (0/300) in patients closed with a combination of surgical wires and polymer cable ties.[46]

A 118-patient, prospective, randomized study found no difference in pain-related outcomes but more sternal and manubrial movement, by ultrasound, when polymer cable ties were used instead of steel wires. In contrast, a larger randomized trial found significantly lower pain scores and rates of sternal dehiscence with the use of cable ties, with similar rates of infection (2.76%).[48] Independent criticism of these conflicting studies has noted that both are limited by lack of definition/standardization of wiring technique, different choice of outcomes, and biases in study design and reporting.[49,50] Given further conflicting results in biomechanical studies comparing conventional versus figure-of-8 wire cerclage, polymer cable ties, and steel bands,[42,43] higher-quality data are required before definitive conclusions can be reached about the appropriate role of polymer cable ties in the sternal closure toolkit. Of key importance, despite their proposed advantages over wires and bands, polymer cable ties also do not provide orthopedic stabilization of the osteotomy and are not considered rigid fixation.

Rigid-Plate Fixation

Sternal fixation with rigid plates, mounted to the sternum with screws (see **Fig. 1**), is specifically noted in the ERAS Cardiac guidelines for its potential to "be useful to improve or accelerate sternal healing and reduce mediastinal wound complications."[14] This guideline is presented as a recommendation with moderate benefit (class IIa), based on evidence from one or more randomized clinical trial (level B-R), as well as from biomechanical studies.

Experimentally, rigid fixation with sternal plates has been shown to reduce the extent of sternal gap development under static load compared with wire cerclage.[28,51] A technique for rigid-plate sternal fixation in humans was first published by Gottlieb and colleagues[52] in 1994 using plates intended for mandibular fixation. Later, Song and colleagues[33] published a report evaluating a commercially available plate system configured specifically for the sternum in 45 patients, each of whom had a minimum of 3 established risk factors for dehiscence and mediastinitis. This system consisted of multiple configurations of titanium plates secured with bicortical screws of various sizes depending on the patient's specific anatomy. Compared with matched controls closed with wire cerclage, these patients experienced significantly lower rates of mediastinitis (14.8% vs 0%, $P = .006$). Use of this system also eliminated emergent sternal reentry as a major obstacle to surgeon comfort with use of rigid plates, because it was designed to be cut easily with wire cutters standard to the operating room.[33]

Since those early reports, the results of several studies of both observational and randomized, controlled designs have been published showing that RPF is associated with earlier extubation,[53] shorter postoperative LOS,[53–55] improved sternal healing,[34,56,57] reduced incidence of early sternal wound complications, mediastinitis and DSWI,[34,54,57–60] less pain and lower utilization of analgesic and narcotic medications,[55,56,58,60,61] less radiographic evidence of sternal displacement during recovery,[55] and similar or lower overall cost of care.[34,59,61] The benefits may especially be significant in patients at high risk of sternal dehiscence.[62]

A recent, prospective, single-blinded, multicenter, randomized trial compared outcomes in patients undergoing median sternotomy for cardiac surgery at 12 US sites, and closed either with rigid plates (n = 116) or wire cerclage (n = 120).[34] Importantly, the study excluded high-risk patients in order to understand the potential benefits of RPF for the general cardiac surgery population. For the primary endpoint of the study, radiographic and clinical evidence of sternal healing, RPF resulted in better sternal healing scores at 3 and 6 months compared with wire cerclage ($P<.0001$ and $P = .0007$, respectively). Sternal union rates were also greater at these time points ($P<.0001$ and $P = .03$), with no sternal complications at 6 months in the RPF group versus 5% in the wire cerclage group ($P = .03$). Overall cost of care was neutral between groups over the total study period.

Furthermore, Allen and colleagues[61] noted a greater proportion of patients treated with RPF reported absence of pain after coughing at 3 and 6 weeks of follow-up ($P = .001$ and $P = .005$), and at rest at 6 weeks and 3 months ($P = .02$ and $P = .03$) compared with wire cerclage. These scores correlated with better sternal healing. Patients in the RPF group also reported significantly better quality of life at 3 weeks, 6 weeks, and 6 months. Additional cost analysis using a 90-day global payment model confirmed RPF improved patient outcomes at both 90 and 180 days without increasing cost to the health care system. These results were in patients with standard risk factors for cardiac surgery and illustrate that RPF is likely to benefit all sternotomy patients regardless of their risk profile.

A potential concern for surgeons new to the use of RPF is whether the additional foreign material from the plates could result in residual dead space above the sternum after closure, and therefore, more superficial wound issues, compared with wiring. Clinical experience has shown that this potential problem can be readily addressed by closure technique. When closing fascia after RFP, bites should be taken so that the suture goes under the plates, thus pulling the fascia down to the plates and obliterating any dead space.

Other Devices and Methods for Sternal Fixation

An assortment of other devices, such as a cabling and plating system, transverse bridging plates, locking plates and screws, j-hook plates, quick-release clamps, and special clasps, have been proposed or developed for sternal closure. Many of these products do not incorporate the orthopedic principle of rigid fixation and lack sufficient randomized evidence to be relevant to this review. In addition, chemical and biologic enhancement of healing using bone cement and other polymerizing agents, resorbable materials, platelet-rich plasma, and hydrogels have been proposed to encourage osteosynthesis; however, these products do not provide rigid fixation, and their use as an adjunct to rigid fixation has not been studied. The authors refer the reader to several excellent reviews that go into greater depth regarding the full spectrum of products and techniques under investigation.[28]

Based on the available evidence, the ERAS Cardiac working group concluded that RPF should be the recommended method of closure after median sternotomy, with benefits that would especially accrue to patients whose comorbidities put them at high risk of sternal dehiscence.[14]

RIGID-PLATE FIXATION AND RAPID MOBILIZATION

The paradigm for managing postsurgical recovery is changing across surgical disciplines, informed by emphasis on evidence over tradition.[1,7,63–65] Evidence shows that deliberate, strategic interventions aimed at safely getting the patient extubated, awake, eating, moving, and home as soon as possible after surgery have positive benefits for the patient's physical, mental, and psychosocial recovery as well as for cost-effective health care delivery.[1–4,7,63–65]

In cardiac surgery, the ERAS Cardiac recommendation for use of RPF to establish sternal stability and promote healing after median sternotomy has enabled a shift in attitudes toward sternal precautions. Historically, physical rehabilitation programs have called for drastic restrictions on activity and upper-body mobility, dictated by the limitations imposed by patient pain and the slow pace of healing associated with the unstable, wired sternum.[17,18,20,22,23] As real-world experience with RPF proves consistent with controlled trials, surgeons are piloting new paths to patient recovery. For example, following 2 years of study participation and data review, in March 2017, Franciscan Health Heart Center (Indianapolis, Indiana, USA) made RPF the standard closure method for all sternotomies. The departments of Cardiac Surgery and Physical Therapy developed a rapid assessment and mobilization protocol (**Table 1**). This aggressive protocol was made possible by stable sternotomies allowing for near-normal upper body mobility. Sternal stability has dramatically diminished pain, and after discharge from ICU, 70% of patients do not receive opioids, including after discharge. Patients are permitted to use their arms immediately after surgery with early freedom to get out of bed, up from a chair, or off the commode unassisted. Patients are now much more likely to be discharged home instead of to a skilled nursing facility, and to return to normal activities and back to work earlier (see **Table 1**).

Table 1
Example of accelerated mobilization protocol for patients with rigid plate fixation

Timing	Allowed Activities
At discharge	• Ride in a car • Walk inside house or in yard • Climb 1 flight of stairs (no carrying)
First week	• Lift 10 pounds each hand • Light household activities: limited cooking, dishwashing, dusting, small repairs
1–2 wk	• Attend religious services • Go out to eat or going to movies • Visit friends
2–3 wk	• Take out trash • Grocery shopping • Mow lawn with a riding mower • Putt golf balls in yard • Evaluation for driving a car at 2-wk office visit
2–4 wk	• Sexual relations
4–8 wk	• Lift 15 pounds each hand (most restrictions lifted by 5 wk) • Heavy household activities: vacuuming, sweeping, mopping, changing bed linens • Gardening or pulling weeds • Mow lawn with a push mower
8–10 wk	• Bowling • Golfing • Fishing

Table created following guidelines of Franciscan Health Heart Center, Departments of Cardiothoracic Surgery and Physical Therapy.

In addition to reducing all forms of sternal wound complications, RPF removes most limitations following sternotomy. Mobilization following RPF is conceptually similar to that for patients treated by minimally invasive approaches, without full sternotomy incisions. Indeed, evidence from studies of recovery after robotic, transcatheter, and other minimally invasive cardiac-surgical procedures supports the assertion that eliminating concern for sternal instability in the postoperative phase of care improves recovery, patient experience, and cost-effectiveness.[8,66–70]

SUMMARY

Evidence supporting best practices throughout the perioperative process has fostered significant changes in attitudes toward postoperative recovery, across a wide range of surgical disciplines. Programs aimed at promoting structured, rapid physical recovery, with the earliest-possible safe return to normal activities have yielded improvements in clinical, economic, and patient-reported outcomes, representing a win-win-win scenario for all stakeholders. Median sternotomy presents specific challenges for recovery after cardiac surgery. However, adoption of evidence-based techniques, including sternal RPF, maximizes adherence to orthopedic principles, minimizes patient pain, reduces opioid use, promotes healing, and can enable downstream implementation of aggressive, rapid mobilization protocols that are consistent with ERAS principles.

ACKNOWLEDGMENTS

Jeanne McAdara, PhD (Biolexica Health Science Communications, Longmont, Colorado) provided professional medical writing assistance. The medical writer worked at the direction of the authors.

DISCLOSURE

MWG discloses a consulting relationship with Zimmer Biomet; KBA discloses a research grant and consulting relationship with Zimmer Biomet; David Cohen, MD, discloses research funding for health economics core laboratory with Zimmer Biomet. All other authors have nothing to disclose with regard to commercial support. The authors maintained full control over this manuscript.

REFERENCES

1. Ljungqvist O, Scott M, Fearon KC. Enhanced recovery after surgery: a review. JAMA Surg 2017;152(3):292–8.
2. Spanjersberg WR, Reurings J, Keus F, et al. Fast track surgery versus conventional recovery strategies for colorectal surgery. Cochrane Database Syst Rev 2011;(2):CD007635.
3. Stone AB, Grant MC, Pio Roda C, et al. Implementation costs of an enhanced recovery after surgery program in the United States: a financial model and sensitivity analysis based on experiences at a quaternary academic medical center. J Am Coll Surg 2016;222(3):219–25.
4. Thiele RH, Rea KM, Turrentine FE, et al. Standardization of care: impact of an enhanced recovery protocol on length of stay, complications, and direct costs after colorectal surgery. J Am Coll Surg 2015;220(4):430–43.
5. Krohn BG, Kay JH, Mendez MA, et al. Rapid sustained recovery after cardiac operations. J Thorac Cardiovasc Surg 1990;100(2):194–7.
6. Engelman RM, Rousou JA, Flack JE, et al. Fast-track recovery of the coronary bypass patient. Ann Thorac Surg 1994;58(6):1742–6.

7. Noss C, Prusinkiewicz C, Nelson G, et al. Enhanced recovery for cardiac surgery. J Cardiothorac Vasc Anesth 2018;32(6):2760–70.

8. Zaouter C, Imbault J, Labrousse L, et al. Association of robotic totally endoscopic coronary artery bypass graft surgery associated with a preliminary cardiac enhanced recovery after surgery program: a retrospective analysis. J Cardiothorac Vasc Anesth 2015;29(6):1489–97.

9. Fleming IO, Garratt C, Guha R, et al. Aggregation of marginal gains in cardiac surgery: feasibility of a perioperative care bundle for enhanced recovery in cardiac surgical patients. J Cardiothorac Vasc Anesth 2016;30(3):665–70.

10. Li M, Zhang J, Gan TJ, et al. Enhanced recovery after surgery pathway for patients undergoing cardiac surgery: a randomized clinical trial. Eur J Cardiothorac Surg 2018;54(3):491–7.

11. Grant MC, Isada T, Ruzankin P, et al. Results from an enhanced recovery program for cardiac surgery. J Thorac Cardiovasc Surg 2020;159(4):1393–402.e7.

12. Williams JB, McConnell G, Allender JE, et al. One-year results from the first US-based enhanced recovery after cardiac surgery (ERAS Cardiac) program. J Thorac Cardiovasc Surg 2019;157(5):1881–8.

13. McConnell G, Woltz P, Bradford WT, et al. Enhanced recovery after cardiac surgery program to improve patient outcomes. Nursing 2018;48(11):24–31.

14. Engelman DT, Ben Ali W, Williams JB, et al. Guidelines for perioperative care in cardiac surgery: enhanced recovery after surgery society recommendations. JAMA Surg 2019;154(8):755–66.

15. Dalton ML, Connally SR, Sealy WC. Julian's reintroduction of Milton's operation. Ann Thorac Surg 1992;53(3):532–3.

16. Nenna A, Nappi F, Dougal J, et al. Sternal wound closure in the current era: the need of a tailored approach. Gen Thorac Cardiovasc Surg 2019;67(11):907–16.

17. Adams J, Lotshaw A, Exum E, et al. An alternative approach to prescribing sternal precautions after median sternotomy, "Keep Your Move in the Tube". Proc (Bayl Univ Med Cent) 2016;29(1):97–100.

18. El-Ansary D, LaPier TK, Adams J, et al. An evidence-based perspective on movement and activity following median sternotomy. Phys Ther 2019;99(12):1587–601.

19. Katijjahbe MA, Granger CL, Denehy L, et al. Standard restrictive sternal precautions and modified sternal precautions had similar effects in people after cardiac surgery via median sternotomy ('SMART' Trial): a randomised trial. J Physiother 2018;64(2):97–106.

20. Katijjahbe MA, Denehy L, Granger CL, et al. The Sternal Management Accelerated Recovery Trial (S.M.A.R.T) - standard restrictive versus an intervention of modified sternal precautions following cardiac surgery via median sternotomy: study protocol for a randomised controlled trial. Trials 2017;18(1):290.

21. Balachandran S, Lee A, Royse A, et al. Upper limb exercise prescription following cardiac surgery via median sternotomy: a web survey. J Cardiopulm Rehabil Prev 2014;34(6):390–5.

22. Cahalin LP, Lapier TK, Shaw DK. Sternal precautions: is it time for change? Precautions versus restrictions - a review of literature and recommendations for revision. Cardiopulm Phys Ther J 2011;22(1):5–15.

23. Pengelly J, Pengelly M, Lin KY, et al. Resistance training following median sternotomy: a systematic review and meta-analysis. Heart Lung Circ 2019;28(10):1549–59.

24. Marsell R, Einhorn TA. The biology of fracture healing. Injury 2011;42(6):551–5.

25. Sathyendra V, Darowish M. Basic science of bone healing. Hand Clin 2013;29(4):473–81.

26. Dabis J, Templeton-Ward O, Lacey AE, et al. The history, evolution and basic science of osteotomy techniques. Strateg Trauma Limb Reconstr 2017;12(3): 169–80.
27. Ilizarov GA. Transosseous osteosynthesis: theoretical and clinical aspects of the regeneration and growth of tissue. Berlin (Germany): Springer Science & Business Media; 2012.
28. Gandhi HS. Rationale and options for choosing an optimal closure technique for primary midsagittal osteochondrotomy of the sternum, part 2: a theoretical and critical review of techniques and fixation devices. Crit Rev Biomed Eng 2019; 47(1):27–57.
29. Raman J, Straus D, Song DH. Rigid plate fixation of the sternum. Ann Thorac Surg 2007;84(3):1056–8.
30. Balachandran S, Lee A, Denehy L, et al. Risk factors for sternal complications after cardiac operations: a systematic review. Ann Thorac Surg 2016;102(6): 2109–17.
31. Imren Y, Selek H, Zor H, et al. The management of complicated sternal dehiscence following open heart surgery. Heart Surg Forum 2006;9(6):E871–5.
32. Yusuf E, Chan M, Renz N, et al. Current perspectives on diagnosis and management of sternal wound infections. Infect Drug Resist 2018;11:961–8.
33. Song DH, Lohman RF, Renucci JD, et al. Primary sternal plating in high-risk patients prevents mediastinitis. Eur J Cardiothorac Surg 2004;26(2):367–72.
34. Allen KB, Thourani VH, Naka Y, et al. Randomized, multicenter trial comparing sternotomy closure with rigid plate fixation to wire cerclage. J Thorac Cardiovasc Surg 2017;153(4):888–96.e1.
35. Losanoff JE, Collier AD, Wagner-Mann CC, et al. Biomechanical comparison of median sternotomy closures. Ann Thorac Surg 2004;77(1):203–9.
36. Vos RJ, Van Putte BP, Kloppenburg GTL. Prevention of deep sternal wound infection in cardiac surgery: a literature review. J Hosp Infect 2018;100(4):411–20.
37. Pinotti KF, Cataneo DC, Rodrigues OR, et al. Closure of the sternum with anchoring of the steel wires: systematic review and meta-analysis. J Thorac Cardiovasc Surg 2018;156(1):178–86.
38. Franco S, Herrera AM, Atehortúa M, et al. Use of steel bands in sternotomy closure: implications in high-risk cardiac surgical population. Interact Cardiovasc Thorac Surg 2009;8(2):200–5.
39. Bhattacharya S, Sau I, Mohan M, et al. Sternal bands for closure of midline sternotomy leads to better wound healing. Asian Cardiovasc Thorac Ann 2007;15(1): 59–63.
40. Riess FC, Awwad N, Hoffmann B, et al. A steel band in addition to 8 wire cerclages reduces the risk of sternal dehiscence after median sternotomy. Heart Surg Forum 2004;7(6):387–92.
41. Grapow MT, Melly LF, Eckstein FS, et al. A new cable-tie based sternal closure system: description of the device, technique of implantation and first clinical evaluation. J Cardiothorac Surg 2012;7:59.
42. Orhan SN, Ozyazicioglu MH. Evaluation of sternum closure methods by means of a nonlinear finite element analysis. Proc Inst Mech Eng H 2019;233(12):1282–91.
43. Orhan SN, Ozyazicioglu MH, Colak A. A biomechanical study of 4 different sternum closure techniques under different deformation modes. Interact Cardiovasc Thorac Surg 2017;25(5):750–6.
44. Marasco SF, Fuller L, Zimmet A, et al. Prospective, randomized, controlled trial of polymer cable ties versus standard wire closure of midline sternotomy. J Thorac Cardiovasc Surg 2018;156(4):1589–95.e1.

45. Samuels L. Sternal closure with tie bands: a word of caution. Ann Thorac Surg 2016;102(2):e121–2.

46. Stelly MM, Rodning CB, Stelly TC. Reduction in deep sternal wound infection with use of a peristernal cable-tie closure system: a retrospective case series. J Cardiothorac Surg 2015;10:166.

47. Melly L, Gahl B, Meinke R, et al. A new cable-tie-based sternal closure device: infectious considerations. Interact Cardiovasc Thorac Surg 2013;17(2):219–23 [discussion: 223].

48. Nezafati P, Shomali A, Kahrom M, et al. ZipFix versus conventional sternal closure: one-year follow-up. Heart Lung Circ 2019;28(3):443–9.

49. Omer S. Polymer cable tie closure of the sternum: is it an acceptable fix. J Thorac Cardiovasc Surg 2018;156(4):1611–2.

50. Tam DY, Fremes SE. Cable ties for chest closure: ZipFix or ZipFail. J Thorac Cardiovasc Surg 2018;156(4):1611.

51. Fawzy H, Alhodaib N, Mazer CD, et al. Sternal plating for primary and secondary sternal closure; can it improve sternal stability. J Cardiothorac Surg 2009;4:19.

52. Gottlieb LJ, Pielet RW, Karp RB, et al. Rigid internal fixation of the sternum in postoperative mediastinitis. Arch Surg 1994;129(5):489–93.

53. Hirose H, Yamane K, Youdelman BA, et al. Rigid sternal fixation improves postoperative recovery. Open Cardiovasc Med J 2011;5:148–52.

54. Snyder CW, Graham LA, Byers RE, et al. Primary sternal plating to prevent sternal wound complications after cardiac surgery: early experience and patterns of failure. Interact Cardiovasc Thorac Surg 2009;9(5):763–6.

55. Matsuyama K, Kuinose M, Koizumi N, et al. Sternal closure by rigid plate fixation in off-pump coronary artery bypass grafting: a comparative study. J Artif Organs 2016;19(2):175–8.

56. Raman J, Lehmann S, Zehr K, et al. Sternal closure with rigid plate fixation versus wire closure: a randomized controlled multicenter trial. Ann Thorac Surg 2012; 94(6):1854–61.

57. Allen KB, Icke KJ, Thourani VH, et al. Sternotomy closure using rigid plate fixation: a paradigm shift from wire cerclage. Ann Cardiothorac Surg 2018;7(5): 611–20.

58. Nazerali RS, Hinchcliff K, Wong MS. Rigid fixation for the prevention and treatment of sternal complications. Ann Plast Surg 2014;72(Suppl 1):S27–30.

59. Park JS, Kuo JH, Young JN, et al. Rigid sternal fixation versus modified wire technique for poststernotomy closures: a retrospective cost analysis. Ann Plast Surg 2017;78(5):537–42.

60. Liao JM, Chan P, Cornwell L, et al. Feasibility of primary sternal plating for morbidly obese patients after cardiac surgery. J Cardiothorac Surg 2019; 14(1):25.

61. Allen KB, Thourani VH, Naka Y, et al. Rigid plate fixation versus wire cerclage: patient-reported and economic outcomes from a randomized trial. Ann Thorac Surg 2018;105(5):1344–50.

62. Tam DY, Nedadur R, Yu M, et al. Rigid plate fixation versus wire cerclage for sternotomy after cardiac surgery: a meta-analysis. Ann Thorac Surg 2018;106(1): 298–304.

63. Brown JK, Singh K, Dumitru R, et al. The benefits of enhanced recovery after surgery programs and their application in cardiothoracic surgery. Methodist Debakey Cardiovasc J 2018;14(2):77–88.

64. Krzych Ł, Kucewicz-Czech E. It is time for enhanced recovery after surgery in cardiac surgery. Kardiol Pol 2017;75(5):415–20.

65. Ljungqvist O. The enhanced recovery after surgery in cardiac surgery revolution. JAMA Surg 2019;154(8):767.

66. Baron S, Reynolds MR, Cohen DJ. Economic considerations for TAVR Vs. SAVR: historical perspective and future predictions. American College of Cardiology website. 2019. Available at: https://www.acc.org/latest-in-cardiology/articles/2019/06/18/07/43/economic-considerations-for-tavr-vs-savr. Accessed: January 10, 2020.

67. Baron SJ, Magnuson EA, Lu M, et al. Health status after transcatheter versus surgical aortic valve replacement in low-risk patients with aortic stenosis. J Am Coll Cardiol 2019;74(23):2833–42.

68. Olds A, Saadat S, Azzolini A, et al. Improved operative and recovery times with mini-thoracotomy aortic valve replacement. J Cardiothorac Surg 2019;14(1):91.

69. Stoliński J, Plicner D, Grudzień G, et al. A comparison of minimally invasive and standard aortic valve replacement. J Thorac Cardiovasc Surg 2016;152(4):1030–9.

70. Tokarek T, Siudak Z, Dziewierz A, et al. Assessment of quality of life in patients after surgical and transcatheter aortic valve replacement. Catheter Cardiovasc Interv 2016;88(3):E80–8.

Postoperative Multimodal Analgesia in Cardiac Surgery

Linda F. Barr, MD[a], Michael J. Boss, MD[b], Michael A. Mazzeffi, MD, MPH, MSc[c],
Bradley S. Taylor, MD[c], Rawn Salenger, MD[c],*

KEYWORDS

- Cardiac surgery • Postoperative pain • Opioids • Multimodal pain management
- Enhanced recovery after surgery (ERAS)

KEY POINTS

- Cardiac surgical pain management is complicated by multiple surgical sites and by the complex hemodynamics of the cardiac surgical patient.
- Surgical pain management by just-in-time opioids has been complicated by side effects that slow surgical recovery. Further, postoperative opioids may predispose to long-term opioid dependence, which is a national crisis.
- A multimodal opioid-sparing approach to postoperative pain management uses several nonopioid medications and techniques to target different pain pathways. This approach is preemptive and involves a collaboration of all of the health care providers, patients, and families. Education, feedback, and continuous evolution are key elements of this strategy.
- Preliminary studies suggest that this multimodal approach for cardiac surgical patients improves pain management and ameliorates side effects to improve functional recovery.

INTRODUCTION

Cardiac surgery is associated with significant postoperative pain, which complicates recovery. The unique aspects of cardiac surgical pain include multiple sites of pain, initial hemodynamic instability, and longer duration of acute postoperative recovery. Sources of pain include those directly related to surgery such as incisional pain, sternotomy, chest retraction, intercostal nerve pain, visceral pain, and leg pain from vein graft harvesting. There is also pain from operative positioning, which is worse for patients with preexisting back or limb issues. Postoperative sources of pain also include

[a] Division of Pulmonary and Critical Care Medicine, Johns Hopkins University School of Medicine, 733 N Broadway, Baltimore, MD 21205, USA; [b] University of Maryland Saint Joseph Medical Center, 7601 Osler Drive, Towson, MD 21204, USA; [c] University of Maryland School of Medicine, 22S Greene St, Baltimore, MD 21201, USA
* Corresponding author. University of Maryland Saint Joseph Medical Center, 7505 Osler Drive, Odea Building Suite 302, Towson, MD 21204.
E-mail address: rawnsalenger@umm.edu
Twitter: @RawnSalenger (R.S.)

Crit Care Clin 36 (2020) 631–651
https://doi.org/10.1016/j.ccc.2020.06.003
0749-0704/20/© 2020 Elsevier Inc. All rights reserved.

pain from the invasion of chest tubes, endotracheal tube, tracheal suctioning, urinary catheter, intravascular lines, nasogastric tube, and possibly postoperative pericarditis and pleuritis.

Multiple studies have demonstrated that pain from cardiac surgery peaks over the first 2 days, then declines daily through postoperative day 6.[1,2] Over the first 2 postoperative days, patients most commonly report discomfort in the legs, shoulders, lower back and abdomen, as well as the midsternum. Chest tubes cause significant pain because they can irritate the parietal pleura, which is sensitive to pain and temperature. Approximately one-half of patients have pain in more than one area. After the first postoperative week there is more reported sternal and osteoarticular pain, as the pain from tubes and the incision recedes.[2] The activity that elicits the most pain for the postcardiac surgery patient is coughing, which is followed in pain intensity by patient movement, turning in bed, getting up, and deep breathing. Activity-related pain scores decrease after the second postoperative day; however, pain from coughing continues to be severe throughout the first week. Removal of chest tubes results in significant pain relief at rest and with activity.[1,2]

Certain subgroups of patients report greater intensity and duration of pain. Younger patients and those with a high body mass index report more pain. The type of cardiac surgery does not affect pain characteristics, although the extent of the saphenous vein harvest wound does correlate with leg pain.[2] Persistent postoperative pain is defined as poststernotomy neuralgia for at least 3 months duration, with other causes of pain excluded. A retrospective analysis of 23 studies involving 11,057 patients found that 37% of patients have pain 6 months after cardiac surgery, and 17% have pain more than 2 years after surgery.[3] Some groups of patients are clearly high risk for difficult postoperative pain management, including patients with chronic opioid use or those with other chronic pain disorders such as fibromyalgia.

The potential complications associated with acute postoperative pain have been well documented[4] and are particularly problematic for cardiac surgical patients who are hemodynamically fragile. The sympathetic response to pain increases myocardial oxygen consumption, and increased myocardial oxygen consumption may predispose to arrhythmia and potentially myocardial injury.[5] Inadequate respiratory effort due to sternotomy and chest tube pain leads to atelectasis and hypoxemia. Inadequate cough translates to retention of sputum in patients who already have an increased pulmonary secretion burden due to chest stasis during cardiopulmonary bypass and may have the added burden of comorbid chronic obstructive pulmonary disease, and this increases the risk of acute bronchitis and pneumonia. All of these issues are associated with increased need for ventilatory support and therefore prolonged intensive care unit (ICU) and hospital stay. Inadequate pain control is also associated with nausea, vomiting, and anorexia, compromising nutritional status. Further, surgery depresses the immune response, and poor pain control compounds this immunosuppression.[6,7] Poor nutrition and immune dysfunction can delay wound healing and predispose to infection.

Another potential complication exacerbated by postoperative pain is delirium. Pain leads to insomnia and exhaustion, which can contribute to the development of delirium. In addition, the decreased quality of life can cause demoralization. These issues decrease patient participation in physical therapy and other recovery strategies, all of which delay hospital discharge. In addition, the subsequent decreased ambulation can increase the risk of venous thromboembolism. Finally, studies in other surgical patients show that inadequate control of immediate postoperative pain increases the risk for prolonged outpatient opioid use.[8]

As is true for postoperative pain in general, the pathophysiology of cardiac surgical pain can be characterized as somatic and neuropathic pain.[9] Somatic pain is initiated by neurogenic inflammation at the surgical site due to mediator release. This subsequently causes peripheral sensitization, activation of sleeping nociceptors, and central sensitization, which leads to primary and secondary hyperalgesia and allodynia.[10] The somatic pain lasts longer than the noxious stimulus, is diffuse and difficult to locate, and can affect a patients' ability to fully mobilize. Neuropathic pain is initiated by irritation of nociceptors in the peripheral nerves, which stimulates the A delta and C fibers. Subsequently, the signal is conducted via cranial nerves V, VII, IX, and X to the dorsal spinal cord and toward the cerebral cortex and limbic system. This neurologic pathway is affected by endogenous opioids, noradrenergic, cholinergic, serotonergic, and gamma-aminobutyric adrenergic systems. Finally, the cerebral cortex responds to this stimulation, and the patient experiences pain. The strategies to modulate postoperative pain target this biological loop.

TRADITIONAL OPIOID ANALGESIA

Historically, the cornerstone of postoperative pain management has been intravenous or oral opioids. However, opioids alone are likely not the most effective means of alleviating pain.[4] In addition, opioid use can be complicated by side effects such as nausea, constipation, ileus, urinary retention, pruritus, sedation, delirium, and respiratory depression.[11] Complications from opioid use impede the quality and timing of patient recovery, prolong hospital stay, and increase costs.[12–14] Of particular relevance to the cardiac surgical patient, opioids have complex effects on cardiovascular dynamics. Opioids can cause vasodilatation, decreased blood pressure, and heart rate. These effects are variable depending on multiple factors including the specific agent, patient volume status, and level of consciousness. Postoperative physiology can also modify the magnitude of these effects through altered interaction with receptors and release of mediators such as histamine.[15]

Perioperative opioids lead to both central and peripheral neural hyperexcitability that may amplify and prolong pain. Some evidence suggests that heavy reliance on opioids postoperatively contributes to analgesic tolerance, hyperalgesia, and the development of chronic pain.[16,17] These phenomena can lead to the need for escalating opioids and contribute to the development of long-term opioid dependence.[8,18,19] Consistent with this pharmacology, the amount of opioids prescribed in the postoperative period correlates with long-term opioid use.[20] Prolonged opioid dependence of patients following surgery has contributed to the current opioid epidemic and has led to an aggressive search to implement effective nonopioid pain management strategies.

MULTIMODAL/OPIOID-SPARING ANALGESIA

The effectiveness of an opioid-sparing strategy in improving cardiac surgical outcomes was first demonstrated by the "Fast Track" approach. These protocols promote multimodal strategies of education, early extubation, prophylactic medications for gastrointestinal complications, accelerated rehabilitation, early discharge, and nonopioid pain management.[21] Many protocols include use of short-acting hypnotic drugs with reduced doses of opioids and the use of short-acting opioids to facilitate rapid extubation. A Cochrane analysis of 28 cardiac surgical trials involving 4438 patients found that opioid sparing reduced time to extubation and length of stay in the ICU, without a change in total length of hospital stay, and was safe.[22]

Current multimodal pain management builds on the "Fast Track" concept. By using multiple agents and techniques that each target a different pain pathway, modern multimodal cardiac surgical protocols hope to create a synergy to improve pain control and decrease opioid dependence. Further, the goal is to use lower doses of each individual agent and decrease the incidence of side effects.[23] Nonopioid agents that have been used for surgical pain management, pharmacologic profiles, and doses are outlined in **Table 1**. The promise of a multimodal pain strategy is that improved pain management and amelioration of side effects will improve functional recovery. Decreased total opioids consumed in the immediate postoperative period have been shown to decrease hospital length of stay, long-term opioid use, and chronic pain.[24,25]

An important element of multimodal pain management is preemptive analgesic dosing rather than reactive medication use. Analgesics are started preoperatively and intraoperatively, and some agents are dosed around-the-clock. Medications are titrated based on effects, mainly altered level of consciousness. Minimal supplemental opioids are added as needed. This preemptive approach can achieve improved pain control with decreased opioid use.[26,27] Regional anesthesia for cardiac surgery is also a promising adjunct.[28]

A multimodal opioid-sparing pain management strategy has proved effective for improving pain control, decreasing opioid use, and improving functional recovery for a variety of noncardiac surgeries including gastrointestinal, gynecologic, and orthopedic.[29–31] Cardiac surgical programs have recently begun adopting multimodal opioid-sparing strategies as part of their Enhanced Recovery After Surgery programs.[32] The elements are similar to those that have proved effective for other surgeries and modified to address the particular challenges of the cardiac surgical patient. Studies that exemplify the cardiac surgical experience with nonopioid pain medications are described in **Table 2**.

REGIONAL ANESTHETICS IN CARDIAC SURGERY

Historically, reliable methods of achieving dense anesthesia or postoperative analgesia to the thoracic wall and surrounding structures were accomplished by placing either a thoracic epidural, a spinal anesthetic, a paravertebral block, or an intercostal block. Because nearly all cardiac surgical patients are anticoagulated and placed on cardiopulmonary bypass, manipulation of the epidural or spinal space can be a risky endeavor. Hemorrhage from needle trauma can result in spinal-epidural hematoma formation, nerve and spinal cord compression, sensory and motor block, bowel and bladder dysfunction, and in rare cases, paraplegia.[33] Pleural puncture and pneumothorax, although uncommon, are potential complications that may occur with intercostal and paravertebral blocks. With greater adoption of ultrasound guidance and the addition of newer regional nerve block techniques, analgesia can be achieved while avoiding the rare but potentially catastrophic complications of neuraxial anesthesia.

For cardiothoracic surgery specifically, ultrasound has allowed for the placement of various regional blocks under direct visualization within neural planes providing significant pain relief to the patient. Although these blocks may offer perceived safety as they are placed under direct visualization, the risks of neural injury, vascular or pleural puncture, infection, and intravascular injection of local anesthetic remain a possibility. When considering analgesia for median sternotomy, bilateral nerve blocks must be placed to achieve adequate analgesic coverage, and one must be mindful of total anesthetic dose and concentration to minimize the risk of local anesthetic toxicity.[34]

Table 1
Nonopioid agents used to manage pain

Medication	Mechanism of Action	Suggested Dosing	Side Effects	Precautions	Comments
Ketamine[51]	NMDA antagonist also acts at: Mu GABA Muscarinic Monoaminergic	Bolus up to 0.35 mg/kg IV. Infusion immediately after loading at 0.1–0.2 mg/kg/h IV	Confusion Delirium Excitement, dreamlike state hallucinations vivid imagery, sialorrhea hyper-/hypotension Increased interocular or intracranial pressure (mainly seen in doses higher than those recommended for analgesia)	• Pregnancy • Should avoid in severe hepatic disease/use cautiously in patients with less severe liver disease • Poorly regulated cardiovascular disease • Active or severe psychosis • Increased intraocular pressure/intracranial pressure (all poorly studied in subanesthetic doses). (Pediatric dose-dependent study does not demonstrate increase in IOP with low-dose ketamine)[52]	• Many studies use higher bolus doses—consensus guidelines acknowledge this. • Infusion rate may be increased or decreased as necessary depending on tolerance/side effects. • Most studies note subanesthetic doses to be 0.5 mg/kg bolus and 0.5 mg/kg/h infusion or less

(continued on next page)

Table 1
(continued)

Medication	Mechanism of Action	Suggested Dosing	Side Effects	Precautions	Comments
Gabapentin/ Pregabalin[53]	α-2δ subunit of presynaptic P/Q-type voltage-gated calcium channels	Gabapentin: preop— 1200 mg PO once 2+ h before incision and postop—300 mg PO TID Pregabalin: preop— 300 mg PO once 2+ h before incision AND postop—150 mg PO BID	Dizziness Visual alterations Headache Sedation Peripheral edema (gabapentin)	• Renal dysfunction • Older age • Combined sedative effect	• Adjustments must be made for decreased CrCl. • Widely varying tolerance regarding sedative effect— decrease dosage for increased age and decreased renal function. • Be mindful of sedative effect in outpatient population • Preoperative dosing not required. All dosing methods shown to reduce postoperative pain.

Dexmedetomidine	• α2 adrenergic receptor agonist • Weak peripheral α1 agonist with rapid loading	• 0.5–1 mcg/kg over 10 min (loading dose after cardiopulmonary bypass) Followed by: 0.4–1.5 mcg/kg/h infusion through extubation	Sedation Hypotension/hypertension Profound bradycardia (most often with loading dose)	• Preadministration presence of bradycardia • High vagal tone • Hemodynamic instability
Lidocaine	Initiation and conduction of nerve impulses blocked via decreasing membrane permeability to Na + ions	1.5–2 mg/kg loading dose Followed by: 1.5–3 mg/kg/h infusion	Tremor Tinnitus Metallic taste in mouth Lightheadedness Nausea/vomiting Seizure at toxic high concentration Bradycardia Asystole (rare)	• More severe degrees of heart block • Wolff-Parkinson-White syndrome Local anesthetic sensitivity	Inconclusive data as to effectiveness of IV lidocaine. Most likely no benefit after 24 h infusion time. Side effects/toxicity poorly studied for prolonged infusions[54]
Magnesium	NMDA antagonist	Varies 50 mg/kg load followed by: 8 mg/kg/h for 48 h[55]	Flushing Hypotension Vasodilation Toxicity (in order of increasing plasma concentration) • Loss of deep tendon reflexes • Respiratory paralysis • Cardiac conduction abnormalities • Cardiac arrest[55]	Use with caution in neuromuscular disease (myasthenia gravis)/renal impairment (increased mag concentrations over time may lead to toxicity)	Reduction in morphine used with improvement in sleep and overall satisfaction[56]

(continued on next page)

Table 1
(continued)

Medication	Mechanism of Action	Suggested Dosing	Side Effects	Precautions	Comments
Acetaminophen	Analgesic effect on descending serotonergic inhibitory pathways in CNS. Not fully understood	1 g every 6 h	Nausea (IV administration)	• No contraindication in mild/moderate hepatic impairment • Contraindicated in severe hepatic impairment	Unclear benefit to IV administration over oral or rectal administration
Ketorolac/NSAID	Reversible COX-1/COX-2 Inhibitor	30 mg single dose OR every 6 h—max daily dosing 120 mg. Consider lower dosing, 10 mg/15 mg, may provide similar analgesic effect[57,58]	Headache Nausea GI pain/dyspepsia	• Contraindicated in severe renal impairment or at risk of renal impairment with hypovolemia • Contraindicated in CABG (US boxed warning) • Contraindicated in heart failure secondary to sodium/fluid retention[56] • GI inflammation	

Abbreviations: CABG, coronary artery bypass grafting; CNS, central nervous system; GABA, gamma aminobutyric acid; GI, gastrointestinal; IV, intravenous; NMDA, N-methyl-D-aspartate; NSAID, nonsteroidal antiinflammatory drug.
Data from Refs.[51–57]

Table 2
Cardiac surgical opioid-sparing, multimodal, and enhanced recovery after surgery pain management studies

Study Type and Reference	Patients (N)	Interventions	Outcomes—Intervention vs Control
Prospective observational Fleming et al,[59] 2016	Pre-ERAS (53) ERAS (52)	Preoperative Gabapentin 600 mg/ondansetron Postoperative Paracetamol/codeine prn/morphine prn/ondansetron x 48 h	Decreased pain scores No change in morphine use Improved nausea and enteral tolerance
Retrospective review Williams et al,[14] 2019	Pre-ERAS (489) ERAS (443)	Preoperative Gabapentin 300 mg/acetaminophen/ anxiolytic Intraoperative Acetaminophen/hydromorphone/ dexmedetomidine or propofol Postoperative Acetaminophen/gabapentin, 300 mg bid x 5 d or 100 mg bid for age >70 y/ oxycodone prn/fentanyl IV prn/ ondansetron	Decreased mean hospital stay/ICU stay/ ileus/reintubation No change in duration of mechanical ventilation
Randomized, double-blind, placebo- controlled Menda et al,[60] 2010	Gabapentin (30) Control (30)	Preoperative Gabapentin, 600 mg	Decreased pain scores at rest and with cough first 12 h after surgery only/ morphine use at 24 h/nausea Increased incidence of oversedation/ duration of mechanical ventilation
Retrospective, case-matched Grant et al,[61] 2019	ERAS compliance: high (84) Low (231)	Preoperative Gabapentin, 600 mg or 300 mg, for age >70 y or creatinine clearance <60 mL/min/ acetaminophen Intraoperative Ketamine/dexmedetomidine/bilateral serratus anterior plane block with bupivacaine/reversal neuromuscular blockade	High compliance Increased early extubation Decreased hospital length of stay (LOS)

(continued on next page)

Table 2
(continued)

Study Type and Reference	Patients (N)	Interventions	Outcomes—Intervention vs Control
Retrospective, case-matched Markham et al,[62] 2019	ERAS (25) Control (25)	Preoperative Gabapentin, 300 mg/acetaminophen Intraoperative Bilateral serratus anterior plane and adductor canal blocks with ropivacaine and dexamethasone/ dexmedetomidine/reversal neuromuscular blockade Postoperative Gabapentin 300 mg x 1/ondansetron/ opioids as needed	Decreased duration of mechanical ventilation/opioid use/intensive care LOS No change hospital LOS/ileus/ arrhythmias/pericarditis
Prospective randomized Li et al,[63] 2018	ERAS (104) Control (105)	Preoperative Paravertebral nerve block T2-3, T5-6 Postoperative Patient-controlled analgesia pump with sufentanil/ropivacaine to incision/ondansetron as needed	Decreased hospital LOS/ICU LOS/duration of mechanical ventilation/hospital cost/ postoperative atrial fibrillation
Randomized, double-blind, placebo-controlled Florkiewicz et al,[64] 2019	Ropivacaine (47) Control (43)	Postoperative Ropivacaine or placebo saline to sternotomy x 48 h/oxycodone and patient-controlled intravenous analgesia/propofol/paracetamol	No change in pain scores/oxycodone use/ nausea and emesis/oversedation/ wound infection
Prospective randomized controlled trial Rafiq et al,[65] 2014	ERAS (77) Control (74)	Postoperative Ketorolac/dexamethasone/ paracetamol before extubation/then gabapentin, 300 mg/paracetamol night of surgery/then gabapentin, 300 mg, bid/ibuprofen/paracetamol/ pantoprazole/magnesium oxide/ morphine needed	Decreased opioid use/pain score/nausea and emesis Increased acute renal injury

Study	Groups (n)	Protocol	Outcomes
Prospective randomized placebo-controlled study Subramaniam et al,[66] 2019	Dexmedetomidine/ acetaminophen Propofol/ acetaminophen Dexmedetomidine/ placebo Propofol/placebo 120 total patients divided into 4 groups (1:1:1:1)	Postoperative acetaminophen/dexmedetomidine or propofol for up to 6 h or extubation	Decreased delirium and opioid use with acetaminophen No difference between dexmedetomidine and propofol
Meta-analysis of randomized controlled trials Peng et al,[67] 2019	9 trials (total 1308)	Intraoperative/postoperative Dexmedetomidine up to first postoperative day	Decreased acute renal injury/prolonged ventilation/pulmonary complications/ delirium/hospital mortality
Meta-analysis Souvik et al,[68] 2017	4 gabapentin trials (total 220) 4 pregabalin trials (total 110)	Gabapentin 800 mg 2 h preoperative + 400 mg 2 h postextubation 600 mg 2 h preoperative 1200 mg 2 h preoperative + 600 mg bid x 2 d Pregabalin 1200 mg 1 h preoperative + 1200 mg daily x 2 d 150 mg 1–2 h preop/2 studies added 75 mg bid x 2 and 5 d postoperatively	Decreased opioid use in 3 gabapentin and 2 pregabalin studies/no difference for 1 gabapentin and 2 pregabalin studies Lower pain scores in 3 gabapentin and 3 pregabalin studies Increased duration of mechanical ventilation in 2 gabapentin studies/no difference in 1 pregabalin study
Prospective randomized double-blind placebo-controlled Lahtinen et al,[69] 2004	Ketamine (44) Placebo (46)	Intraoperative Ketamine continued x 48 h Postoperative Oxycodone patient-controlled analgesia (PCA)	Decreased opioid use Improved patient satisfaction No change in pain scores/nausea and emesis
Prospective randomized controlled Qazi et al,[70] 2015	Ibuprofen (93) Oxycodone SR (89)	Postoperative Ibuprofen SR 800 mg oral bid plus lansoprazole daily (versus oxycodone SR) x 7 d/paracetamol 1 g qid/PRN oxycodone IR	Increased acute renal injury (creatinine doubled in all ibuprofen patients, then normalized in most over 14 d, no dialysis) No change in sternal wound healing/ myocardial infarction/GI bleeding

(continued on next page)

Table 2
(continued)

Study Type and Reference	Patients (N)	Interventions	Outcomes—Intervention vs Control
Retrospective analysis of pooled data from 2 multicenter randomized controlled trials De Souza et al,[71] 2017	NSAID preoperative and postoperative (289) NSAID preop only (257) No NSAID (3519)	Nonsteroidal antiinflammatory drug (NSAID)	No difference in mortality/myocardial infarction/stroke/renal injury/mediastinitis/reoperation for bleeding
Prospective randomized placebo-controlled, double-blind study Vrooman et al,[72] 2015	Lidocaine patch (39) Placebo patch (39)	Postoperative Lidocaine (or placebo) patch 5%—up to 3 for up to 6 mo/fentanyl PCA x 3 d/oral narcotics	No difference in opioid use/pain scores/patient satisfaction Mean pain scores were baseline for both groups by 90 d

Abbreviation: ERAS, enhanced recovery after surgery.
Data from Refs.[14,59–72]

Erector Spinae Plane Block

The erector spinae plane (ESP) block can be placed bilaterally as a single shot or by inserting catheters for continuous postoperative infiltration. The block is placed by injecting local anesthetic at the T5 level between the transverse process and the erector spinae muscle. Local anesthetic spread is 3 to 4 levels above and below the site of injection ultimately covering the T2-T9 dermatomal distribution. The ESP block functions through blockade of the dorsal and ventral rami of spinal nerve roots.[30] Krishna and colleagues[35] showed that the ESP block provided superior analgesia and duration of analgesia postoperatively when compared with intravenous paracetamol/tramadol.

Transversus Thoracis Plane Block/Pecto-intercostal Block

The transversus thoracis plane block and pecto-intercostal block achieve analgesia through blocking the anterior branches of the intercostal nerves. The transversus thoracis plane block is placed by injecting local anesthetic under ultrasound guidance between the internal intercostal muscle and the transversus thoracis muscle lateral to the sternum at the level of the 3rd to 4th or 4th to 5th ribs. Local anesthetic spread then provides analgesia at multiple levels. The pecto-intercostal block can be placed in the surgical field by the surgeon or under ultrasound guidance by injecting local anesthetic just below the pectoralis major muscle at multiple levels or in a single injection in the midsternum. **Fig. 1** shows the common quantitative pain scales. The authors' approach for this block and the pertinent ultrasound anatomy are shown in **Fig. 1**. Continuous catheter infiltration to the sternal wound may also be used; however, concerns surrounding local infection and efficacy may dissuade the clinician from this approach.[34] For both the transversus thoracis plane block and the pecto-intercostal block, large volumes of local anesthetic (approximately 20 mL per side) are preferable so that local anesthetic can spread to multiple nerve levels. Typically, these blocks are performed with bupivacaine, 0.25%, or ropivacaine, 0.25%. Ropivacaine offers the advantage of less cardiac toxicity.

Paravertebral Block

The paravertebral block is achieved by injecting local anesthetic in the paravertebral space with local anesthetic spread covering multiple dermatomal levels. This block can be performed under ultrasound guidance with direct visualization of the

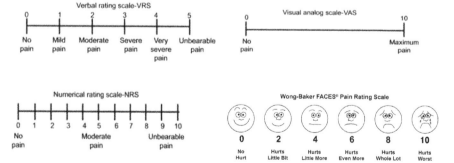

Fig. 1. Common quantitative pain scales: Verbal Rating Scale (VRS), Visual Analog Scale (VAS), Numerical Rating Scale (NRS), Faces Pain Rating Scale. (*From* Zubrzycki M, Liebold A, Skrabal C, et al. Assessment and pathophysiology of pain in cardiac surgery. J Pain Res 2018; 11:1599 – 1611. https://doi.org/10.2147/JPR.S162067. eCollection 2018. And Wong-Baker FACES Foundation (2019). Wong-Baker FACES® Pain Rating Scale. Retrieved 12/6/2019 with permission from http://www.WongBakerFACES.org.)

paravertebral space and the pleura, thus reducing the risk of pleural puncture and pneumothorax. A catheter may be left for continuous infusion. El Shora and colleagues[36] demonstrated the efficacy and safety of bilateral paravertebral blocks in providing postoperative analgesia for median sternotomy pain. Results were similar but not superior to the analgesia provided by a thoracic epidural.

Pectoralis Block (PECS I and II)/Serratus Anterior Plane Block

Although the PECS blocks and serratus anterior plane block cannot be expected to completely provide analgesia for cardiac surgical procedures involving median sternotomy, the blocks should remain in the anesthesiologist's armamentarium to provide pain control during minimally invasive cardiac surgical procedures, thoracotomy, and subclavian cutdowns for vascular access, whether it be axillary cannulation for cardiopulmonary bypass or an axillary approach for a transcatheter aortic valve replacement. In addition, Kumar and colleagues[37] described improved postoperative patient comfort and satisfaction as well as improved pulmonary rehabilitation with the placement of bilateral PECS I and II blocks under ultrasound guidance.

Although regional blocks for intraoperative and postoperative analgesia are a developing area to be considered for a multimodal pain management approach, data remain rather sparse when attempting to evaluate their overall effectiveness and safety in a larger patient population. They are, nonetheless, a promising approach to pain management offering a potential reduction of complications and side effects than may be found with the use of neuraxial anesthesia/analgesia and parenteral analgesia. Additional prospective trials with larger patient populations are needed to better elucidate the true benefit and safety of regional blocks in cardiac surgery.

ALTERNATIVE ANALGESIC THERAPIES

Alternative pain management therapies include physical and cognitive modalities. Overall evidence for most of these modalities is mixed but there is weak to moderate evidence to support their adjunctive use,[38,39] and the risks are low. Transcutaneous electrical nerve stimulation has moderate quality evidence regarding its utility as an adjunct after surgery. This modality sends low voltage electrical signals through the skin, which are believed to activate opioid receptors and decrease central nervous excitability.[40] Acupuncture, cold therapy, and massage all have been studied with mixed results. Cognitive behavioral therapy has also been well studied and has moderate evidence supporting adjunctive use for postoperative pain alleviation. Meditation, guided imagery, and music therapy are popular alternative modalities with no risk of harm. Hypnosis and intraoperative suggestion have been used less frequently.[41–44] Consideration of using more than one modality when implementing alternative therapy allows patients to individualize their treatment plan.

PAIN ASSESSMENT

As discussed, an effective enhanced recovery after surgery opioid-sparing multimodal pain regimen can be composed of a variety of therapeutic strategies. In order to confirm efficacy, results must be audited and analyzed regularly. The most common way to measure opioid consumption is to calculate morphine milligram equivalents (MMEs) to arrive at the total opioid dose. The MME conversion chart (**Table 3**) provides the recommended conversion from other opioids to morphine, as updated in 2018.[45] MMEs can be tracked during the inpatient postoperative recovery via the electronic health record, and specific auditing tools are being developed to facilitate gathering these data. Once a program's baseline amount of opioid use is established, the effect

Table 3
Conversion chart to calculate morphine milligram equivalents

Opioid	Conversion Factor
Codeine	0.15
Fentanyl (IV)	100
Hydrocodone	1
Hydromorphone	4
Methadone	
1–20 mg	4
21–40 mg	8
41–60 mg	10
>60 mg	12
Morphine	1
Oxycodone	1.5
Oxymorphone	3

From Centers for Disease Control and Prevention. 2018 Annual Surveillance Report of Drug-Related Risks and Outcomes — United States. Surveillance Special Report 2pdf icon. Centers for Disease Control and Prevention, U.S. Department of Health and Human Services. Published August 31, 2018. With permission.

of a multimodal opioid-sparing analgesic regimen can be assessed and changes implemented as indicated. Multidisciplinary buy-in, especially from bedside nursing, is essential.

The corollary metric that must be tracked along with MMEs to gauge the success of an opioid reduction strategy is patient pain perception during the postoperative period. This is commonly accomplished by setting individualized goals for each patient and then guiding the patient to self-report quantitative pain scores. The challenges around quantitating pain scores are numerous and include individualized patient perception of pain severity, individualized nursing interpretation of patient reports, varying levels of patient consciousness, intubated patients, delirium, and the use of multiple different methods to report quantitative pain levels. Clinicians' and patients' education levels and cultural backgrounds can have a great impact on how pain is communicated and interpreted. Further, patients may be experiencing significant pain without displaying classic physiologic signs or facial expressions.[46,47]

A variety of validated objective assessment scales can be used. Specific scales are tailored depending on patients' condition, level of consciousness, and consequent ability to communicate. The most frequently used postoperative scales include the verbal rating scale (VRS), numeric rating scale (NRS), visual analog scale (VAS), and the face pain rating scale (see **Fig. 1**). Each scale allows self-assessment of pain intensity by the patient. The VAS is the most challenging for patients, especially those with cognitive impairment. The VRS is the easiest for patients but tends to group answers in the middle with the least discriminatory capacity. The NRS is ordinal with balanced sensitivity to the extremes and easy for patients to use, leading many experts to recommend this scale.[9] The face rating scale is well suited for patients who are intubated or otherwise unable to communicate verbally.

SUCCESS WITH MULTIMODAL THERAPY

The multimodal pain management strategy for cardiac surgery involves a collaboration of cardiac surgeons, cardiac anesthesiologists, critical care physicians, cardiac intensive care nurses, physical therapists, respiratory therapists, pharmacists, patients, and families. This strategy includes the elements outlined in **Box 1.**

Education of nursing staff, nursing assistants, and allied health professionals before the introduction of a multimodal opioid-sparing analgesic program helps ensure success with minimal side effects. Nursing education should include reviewing the mechanism of action, pharmacokinetics, and side effects for opioids as well as multimodal agents. Aspects of a successful educational program include reviewing the institution's preferred pain intensity scales for each specific patient population. Bedside staff will routinely establish a patient's expectations regarding pain and their individualized acceptable pain threshold. The care team will need to assess the patient's comorbidities and physiologic state that can affect the safety and efficacy of opioids as well as adjuvant therapies. These factors can include level of consciousness, respiratory status, cardiovascular stability, and overall strength. Patient history of chronic pain and prior opioid use will also have a significant impact on efficacy and patient expectations. The care plan should clearly delineate when to consider dose escalation or consideration of alternate agents. Staff must reassess pain regularly at intervals adjusted to the needs and sleep patterns of individual patients. Pain should also be assessed during periods of activity such as deep breathing, coughing, and ambulation to help encourage early mobility.[48] Patient and family education regarding goals and expectations facilitates communication, reduces opioid utilization, improves outcomes.[49]

Another important area of increasing focus includes the amount of opioids prescribed at discharge. Recent studies have indicated that US providers prescribe a much higher dosing of opioids for patients going home after surgery than providers in other countries.[50] Discharge MMEs are currently tracked by Centers of Medicare and Medicaid Services, and efforts are underway to reduce the amount of opioids being prescribed for patients at home. Excess discharge opioids can lead to increasing risk of opioid dependence for patients as well as others in their household.[50] Reducing opioid use at home will require discussion with patients and their families and likely continuation of alternative agents postdischarge. The ideal standard regimen for

---

Box 1
Keys to success with multimodal therapy

Education and Planning
1. Education of front-line providers and allied staff
2. Education of patients and families
3. Set realistic, specific goals
4. Quantitative pain assessments

Interventions:
1. Multimodal analgesic strategy that targets different parts of pain pathways
2. Use of preemptive, scheduled nonopioid analgesics
3. Regional anesthetic techniques
4. Minimize opioids
5. Nausea prophylaxis
6. Remove lines and tubes as soon as possible
7. Early extubation
8. Early mobilization
9. Integration of pain management and recovery pathways into discharge planning

Continuous Improvement:
1. Longitudinal data capture for program assessment
2. Obtain feedback from providers and patients to modify program

cardiac surgery patients postdischarge is an area that requires further study. The overall goal following surgery is to use lower doses of opioids with the same or better pain control.

DISCLOSURE

The authors have no relevant financial disclosures.

REFERENCES

1. Milgrom LB, Brooks JA, Qi R, et al. Pain levels experienced with activities after cardiac surgery. Am J Crit Care 2004;13(2):116–25.
2. Mueller XM, Tinguely F, Tevaearai HT, et al. Pain location, distribution, and intensity after Cardiac surgery. Chest 2000;118(2):391–6.
3. Guimaraes-Pereira L, Reis P, Abelha F, et al. Persistent postoperative pain after cardiac surgery: a systematic review with meta-analysis regarding incidence and pain intensity. Pain 2017;158(10):1869–85.
4. Gan TJ. Poorly controlled postoperative pain: prevalence, consequences and prevention. J Pain Res 2017;10:2287–98.
5. Remme WJ. The sympathetic nervous system and ischemic heart disease. Eur Heart J 1998;(Suppl F):F62–71.
6. Baral P, Udit S, Chiu IM. Pain and immunity: implications for host defense. Nat Rev Immunol 2019;19(7):433–47.
7. Amodeo G, Bugada D, Franchi S, et al. Immune function after major surgical interventions: the effect of postoperative pain treatment. J Pain Res 2018;11:1297–305.
8. Goesling J, Moser SE, Zaidi B, et al. Trends and predictors of opioid use following total knee and total hip arthroplasty. Pain 2016;157(6):1259–65.
9. Zubrzycki M, Liebold A, Skrabal C, et al. Assessment and pathophysiology of pain in cardiac surgery. J Pain Res 2018;11:1599–611.
10. de Goeij M, van Eijk LT, Vanelderen P, et al. Systemic inflammation decreases pain threshold in humans in vivo. PLoS One 2013;8(12):e84159.
11. Nagappa M, Weinarten TN, Montandon G, et al. Opioids, respiratory depression, and sleep – disordered breathing. Best Pract Res Clin Anaesthesiol 2017;31(4):469–85.
12. Oberda GM, Evans RS, Lloyd J, et al. Cost of opioid-related adverse drug events in surgical patients. J Pain Symptom Manage 2003;25(3):276–83.
13. Barletta JF. Clinical and economic burden of opioid use for post-surgical pain: focus on ventilator impairment and ileus. Pharmacotherapy 2012;32(9 Suppl):12S–8S.
14. Williams JB, McConnell G, Allendra JE, et al. One – year results from the first US-based enhanced recovery after cardiac surgery (ERAS Cardiac) program. J Thorac Cardiovasc Surg 2019;157(5):1881–8.
15. Feuerstein G. The opioid system and central cardiovascular control: analysis of controversies. Peptides 1985;6(Suppl 2):51–6.
16. Hayhurst CJ, Durieux MD. Differential opioid tolerance and opioid induced hyperalgesia: a clinical reality. Anesthesiology 2016;124(2):216, 483–88.
17. van Gulik L, Ahlers SJ, van deGarde EM, et al. Remifentanil during cardiac surgery is associated with chronic thoracic pain a year after sternotomy. Br J Anesth 2012;109(4):616–22.
18. Alam A, Gomes T, Zheng H. Long-term analgesic use after low risk surgery: a retrospective cohort study. Arch Intern Med 2012;172(5):425–30.

19. Steyaert A, Forget P, Dubois V, et al. Does the perioperative analgesic/anesthetic regimen influence the prevalence of long-term chronic pain after mastectomy? J Clin Anesth 2016;33:20–5.
20. Deyo RA, Hallvik SE, Hildebran C, et al. Use of prescription opioids before and after an operation for chronic pain (Lumbar fusion surgery). Pain 2018;159(6): 1147–54.
21. Engelman RM, Rousou JA, Flack JE, et al. Fast track recovery of the coronary bypass patient. Ann Thorac Surg 1994;58(6):1742–6.
22. Wong W-T, Lai VKW, Chee YI, et al. Fast-track cardiac care for adult cardiac surgical patients. Cochrane Database Syst Rev 2016;(9):CD003587.
23. Kehlet H, Dahl JB. The value of "multimodal" or "balanced analgesia" in post-operative pain treatment. Anesth Analg 1993;77(5):1048–56.
24. Weinbroum AA. Non-opiod IV adjuvants in the perioperative period: pharmacological and clinical aspects of ketamine and gabapentinoids. Pharmacol Res 2012;65(4):411–29.
25. Mauermann E, Ruppen W, Bandschapp O. Different protocols used today to achieve total opioid-free general anesthesia without locoregional blocks. Best Pract Res Clin Anaesthesiol 2017;31(4):533–45.
26. Doleman B, Read D, Lund JN. Preventive acetaminophen reduces post-operative opioid consumption, vomiting and pain scores after surgery: systematic review and meta-analysis. Reg Anesth Pain Med 2015;40(6):706–12.
27. Nir RR, Nahman N, Averbach, et al. Preoperative preemptive drug administration for acute postoperative pain: a systematic review and meta-analysis. Eur J Pain 2016;20(7):1025–43.
28. Caruso TJ, Lawrence K, Tsui BCH. Regional anesthesia for cardiac surgery. Curr Opin Anaesthesiol 2019;32(5):674–82.
29. Starkweather A, Perry M. Enhanced Recovery programs and pain management. Top Pain Manag 2017;32(8):1–9.
30. Wick EC, Grant MC, Wu CL. Postoperative multimodal analgesia pain management with nonopioid analgesics and techniques. JAMA Surg 2017;152(7):691–7.
31. Ljungqvist O, Scott M, Fearon KC. Enhanced recovery after surgery: a review. JAMA Surg 2017;152(3):292–8.
32. Engelman DT, Ben AW, Williams JB, et al. Guidelines for preoperative care in cardiac surgery: enhanced Recovery after Surgery Society recommendations. JAMA Surg 2019;154(8):755–66.
33. Allen DJ, Chae-Kim SH, Trousdale DM. Risks and complications of neuraxial anesthesia and the use of anticoagulation in the surgical patient. Proc (Bayl Univ Med Cent) 2002;15(4):369–73.
34. Mittnacht AJC, Shariat A, Weiner MM, et al. Regional techniques for cardiac and cardiac-related procedures. J Cardiothorac Vasc Anesth 2019;33(2):532–46.
35. Krishna SN, Chauhan S, Bhoi D, et al. Bilateral erector spinae plane block for acute post-surgical pain in adult cardiac surgical patients: a randomized controlled trial. J Cardiothorac Vasc Anesth 2019;33(2):368–75.
36. El Shora HA, El Beleehy AA, Adbdelwahab AA, et al. Bilateral paravertebral block verses thoracic epidural analgesia for pain control post-cardiac surgery: a randomized controlled trial. Thorac Cardiovasc Surg 2018. https://doi.org/10.1055/2-0038-1668496.
37. Kumar KN, Kalyane RN, Singh NG, et al. Efficacy of bilateral pectoralis nerve block for ultrafast tracking and postoperative pain management in cardiac surgery. Ann Card Anaesth 2018;21(3):333–8.

38. Chou R, Gordon DB, deLeon-Casasola OA, et al. Management of postoperative pain: a clinical practice guideline from the American Pain Society, the American Society of Regional Anesthesia and Pain Medicine, and te American Society of Anesthesiologists' Committee on Regional Anesthesia, Executive Committee, and Administrative Council. J Pain 2016;17(2):131–57.
39. Anderson EA. Preoperative preparation for cardiac surgery facilitates recovery, reduces psychological distress, and reduces the incidence of acute postoperative hypertension. J Consult Clin Psychol 1987;55(4):513–20.
40. Benedetti F, Amanzio M, Casadio C, et al. Control of postoperative pain by transcutaneous electrical nerve stimulation after thoracic operations. Ann Thorac Surg 1997;63(3):773–6.
41. Block RI, Ghoneim MM, Sum Ping ST, et al. Efficacy of therapeutic suggestions for improved postoperative recovery presented during general anesthesia. Anesthesiology 1991;75(5):746–55.
42. Ashton C Jr, Whitworth GC, Seldomridge JA, et al. Self-hypnosis reduces anxiety following coronary artery bypass surgery: a prospective randomized trial. J Cardiovasc Surg 1997;38(1):69–75.
43. Hattan J, King L, Griffiths P. The impact of foot massage and guided relaxation following cardiac surgery: a randomized controlled trial. J Adv Nurs 2002; 37(2):199–207.
44. Antall GF, Krevic D. The use of guided imagery to manage pain in the elderly orthopedic population. Orthop Nurs 2004;23(5):335–40.
45. Centers for Disease Control and Prevention. 2018 annual surveillance report of drug-related risks and outcomes — United States. Surveillance special report 2pdf icon. Centers for Disease Control and Prevention, U.S. Department of Health and Human Services; 2018.
46. Bignami E, Castella A, Pota V, et al. Perioperative pain management in cardiac surgery: a systematic review. Minerva Anesthesiol 2018;84(4):488–503.
47. Cogan J, Ouimette MF, Yegin Z, et al. Perioperative pain management barriers in cardiac surgery: should we persevere? Appl Nurs Res 2017;35:6–12.
48. Watt-Watson J, Stevens B, Garfinkel P, et al. Relationship between nurses' pain knowledge and pain management outcomes for their postoperative cardiac patients. J Adv Nurs 2001;36(4):535–45.
49. Bjornnes AK, Parry M, Lie I, et al. The impact of an educational pain management booklet intervention on postoperative pain control after cardiac surgery. Eur J Cardiovasc Nurs 2017;16(1):18–27.
50. Ladha KS, Neuman MD, Broms G, et al. Opioid prescribing after surgery in the United States, Canada, and Sweden. JAMA Netw Open 2019;2(9):e1910734.
51. Schwenk ES, Viscusi ER, Buvanendran A, et al. Consensus guidelines on the use of intravenous ketamine infusions for acute pain management from the American Society of Regional Anesthesia and Pain Medicine, the American Academy of Pain Medicine, and the American Society of Anesthesiologists. Reg Anesth Pain Med 2018;43(5):456–66.
52. Naqdeve NG, Yaddanapudi S, Pandav SS. The effect of different doses of ketamine on intraocular pressure in anesthetized children. J Pediatr Ophthalmol Strabismus 2006;43(4):219–23.
53. Schmidt PC, Ruchelli G, Mackey SC, et al. Choice of agent, dose, timing, and effects on chronic postsurgical pain. Anesthesiology 2013;119(5):1215–21.
54. Weibel S, Jelting Y, Helf A, et al. Continuous intravenous perioperative lidocaine infusion for postoperative pain and recovery in adults. Cochrane Database Syst Rev 2018;(6):CD009642.

55. Lu JF, Nightingale CH. Magnesium sulfate in pre-eclampsia: pharmacokinetic principles. Clin Pharmacokinet 2000;38(4):305–14.

56. Jabbour HJ, Naccache NM, Jawish RJ, et al. Ketamine and magnesium association reduces morphine consumption after scoliosis surgery: prospective randomised double-blind study. Acta Anaesthesiol Scand 2014;58(5):572–9.

57. Motov S, Yasavolian M, Likourezos A, et al. Comparison of intravenous Ketorolac at three single-dose regimens for treating acute pain in the emergency department: a randomized controlled trial. Ann Emerg Med 2017;70(2):177–84.

58. Yancy CW, Jessup M, Bozkurt B, et al. American College of Cardiology Foundation/American Heart Association task force on practice guidelines. 2013 ACCF/AHA guideline for the management of heart failure: a report of the American College of Cardiology Foundation/American Heart Association Task Force on practice guidelines. Circulation 2013;128(16):e240–327.

59. Fleming IO, Garratt C, Guha R, et al. Aggregation of marginal gains in cardiac surgery: feasibility of a perioperative care bundle for enhanced recovery in cardiac surgical patients. J Cardiothorac Vasc Anesth 2016;30(3):665–70.

60. Menda F, Koner O, Sayin M, et al. Effects of single-dose gabapentin on postoperative pain and morphine consumption after cardiac surgery. J Cardiothorac Vasc Anesth 2010;24(5):808–13.

61. Grant MC, Isada T, Ruzankin P, et al. Results from an enhanced recovery program for cardiac surgery. J Thorac Cardiovasc Surg 2019. https://doi.org/10.1016/j.jtcvs.2019.05.035.

62. Markham T, Wegner R, Hernandez N, et al. Assessment of a multimodal analgesia protocol to allow the implementation of enhanced recovery after cardiac surgery: retrospective analysis of patient outcomes. J Clin Anesth 2019;54:76–80.

63. Li M, Zhang J, Gan TJ, et al. Enhanced recovery after surgery pathway for patients undergoing cardiac surgery: a randomized clinical trial. Eur J Cardiothorac Surg 2018;54(3):491–7.

64. Florkiewicz P, Musialowicz T, Hippelainen M, et al. Continuous ropivacaine infusion offers no benefit in treating postoperative pain after cardiac surgery. J Cardiothorac Vasc Anesth 2019;33(2):378–84.

65. Rafiq S, Steinbruchel DA, Wanscher MJ, et al. Multimodal analgesia versus traditional opiate based analgesia after cardiac surgery, a randomized controlled trial. J Cardiothorac Surg 2014;9:52.

66. Subramaniam B, Shankar P, Shaefi S, et al. Effect of intravenous acetaminophen vs placebo combined with propofol or dexmedetomidine on postoperative delirium among older patients following cardiac surgery: the DEXACET randomized clinical trial. JAMA 2019;321(7):686–96.

67. Peng K, Li D, Applegate RL, et al. Effect of dexmedetomidine on cardiac surgery-associated acute kidney injury: a meta-analysis with trial sequential analysis of randomized controlled trials. J Cardiothorac Vasc Anesth 2019. https://doi.org/10.1053/j.jvca.2019.09.011.

68. Souvik M, Baidya DK, Bhattacharjee S, et al. Perioperative gabapentin and pregabalin in cardiac surgery: a systematic review and meta-analysis. Rev Bras Anestesiol 2017;67(3):294–304.

69. Lahtinen P, Kokki H, Hakala T, et al. S(+)-ketamine as an analgesic adjunct reduces opioid consumption after cardiac surgery. Anesth Analg 2004;99(5):1295–301.

70. Qazi SM, Sindby EJ, Norgaard MA. Ibuprofen- a safe analgesic during cardiac surgery recovery? A randomized controlled trial. J Cardiovasc Thorac Res 2015;7:141–8.

71. De Souza BF, Mehta RH, Lopes RD, et al. Nonsteroidal anti-inflammatory drugs and clinical outcomes in patients undergoing coronary artery bypass surgery. Am J Med 2017;130(4):462–8.
72. Vrooman B, Kapural L, Sarwar S, et al. Lidocaine 5% patch for treatment of acute pain after robotic cardiac surgery and prevention of persistent incisional pain: a randomized, placebo-controlled, double-blind trial. Pain 2015;16(8):1610–21.

Goal-Directed Therapy for Cardiac Surgery

Kevin W. Lobdell, MD[a],*, Subhasis Chatterjee, MD[b,c], Michael Sander, MD[d,e]

KEYWORDS

- Goal-directed therapy • Cardiac surgery • Acute kidney injury • Monitoring
- Biomarkers

KEY POINTS

- Enhanced recovery after surgery efforts aim to decrease surgical stress, maintain physiologic functional capacity, and facilitate postoperative recovery through standardized use of best practices.
- Goal-directed therapy is a recommended component of cardiac surgical enhanced recovery.
- Goal-directed therapy is associated with favorable results in heterogeneous patient populations (both surgical and nonsurgical), despite differing goals and variations in monitoring and therapeutic strategies.
- Novel data sources, along with advanced data management and analytics such as artificial intelligence, will converge to extend our insight into risk assessment and mitigation strategies.

INTRODUCTION

Enhanced recovery after surgery efforts use evidence-based practice methods to decrease surgical stress, maintain physiologic functional capacity, and facilitate postoperative recovery.[1] The importance of attempting to achieve these goals is underscored by the high rate of complications after surgery. According to the World Health Organization's most recent update,[2] an estimated 313 million surgical procedures were performed worldwide in 2012. Depending on the type of surgery and presurgical comorbidities, 30% to 40% of patients will develop complications; in as many as 20% of patients, these complications will be severe

[a] Atrium Health Cardiothoracic Surgery, Atrium Health's Carolinas Medical Center, PO Box 32861, Charlotte, NC 28232, USA; [b] Department of Surgery, Baylor College of Medicine, One Baylor Plaza, MS: BCM 390, Houston, TX 77030, USA; [c] Division of Cardiovascular Surgery, Texas Heart Institute, Houston, TX, USA; [d] Department of Anesthesiology, Intensive Care Medicine and Pain Therapy, University Hospital Giessen, Justus-Liebig University Giessen, Rudolf-Buchheim-Strasse 7, Giessen 35392, Germany; [e] Charity Medical University, Berlin, Germany
* Corresponding author.
E-mail address: kevin.lobdell@atriumhealth.org
Twitter: @Perfect_Care_ (K.W.L.); @SXC71 (S.C.); @Mich_San_d (M.S.)

Crit Care Clin 36 (2020) 653–662
https://doi.org/10.1016/j.ccc.2020.06.004
0749-0704/20/© 2020 Elsevier Inc. All rights reserved.

and possibly life threatening.[3–5] This is especially true for cardiac procedures. The results of the International Surgical Outcomes Study showed that complication rates were greatest (57%) for patients who underwent cardiac surgery.[6] Thus, making even small decreases in the frequency of complications can affect thousands of patients.

A long history of related experience, research, and evaluation of the physiologic, metabolic, and inflammatory insults of surgery, trauma, and shock provide important perspectives for understanding enhanced recovery after surgery efforts. Goal-directed therapy (GDT) is a strongly recommended component of cardiac surgical enhanced recovery.[7] With its focus on such concepts as physiologic reserve, negative base excess,[8] oxygen debt and debt repayment,[9,10] potential downregulation of oxygen demand, and tissue oxygenation, GDT aims to provide clinicians with a guide to targeted resuscitation.[11] Although most GDT studies emphasize physiologic metrics such as cardiac output, systemic blood pressure, and right and left heart filling pressures, it is also important to acknowledge the complex interplay of surgical insult on metabolism, inflammation, and coagulation.[12]

GOAL-DIRECTED THERAPY OUTCOMES

Early GDT for the treatment of sepsis was popularized in response to the landmark 2001 Rivers trial[13] in which 263 patients in a single urban Detroit emergency department with severe sepsis or septic shock were randomized to early GDT, with resuscitation based on achieving hemodynamic (central venous pressure, mean arterial pressure, central venous oxygen saturation) and physiologic (urine output) goals achieved with fluid boluses, transfusions, vasopressors, and inotropes, versus standard management. There was a striking reduction in hospital mortality in the GDT-treated group compared with the standard-treatment group (30.5% vs 46.5%; relative risk, 0.58; 95% confidence interval, 0.38–0.87; $P = .009$). Subsequent large multicenter studies, however, could not corroborate the value of GDT in preventing sepsis-associated mortality. Most observers attribute this to the generalized adoption of much of GDT in the standard management group, such that striking differences in mortality between protocolized GDT and current standard care could not be found.[14–16] In other words, standard treatment has improved over time in the 2 decades since the Rivers trial. Indeed, many other GDT algorithms have been introduced, with evidence pointing toward the benefits of an individualized early GDT protocol.

GDT has produced favorable results in noncardiac surgery, including fewer complications, decreased length of stay (LOS), and improvements in short- and long-term survival.[17–25] On the basis of the existing evidence, the European Society of Anesthesiology's guideline for the cardiovascular assessment and management of patients undergoing noncardiac surgery[26] recommends GDT for those patients at high cardiac or surgical risk. GDT includes predefined hemodynamic treatment goals targeting normal or supranormal levels of oxygen delivery and focuses on optimizing fluid management and inotropic support. Nevertheless, a systematic review of 112 randomized perioperative GDT trials found conflicting results caused by the large heterogeneity within the patient cohorts, types of monitoring, targeted hemodynamic variables, and interventions performed. There was also a wide variety of surgical procedures along with a high overall risk for bias, such that a planned meta-analysis could not be completed.[27] After decades of investigation in these other areas, the evidence for using GDT in cardiac surgery has solidified.[28]

QUALITY AND VALUE CONSIDERATIONS

Risk assessment is fundamental to contemporary cardiac surgical practice. Surgical risk is conferred through a combination of patient-specific factors, the surgical procedure itself, and the perioperative care provided.[29,30] In addition to standard preoperative cardiac surgery risk assessment models,[31,32] examinations of the risks associated with perfusion,[33] cardiac intensive care,[34] and organ-specific reserve[35] have been undertaken. Examples of commonly accepted risk factors associated with acute kidney injury (AKI)—whose prevention is integrally associated with GDT—include age, female sex, impaired ventricular function, diabetes mellitus, chronic kidney disease, systemic hypertension, anemia, emergency status, and preoperative intra-aortic balloon pump use, among others. Advanced risk models may include the measurement of physiologic reserve, a focus on all phases of care, and even artificial intelligence,[36] although these are not commonly used at this time.

Risk stratification may also refine our therapeutic approach to GDT and its associated value.[37] A deeper understanding of risk assessment and the benefits associated with GDT requires additional investigation and consensus on definitions, along with the associated monitoring of creatinine, glomerular filtration rate, urine output, and renal replacement therapy details. Various classification schemes, such as Risk, Injury, Failure, Loss of Kidney Function, and End-Stage Kidney Disease (RIFLE), Acute Kidney Injury Network (AKIN), and Kidney Disease Improving Global Outcomes (KDIGO), offer standardized criteria for defining AKI severity. In addition, timing, duration, and compliance with GDT strategies must be monitored to develop meaningful insight into interventions that are effective in preventing or mitigating AKI. Follow-up duration also is crucial for understanding the longer term impact that GDT may have on AKI, the subsequent development of chronic kidney disease, and late mortality.

Goals commonly associated with GDT may be conveniently categorized as "macro" and "micro." Macro goals, which are generally derived from hemodynamic measurements that are immediately available, include improving cardiac output and index, systemic blood pressure, and various derivatives of those parameters, such as mean arterial pressure, pulse pressure, perfusion pressure, diastolic pressure,[38] blood pressure lability,[39,40] central venous pressure,[41] systemic venous oxygen saturation, and urine output.[42,43] Micro goals, which are generally laboratory parameters that reflect biochemical processes, include increasing oxygen delivery and consumption, clearance of lactate, inflammatory, and AKI biomarkers,[44–51] as well as preserving intestinal mucosal pH.[52]

Salient methodologic considerations associated with GDT include the domains of people, technology, and process. For example, anesthesia and perfusion GDT efforts in cardiac surgery have been shown to be beneficial.[53–58] Similarly, a nurse-driven GDT protocol in an intensive care unit was found to be feasible and was favorably associated with a shortened LOS.[59] Various technologies are available for cardiac output monitoring, including pulmonary artery catheters with and without systemic venous oxygen saturation monitoring, waveform analysis with peripheral arterial catheters, Doppler analysis, and bioimpedance, among others.[60] Minimally invasive technologies for monitoring cardiac output are evolving, and continued refinements should bring this to the forefront in the near future.[61,62]

Process variables include, but are not limited to, volume expansion with crystalloid and colloid solutions,[63] erythrocyte transfusion,[64] and adjustment of the amount and rate of administration of any of these fluids. The use of inotropes—for example, dopamine, dobutamine, levosimendan, or norepinephrine—and vasopressin has been

Table 1
Notable cardiac surgery GDT studies

Reference	Location	Design	No. of Patients	Intervention	Primary End Point	Major Findings
Pölönen et al,[72] 2000	Kuopio, Finland	Randomized controlled trial	N = 393 (196 in protocol group; 197 in control group)	GDT guided by lactate and hemodynamics	Hospital and ICU LOS	Median hospital LOS reduced in the protocol group (6 d vs 7 d; P<.05) Less-frequent morbidity in the protocol group (1.1% vs 6.1%, P<.01)
Meersch et al,[67] 2017	Münster, Germany	Randomized controlled trial	N = 276 (138 in intervention group; 138 in control group)	KDIGO bundle, urinary biomarkers after cardiac surgery	AKI within 72 h after cardiac surgery	AKI reduced in intervention group (55% vs 72%, P = .004)
Kapoor et al,[73] 2017	New Delhi and Gurgaon, India	Randomized, prospective; 2 centers	N = 163 (75 in GDT group; 88 in control group)	GDT with hemodynamic management	Duration of mechanical ventilation, inotropic support, and ICU and hospital LOS	ICU LOS (2.5 d vs 4.2 d, P<.001) and hospital LOS (5.6 d vs 7.4 d, P<.001) reduced in GDT group Duration of inotropes (2.9 h vs 3.2 h, P = .005) reduced in GDT group
Goepfert et al,[74] 2007	Munich, Germany	Prospective vs historical control	N = 80 (40 in GDT group; 40 in control group)	GDT hemodynamic management guided by GEDVI	Vasopressors, catecholamines, fluid administration, mechanical ventilation, LOS	GDT decreased the need for vasopressors (187 min vs 1458 min, P<.01), catecholamines (0.01 mg vs 0.8 mg, P<.01), mechanical ventilation (12.6 h vs 15.4 h, P = .002), and reduced ICU LOS (25 h vs 33 h, P = .03)
Johnston et al,[75] 2019	Virginia, USA	Observational, retrospective; multicenter	N = 1979 (725 in pre-QI group; 1254 in post-QI group)	QI initiative: GDT volume resuscitation	Rate of AKI by RIFLE criteria	GDT group had less renal injury or failure (7.8% vs 12.4%, P = .001)

Abbreviations: GEDVI, Global End-Diastolic Volume Index; ICU, intensive care unit; KDIGO, Kidney Disease Improving Global Outcomes; QI, quality improvement; RIFLE, Risk, Injury, Failure, Loss of Kidney Function, and End-Stage Kidney Disease.
Data from Refs.[67,72–75]

associated with improved outcomes.[65] Moreover, a combination of volume expansion and inotropic support has improved outcomes beyond volume expansion alone.[66] Care "bundles" of supportive measures aimed at reducing AKI, such as the KDIGO-based bundle (which included GDT) tested in the PrevAKI trial, have been developed and correlate with improved outcomes.[67-69] With regard to renal replacement therapy, a study showed that a GDT approach focused on solutes, volume, electrolytes, pH, and hemodynamics was superior to standard management of daily hemofiltration with respect to improving renal recovery, LOS, and costs.[70,71]

Finally, the enhanced recovery after surgery cardiac surgery guidelines recently recommended GDT for reducing postoperative complications (Class 1 and Level of Evidence B).[1] Key cardiac single-institution and multicenter surgical studies evidencing benefits from GDT are noted in **Table 1**.[67,72-75] Meta-analyses of GDT in cardiac surgery also have corroborated its favorable impact on complications and LOS.[76-78] Any comprehensive evaluation of GDT efforts should include perspectives on long-term mortality, morbidity (including chronic kidney disease),[79,80] LOS, and readmissions. By mitigating the likelihood of complications, GDT may have a significant economic impact, given that postoperative complications are costly.[81,82]

INNOVATION AND RESEARCH

Novel data sources, improved data management, and advanced analytics offer the opportunity to converge and extend our insight into risk-assessment and mitigation strategies. For example, DeepMind's artificial intelligence AKI research study investigated 703,782 patients and developed a model that could provide up to 48 hours of advance warning (albeit with 2 false warnings for every true alert) and predicted 55.8% of AKIs overall and 90.2% of AKIs that required dialysis.[83-85]

SUMMARY

Comprehensively and dynamically quantifying risk to include cellular and organ-specific reserve, decreasing the stress of the surgical insult, and mitigating modifiable risk factors are vital to the success of surgery and GDT efforts. Much work remains for GDT to be both personalized and comprehensive. We must also recognize and value the ability of quality-of-care improvement studies, as opposed to a traditional focus that relies exclusively on randomized clinical trials.[75,86] Information technology is evolving quickly, with novel biosensors, big data, and analytical and decision support capabilities. This technology will accelerate learning about GDT outcomes and associated risk modeling and mitigation strategies.

ACKNOWLEDGMENTS

The authors appreciate the editorial support provided by Jeanie F. Woodruff, BS, ELS, of the Texas Heart Institute's Department of Scientific Publications.

DISCLOSURE

Dr K.W. Lobdell is an independent quality consultant for Medtronic and Abbott Nutrition and has received a grant from The Duke Endowment. The remaining authors have disclosed that they have no conflicts of interest.

REFERENCES

1. Engelman DT, Ben Ali W, Williams JB, et al. Guidelines for perioperative care in cardiac surgery: Enhanced Recovery After Surgery Society recommendations. JAMA Surg 2019;154(8):755–66.
2. Weiser TG, Haynes AB, Molina G, et al. Size and distribution of the global volume of surgery in 2012. Bull World Health Organ 2016;94(3):201–209F.
3. Ghaferi AA, Birkmeyer JD, Dimick JB. Variation in hospital mortality associated with inpatient surgery. N Engl J Med 2009;361(14):1368–75.
4. Schilling PL, Dimick JB, Birkmeyer JD. Prioritizing quality improvement in general surgery. J Am Coll Surg 2008;207(5):698–704.
5. Kahan BC, Koulenti D, Arvaniti K, et al. Critical care admission following elective surgery was not associated with survival benefit: prospective analysis of data from 27 countries. Intensive Care Med 2017;43(7):971–9.
6. International Surgical Outcomes Study (ISOS) Group. Global patient outcomes after elective surgery: prospective cohort study in 27 low-, middle- and high-income countries. Br J Anaesth 2017;119(3):553.
7. Desborough JP. The stress response to trauma and surgery. Br J Anaesth 2000; 85(1):109–17.
8. Dunham CM, Siegel JH, Weireter L, et al. Oxygen debt and metabolic acidemia as quantitative predictors of mortality and the severity of the ischemic insult in hemorrhagic shock. Crit Care Med 1991;19(2):231–43.
9. Barbee RW, Reynolds PS, Ward KR. Assessing shock resuscitation strategies by oxygen debt repayment. Shock 2010;33(2):113–22.
10. Rixen D, Siegel JH. Bench-to-bedside review: oxygen debt and its metabolic correlates as quantifiers of the severity of hemorrhagic and post-traumatic shock. Crit Care 2005;9(5):441–53.
11. Lima A, van Bommel J, Jansen TC, et al. Low tissue oxygen saturation at the end of early goal-directed therapy is associated with worse outcome in critically ill patients. Crit Care 2009;13(Suppl 5):S13.
12. Warren OJ, Smith AJ, Alexiou C, et al. The inflammatory response to cardiopulmonary bypass: part 1–mechanisms of pathogenesis. J Cardiothorac Vasc Anesth 2009;23(2):223–31.
13. Rivers E, Nguyen B, Havstad S, et al. Early goal-directed therapy in the treatment of severe sepsis and septic shock. N Engl J Med 2001;345(19):1368–77.
14. ProCESS Investigators, Yealy DM, Kellum JA, et al. A randomized trial of protocol-based care for early septic shock. N Engl J Med 2014;370(18):1683–93.
15. ARISE Investigators, ANZICS Clinical Trials Group, Peake SL, et al. Goal-directed resuscitation for patients with early septic shock. N Engl J Med 2014;371(16): 1496–506.
16. PRISM Investigators, Rowan KM, Angus DC, et al. Early, goal-directed therapy for septic shock - a patient-level meta-analysis. N Engl J Med 2017;376(23): 2223–34.
17. Shoemaker WC. Cardiorespiratory patterns of surviving and nonsurviving postoperative patients. Surg Gynecol Obstet 1972;134(5):810–4.
18. Shoemaker WC, Appel PL, Kram HB, et al. Prospective trial of supranormal values of survivors as therapeutic goals in high-risk surgical patients. Chest 1988;94(6):1176–86.
19. Shoemaker WC, Patil R, Appel PL, et al. Hemodynamic and oxygen transport patterns for outcome prediction, therapeutic goals, and clinical algorithms to

improve outcome. Feasibility of artificial intelligence to customize algorithms. Chest 1992;102(5 Suppl 2):617S–25S.

20. Sinclair S, James S, Singer M. Intraoperative intravascular volume optimisation and length of hospital stay after repair of proximal femoral fracture: randomised controlled trial. BMJ 1997;315(7113):909–12.

21. Pearse R, Dawson D, Fawcett J, et al. Early goal-directed therapy after major surgery reduces complications and duration of hospital stay. A randomised, controlled trial [ISRCTN38797445]. Crit Care 2005;9(6):R687–93.

22. Lees N, Hamilton M, Rhodes A. Clinical review: goal-directed therapy in high risk surgical patients. Crit Care 2009;13(5):231.

23. Rhodes A, Cecconi M, Hamilton M, et al. Goal-directed therapy in high-risk surgical patients: a 15-year follow-up study. Intensive Care Med 2010;36(8):1327–32.

24. Suehiro K, Joosten A, Alexander B, et al. Guiding goal-directed therapy. Curr Anesthesiol Rep 2014;4(4):360–75.

25. Giglio M, Dalfino L, Puntillo F, et al. Hemodynamic goal-directed therapy and postoperative kidney injury: an updated meta-analysis with trial sequential analysis. Crit Care 2019;23(1):232.

26. Kristensen SD, Knuuti J, Saraste A, et al. 2014 ESC/ESA Guidelines on non-cardiac surgery: cardiovascular assessment and management: the Joint Task Force on non-cardiac surgery: cardiovascular assessment and management of the European Society of Cardiology (ESC) and the European Society of Anaesthesiology (ESA). Eur Heart J 2014;35(35):2383–431.

27. Kaufmann T, Clement RP, Scheeren TWL, et al. Perioperative goal-directed therapy: a systematic review without meta-analysis. Acta Anaesthesiol Scand 2018;62(10):1340–55.

28. Fergerson BD, Manecke GR Jr. Goal-directed therapy in cardiac surgery: are we there yet? J Cardiothorac Vasc Anesth 2013;27(6):1075–8.

29. Lobdell KW, Fann JI, Sanchez JA. What's the risk?" Assessing and mitigating risk in cardiothoracic surgery. Ann Thorac Surg 2016;102(4):1052–8.

30. Lobdell KW, Rose GA, Mishra AK, et al. Decision making, evidence, and practice. Ann Thorac Surg 2018;105(4):994–9.

31. The Society of Thoracic Surgeons. STS online risk calculator. Available at: http://riskcalc.sts.org/stswebriskcalc/calculate. Accessed February 18, 2020.

32. EuroSCORE Study Group. EuroSCORE interactive calculator. 2011. Available at: http://euroscore.org/calc.html. Accessed February 18, 2020.

33. Rubino AS, Torrisi S, Milazzo I, et al. Designing a new scoring system (QualyP Score) correlating the management of cardiopulmonary bypass to postoperative outcomes. Perfusion 2015;30(6):448–56.

34. Hekmat K. Online calculation of the cardiac intensive care score. Available at: http://www.cardiac-icu.org/Online-Calculation.html. Accessed February 19, 2020.

35. Husain-Syed F, Ferrari F, Sharma A, et al. Persistent decrease of renal functional reserve in patients after cardiac surgery-associated acute kidney injury despite clinical recovery. Nephrol Dial Transplant 2019;34(2):308–17.

36. Meyer A, Zverinski D, Pfahringer B, et al. Machine learning for real-time prediction of complications in critical care: a retrospective study. Lancet Respir Med 2018;6(12):905–14.

37. Zarbock A, Engelman DT. Commentary: should goal-directed fluid therapy be used in every cardiac surgery patient to prevent acute kidney injury? J Thorac Cardiovasc Surg 2020;159(5):1878–9.

38. Weir MR, Aronson S, Avery EG, et al. Acute kidney injury following cardiac surgery: role of perioperative blood pressure control. Am J Nephrol 2011;33(5): 438–52.

39. Aronson S, Dyke CM, Levy JH, et al. Does perioperative systolic blood pressure variability predict mortality after cardiac surgery? An exploratory analysis of the ECLIPSE trials. Anesth Analg 2011;113(1):19–30.

40. Aronson S, Levy JH, Lumb PD, et al. Impact of perioperative blood pressure variability on health resource utilization after cardiac surgery: an analysis of the ECLIPSE trials. J Cardiothorac Vasc Anesth 2014;28(3):579–85.

41. Gambardella I, Gaudino M, Ronco C, et al. Congestive kidney failure in cardiac surgery: the relationship between central venous pressure and acute kidney injury. Interact Cardiovasc Thorac Surg 2016;23(5):800–5.

42. Engoren M, Maile MD, Heung M, et al. The association between urine output, creatinine elevation, and death. Ann Thorac Surg 2017;103(4):1229–37.

43. Lobdell KW. Invited commentary. Ann Thorac Surg 2017;103(4):1237–8.

44. Bakker J, Nijsten MW, Jansen TC. Clinical use of lactate monitoring in critically ill patients. Ann Intensive Care 2013;3(1):12.

45. Hajjar LA, Almeida JP, Fukushima JT, et al. High lactate levels are predictors of major complications after cardiac surgery. J Thorac Cardiovasc Surg 2013; 146(2):455–60.

46. Schumacher KR, Reichel RA, Vlasic JR, et al. Rate of increase in serum lactate level risk-stratifies infants after surgery for congenital heart disease. J Thorac Cardiovasc Surg 2014;148(2):589–95.

47. Koyner JL, Parikh CR. Clinical utility of biomarkers of AKI in cardiac surgery and critical illness. Clin J Am Soc Nephrol 2013;8(6):1034–42.

48. Wyler von Ballmoos M, Likosky DS, Rezaee M, et al. Elevated preoperative Galectin-3 is associated with acute kidney injury after cardiac surgery. BMC Nephrol 2018;19(1):280.

49. Lobdell KW, Parker DM, Likosky DS, et al. Preoperative serum ST2 level predicts acute kidney injury after adult cardiac surgery. J Thorac Cardiovasc Surg 2018; 156(3):1114–11123.e2.

50. Polineni S, Parker DM, Alam SS, et al. Predictive ability of novel cardiac biomarkers ST2, Galectin-3, and NT-ProBNP before cardiac surgery. J Am Heart Assoc 2018;7(14):e008371.

51. Engelman DT, Crisafi C, Germain M, et al. Using urinary biomarkers to reduce acute kidney injury following cardiac surgery. J Thorac Cardiovasc Surg 2019;1–12.

52. Mythen MG, Webb AR. Perioperative plasma volume expansion reduces the incidence of gut mucosal hypoperfusion during cardiac surgery. Arch Surg 1995; 130(4):423–9.

53. Ranucci M, Romitti F, Isgrò G, et al. Oxygen delivery during cardiopulmonary bypass and acute renal failure after coronary operations. Ann Thorac Surg 2005;80(6):2213–20.

54. de Somer F, Mulholland JW, Bryan MR, et al. O_2 delivery and CO_2 production during cardiopulmonary bypass as determinants of acute kidney injury: time for a goal-directed perfusion management? Crit Care 2011;15(4):R192.

55. Newland RF, Baker RA. Low oxygen delivery as a predictor of acute kidney injury during cardiopulmonary bypass. J Extra Corpor Technol 2017;49(4):224–30.

56. Magruder JT, Crawford TC, Harness HL, et al. A pilot goal-directed perfusion initiative is associated with less acute kidney injury after cardiac surgery. J Thorac Cardiovasc Surg 2017;153(1):118–25.e1.

57. Ranucci M, Johnson I, Willcox T, et al. Goal-directed perfusion to reduce acute kidney injury: a randomized trial. J Thorac Cardiovasc Surg 2018;156(5): 1918–27.e2.

58. Newland RF, Baker RA, Woodman RJ, et al. Predictive capacity of oxygen delivery during cardiopulmonary bypass on acute kidney injury. Ann Thorac Surg 2019;108(6):1807–14.

59. McKendry M, McGloin H, Saberi D, et al. Randomised controlled trial assessing the impact of a nurse delivered, flow monitored protocol for optimisation of circulatory status after cardiac surgery. BMJ 2004;329(7460):258.

60. Kobe J, Mishra N, Arya VK, et al. Cardiac output monitoring: technology and choice. Ann Card Anaesth 2019;22(1):6–17.

61. Joosten A, Desebbe O, Suehiro K, et al. Accuracy and precision of non-invasive cardiac output monitoring devices in perioperative medicine: a systematic review and meta-analysis. Br J Anaesth 2017;118(3):298–310.

62. Metz R. Soon your doctor will be able to wirelessly track your health–even through walls. 2018. Available at: https://www.technologyreview.com/s/612055/dina-katabi-emerald-walls/amp/. Accessed February 18, 2020.

63. Holte K. Pathophysiology and clinical implications of peroperative fluid management in elective surgery. Dan Med Bull 2010;57(7):B4156.

64. Karkouti K, Wijeysundera DN, Yau TM, et al. Influence of erythrocyte transfusion on the risk of acute kidney injury after cardiac surgery differs in anemic and non-anemic patients. Anesthesiology 2011;115(3):523–30.

65. Hajjar LA, Vincent JL, Barbosa Gomes Galas FR, et al. Vasopressin versus norepinephrine in patients with vasoplegic shock after cardiac surgery: the VANCS randomized controlled trial. Anesthesiology 2017;126(1):85–93.

66. Prowle JR, Chua HR, Bagshaw SM, et al. Clinical review: volume of fluid resuscitation and the incidence of acute kidney injury - a systematic review. Crit Care 2012;16(4):230.

67. Meersch M, Schmidt C, Hoffmeier A, et al. Prevention of cardiac surgery-associated AKI by implementing the KDIGO guidelines in high risk patients identified by biomarkers: the PrevAKI randomized controlled trial. Intensive Care Med 2017;43(11):1551–61.

68. Meersch M, Schmidt C, Hoffmeier A, et al. Erratum to: prevention of cardiac surgery-associated AKI by implementing the KDIGO guidelines in high risk patients identified by biomarkers: the PrevAKI randomized controlled trial. Intensive Care Med 2017;43(11):1749.

69. de Geus HRH, Meersch M, Zarbock A. Discussion on "Prevention of cardiac surgery-associated AKI by implementing the KDIGO guidelines in high risk patients identified by biomarkers: the PrevAKI randomized controlled trial". Intensive Care Med 2018;44(2):273–4.

70. Mehta RL. Continuous renal replacement therapy in the critically ill patient. Kidney Int 2005;67(2):781–95.

71. Xu J, Ding X, Fang Y, et al. New, goal-directed approach to renal replacement therapy improves acute kidney injury treatment after cardiac surgery. J Cardiothorac Surg 2014;9:103.

72. Pölönen P, Ruokonen E, Hippeläinen M, et al. A prospective, randomized study of goal-oriented hemodynamic therapy in cardiac surgical patients. Anesth Analg 2000;90(5):1052–9.

73. Kapoor PM, Magoon R, Rawat RS, et al. Goal-directed therapy improves the outcome of high-risk cardiac patients undergoing off-pump coronary artery bypass. Ann Card Anaesth 2017;20(1):83–9.

74. Goepfert MS, Reuter DA, Akyol D, et al. Goal-directed fluid management reduces vasopressor and catecholamine use in cardiac surgery patients. Intensive Care Med 2007;33(1):96–103.

75. Johnston LE, Thiele RH, Hawkins RB, et al. Goal-directed resuscitation following cardiac surgery reduces acute kidney injury: a quality initiative pre-post analysis. J Thorac Cardiovasc Surg 2019;159(5):1868–1877.e1.

76. Giglio M, Dalfino L, Puntillo F, et al. Haemodynamic goal-directed therapy in cardiac and vascular surgery. A systematic review and meta-analysis. Interact Cardiovasc Thorac Surg 2012;15(5):878–87.

77. Aya HD, Cecconi M, Hamilton M, et al. Goal-directed therapy in cardiac surgery: a systematic review and meta-analysis. Br J Anaesth 2013;110(4):510–7.

78. Osawa EA, Rhodes A, Landoni G, et al. Effect of perioperative goal-directed hemodynamic resuscitation therapy on outcomes following cardiac surgery: a randomized clinical trial and systematic review. Crit Care Med 2016;44(4):724–33.

79. Legouis D, Galichon P, Bataille A, et al. Rapid occurrence of chronic kidney disease in patients experiencing reversible acute kidney injury after cardiac surgery. Anesthesiology 2017;126(1):39–46.

80. Cho JS, Shim JK, Lee S, et al. Chronic progression of cardiac surgery associated acute kidney injury: intermediary role of acute kidney disease. J Thorac Cardiovasc Surg 2019. https://doi.org/10.1016/j.jtcvs.2019.10.101.

81. Speir AM, Kasirajan V, Barnett SD, et al. Additive costs of postoperative complications for isolated coronary artery bypass grafting patients in Virginia. Ann Thorac Surg 2009;88(1):40–5 [discussion: 45–6].

82. Manecke GR, Asemota A, Michard F. Tackling the economic burden of postsurgical complications: would perioperative goal-directed fluid therapy help? Crit Care 2014;18(5):566.

83. Tomašev N, Glorot X, Rae JW, et al. A clinically applicable approach to continuous prediction of future acute kidney injury. Nature 2019;572(7767):116–9.

84. Suleyman M, King D. Using AI to give doctors a 48-hour head start on life-threatening illness. In: DeepMind blog. 2019. Available at: https://deepmind.com/blog/article/predicting-patient-deterioration. Accessed February 19, 2020.

85. Olson P, Abbott B. Google algorithm aims to identify at-risk kidney injury patients. In: The Wall Street Journal. 2019. Available at: https://www.wsj.com/articles/google-algorithm-aims-to-identify-at-risk-kidney-injury-patients-11564592448. Accessed February 19, 2020.

86. Niven AS, Herasevich S, Pickering BW, et al. The future of critical care lies in quality improvement and education. Ann Am Thorac Soc 2019;16(6):649–56.

Early Extubation in Enhanced Recovery from Cardiac Surgery

Ciana McCarthy, MB, FCAI, JFICMI, EDIC, MEd[a],*,
Nick Fletcher, MBBS, FRCA, FFICM[b,c,1]

KEYWORDS

- Cardiac surgery • Early extubation • Ventilation • Enhanced recovery
- Fast-track recovery

KEY POINTS

- Early extubation is a key component of the enhanced recovery from cardiac surgery pathway, enabling early mobilization and oral nutrition.
- An effective nurse-led early extubation protocol will define prompt time points for cessation of sedation and return to spontaneous ventilation modes.
- Successful early extubation strategies are also associated with reduced intensive care unit and hospital length of stays.
- A focus on reduced dosages of shorter-acting opiates together with multimodal analgesia, including local anesthetic blockade, can reduce ventilatory weaning times.
- The strategy for an early extubation pathway starts from the moment the patient is scheduled for surgery with a prehabilitation program and respiratory testing and optimization.

INTRODUCTION

Enhanced recovery after surgery (ERAS) is a multimodal, multidisciplinary approach to the care of the patient throughout their perioperative stay using bundles of evidence-based best practice.[1] ERAS protocols have been associated with reductions in overall complications, length of stays (LOS) of up to 50%, improved patient satisfaction, and cost-effectiveness.[2] Enhanced recovery cardiac anesthesia techniques have been in development since the early 1990s.[3] Labeled "Fast-Track cardiac surgery," these techniques included the use of short-acting hypnotic drugs, reduced doses of opioids or the use of ultrashort-acting opioids, the use of antifibrinolytic drugs and drugs to prevent atrial fibrillation,[4] and early extubation.[5] Earlier this year the ERAS cardiac

[a] Guys and St Thomas Hospital, Westminster Bridge Road, London SE1 7EH, UK; [b] St Georges University Hospital, London, UK; [c] Cleveland Clinic, London, UK
[1] Present address: 8 Fitzwilliam Road, London SW4 0DN, UK.
* Corresponding author.
E-mail address: cianamccarthy@gmail.com
Twitter: @Echotrainer (N.F.)

Crit Care Clin 36 (2020) 663–674
https://doi.org/10.1016/j.ccc.2020.06.005
0749-0704/20/Crown Copyright © 2020 Published by Elsevier Inc. All rights reserved.

group published evidence-based guidelines,[6] which were the first consensus recommendations for the optimal perioperative management of patients undergoing cardiac surgery.

Prolonged intubation and mechanical ventilation postcardiac surgery have been demonstrated to be associated with increased hospital and intensive care unit (ICU) length of stays; higher health care costs; and morbidity resulting from atelectasis, intrapulmonary shunting, and pneumonia.[7] In contrast, enhanced recovery programs have become a popular and accepted standard, as they benchmark early extubation within 6 hours from the conclusion of surgery and consequently reduced LOS in the ICU and hospital.[8] The safety of this significant reduction in time to extubation has been demonstrated in systematic reviews.[8]

BACKGROUND

An enhanced recovery program in cardiac surgery was suggested in a 1980 study[9] with promising results. The "fast-track protocol" in 1994[3] was one of the first multimodal bundles that consisted of 8 key principles: (1) preoperative education, (2) early extubation, (3) methylprednisolone, (4) prophylactic digitalization, metoclopramide HCl, docusate sodium, and ranitidine Hcl; (5) accelerated rehabilitation, (6) early discharge; (7) a dedicated fast-track coordinator to perform both daily telephone contact and a 1-week postoperative examination; and (8) a routine 1-month postoperative visit.[3] Interestingly, the duration of endotracheal intubation in this study decreased from 22 hours to 15 hours in the intervention group. This early work demonstrates how far recovery from cardiac surgery has traveled from these beginnings. Fifteen hours would universally be viewed as a prolonged intubation time in 2019. From the beginning of enhanced recovery protocols in cardiac surgery, the benchmarking of early extubation at 4 to 8 hours following surgery has been a key recommendation. This was achieved by a focus on lower dose opiates, limited perioperative fluids, and accelerated physical rehabilitation the morning after the operation. The key outcomes were defined as a shorter time to extubation, shorter ICU stay, and shorter overall hospital stay with no change in morbidity or mortality.[3]

Reyes in 1997 again demonstrated the feasibility and benefits of fast-track cardiac anesthesia, achieving success in these key outcome measures.[5] This led to the development of new paradigms of cardiac anesthesiology philosophies in the 1990s as new short-acting intravenous anesthesia agents and opiates became commercially available, which allowed faster recovery.[9,10] Other benefits that powered this trajectory were new types of ventilators and modes that promoted early return to spontaneous breathing and the accompanying cost/benefit analysis of enhanced recovery and reduced length of ICU stay.[11]

Systematic reviews of fast-track cardiac anesthesia have consistently demonstrated the methodology to be safe and effective.[4,12] Cochrane reviews in 2016 demonstrated low-dose opioid-based general anesthesia and time-directed extubation protocols for fast-track interventions have risks of mortality and major postoperative complications similar to those of conventional (not fast-track) care in patients considered to be at low to moderate risk of death after surgery.[8] A summary of the evidence around early extubation studies is presented in **Table 1**.

Identifying the appropriate patients for enhanced recovery protocols is a key factor for the success of a program. This is especially true as patient demographics have increased in age, frailty, and comorbidities[13] prompting the development of cardiac prehabilitation.[14] In selected patients awaiting cardiac surgery, a structured physical

Table 1
Summary of studies investigating early extubation following cardiac surgery

Study & Year	N Participants Early Extubation	N Participants Usual Care	Randomized Y/N	Extubn Time (h) Early Mean (SD)	Extubn Time Usual Care Mean (SD)	P Value	ICU Stay Hrs Early/Usual	Hosp Stay Days Early/Usual	N Reintubation Early	N Reintubation Usual Care
Engelman et al,[3] 1994	280	282	N	15	22	<.01	45/57	6.8/8.3		
Reyes et al,[5] 1997	201	203	Y	10 (169)	21 (308)	.008	27/44		13	7
Berry et al,[48] 1998	43	42	Y	1.83 (1.05)	12.62 (3.09)		48/48	8/8		0
Cheng et al,[11] 1996	51	51	Y	4.1 (1.1)	18.9 (1.4)	<.001	29/30	7/9	1	0
Engoren et al,[49] 1998	35	35	Y	7.48 (4.2)	6.46 (3.36)	>.05	23/21	6/5	0	10
Probst et al,[19] 2014	100	100	Y	1.5 (1.11)	7.97 (4.17)	<.001	3.3/17	9/9	5	0
Zhu et al,[50] 2015	29	30	Y	6.51 (5.76)	8.85 (6.64)	.013	20/22	12/13	2	
Pettersson et al,[51] 2004	30	27	N	3.3 (1.7)	6.7 (1.4)			7/8		0
Michalopoulos et al,[52] 1998	72	72	Y	7.3 (0.7)	11.6 (1.3)	.0001	16/23	7/8	0	0
Nicholson et al,[53] 2002	16	16	Y	0.76 (0.46)	3.36 (0.35)	.01			1	0
Quasha et al,[9] 1980	16	20	Y	2 (2)	18 (3)	.01	46/57		1	12
Fitch et al,[26] 2014	1174	631	N	8	11				0	0
Salah et al,[54] 2015	26	26	Y	0.23 (1.18)	12.94 (5.03)	.001	57/95		2	0
Simeone et al,[55] 2002	24	25	Y	6.5 (3.8)	8.6 (3.5)	.05	29/46		1	1
Gruber et al,[56] 2008	23	25	Y	5 (1.98)	9 (1.46)	<.05	22/22		0	

activity program designed to improve preoperative aerobic capacity has been shown to be safe and may similarly lead to a decrease in postoperative complications and hospital LOS.[15]

Early extubation is a key component to enhanced recovery programs, with numerous studies validating early extubation within 8 hours, resulting in no difference in morbidity or mortality and reduced LOS.[12] Early extubation went one step further with Straka[16] reporting immediate on-table extubation in patients after off-pump coronary artery bypass grafting without thoracic epidural analgesia.[16] Montes reporting on-table extubation was accompanied by a moderate rate of reintubation and no significant reduction in the ICU or hospital LOS when compared with early extubation at 1 to 6 hours.[17]

"Leipzig fast-track concept" was introduced by Ender[18] and Probst[19] who took an alternative approach to postanesthesia care unit (PACU)-led fast-track surgery, with better physician to patient ratios (1:3), allowing for more focused, early postoperative management, and better adherence to an established fast-track protocol. Physically removing the patient from the ICU environment helped to achieve the recovery milestones. Delaying the decision regarding patient suitability for fast-track treatment until the end of surgery was shown to be feasible, which led to earlier extubation and quicker discharge to a step-down unit compared with an ICU-led fast-track program.[19]

EARLY EXTUBATION

There is no standard definition of early extubation but a consensus from early publications and systematic reviews defined this as less than 8 hours, although no physiologic or pathologic criteria have been advanced to explain why this time point was adopted.[8,12] It makes comparison of studies across differing time points somewhat problematic. There are many presumed benefits of early extubation, balanced by discrete risks that can be identified for the individual patient, which are listed in **Box 1**. The effect of mechanical ventilation on cardiovascular hemodynamics, particularly in relation to an undesirable influence on venous return and right ventricular afterload and function has been widely published.[20] Tracheal intubation is

---

Box 1
Benefits and risks of early extubation

Benefits of early extubation
1. Reduced duration and dose of sedative agent with reduced incidence of delirium and cognitive recovery and reduced cardiovascular depression
2. Earlier mobilization
3. Improved hemodynamics with absent risk of ventilator dyssynchrony and straining
4. Earlier return to normal feeding
5. Reduced risk of ventilator-associated pneumonia
6. Reduced need for ICU stay

Risks of early extubation
1. Increased work of breathing with increased oxygen demand
2. Increased demand on the cardiovascular system
3. Loss of extrinsic PEEP with resulting atelectasis
4. Reduced ability to suction and clear secretions
5. Risk of aspiration
6. Risk of reintubation

poorly tolerated by awake patients immediately following cardiac surgery, which normally mandates the continuation of sedation. Sedative agents, most frequently propofol, have widespread undesirable effects on cardiovascular stability, commonly requiring increased fluid infusion or vasoconstrictor agents to counteract vasodilation and hypotension. In addition, higher doses of sedation, particularly in elderly patients, may contribute to delirium, confusion, and the delayed return of cognitive function.

The benefits of early mobilization of cardiac surgery patients have been identified and are a core item in most ERAS protocols. Clearly, this is not possible in patients with mechanical ventilation. The risks of early extubation have not been substantiated in studies. These risks often relate to the perceived threat of failure of extubation and the risk of subsequent reintubation. This risk may be perceived as significant in centers where prompt attendance by an airway-trained physician is limited. Overnight ventilation is sometimes required where such physicians are not available. Current practice considerations would dictate that in a center where cardiac surgery is performed, services should be organized in a way to navigate this risk without using overnight ventilation as a strategy. As discussed, early endotracheal extubation after surgery is a key component of fast-track cardiac management to reduce the patient's LOS in the ICU and in the hospital. In addition to benefiting the patient, this may reduce hospital costs and improve hospital efficiency.[21] A time-directed extubation protocol improves efficiency of practice by following an expert consensus guideline to reduce variations in (1) decisions about when the patient is ready for weaning, (2) the process of reducing ventilatory support, and (3) criteria for deciding whether patients are ready to be extubated.[22]

High-risk patients with preoperative American Society of Anaesthesiologists' Physical Status score greater than 3, New York Heart Association (NYHA) class greater than III, and operative time greater than 267 minutes required significantly longer time to extubation than low-risk patients when the same fast-track cardiac anesthesia technique was used.[23] This highlights the consideration that an early extubation strategy is not suitable for every patient. Those undergoing long procedures and those with poor preoperative cardiorespiratory function may not necessarily benefit but equally should not be disqualified. The Cochrane review found no differences in the risk of death within the first year after surgery between low-dose and high-dose opioid-based general anesthesia groups and between an early extubation protocol versus the usual care groups. Comparison with usual care revealed no significant differences in risk of postoperative complications associated with a time-directed extubation protocols such as myocardial infarction, reintubation, acute renal failure, major bleeding, stroke, major sepsis, and wound infection.[12] This finding is commonly present throughout the available literature, which is not surprising. An early extubation strategy is an intervention aligned with the process of an accelerated surgical recovery rather than a strategy to prevent catastrophic events.

Infrastructure and staffing investment are required to implement enhanced recovery programs and require the investment of time in the formation of a multidisciplinary team, which should include surgical, anesthesia, and nursing membership. Additional important members include nutritionists, physicians, physical and occupational therapists, and social workers. Once formulated, written protocols must be made available to all those involved.[24] This need for initial investment and multidisciplinary buy-in may be an obstacle to building and implementing a program. Another limitation to starting an enhanced recovery program is compliance to the protocols; even in large multicenter trials, adherence of only approximately 65% has been observed.[25]

PERIOPERATIVE JOURNEY

Enhanced recovery pathways consist of several individual components that facilitate the complete patient pathway. At the same time, each of these components should be positively affected by the whole. In the following sections the authors examine how this relates to early extubation and enhanced recovery for the cardiac surgical patient along the entire perioperative pathway (**Box 2**).

PREOPERATIVE PHASE

Structured preoperative information and engagement of the patient and relatives with nursing, anesthesia, and surgical preoperative assessment is key. An education program relating to the process and a forum to address the expectations and concerns of the patient (and staff) are crucial to the success of an enhanced pathway.

The identification of appropriate patients for early extubation while differentiating those who may present a high risk of prolonged intubation times is essential. Studies have shown a trend toward lower likelihood of early extubation for patients with peripheral vascular disease, urgent surgical status, chronic obstructive pulmonary disease, congestive heart failure, Euroscore greater than 10,[19] recent myocardial infarction, and an increase in preoperative serum creatinine.[26] Therefore, addressing these modifiable risk factors improves extubation times, LOS, and prevents postoperative complications such as sternal wound infections.[15,27]

Optimizing perioperative nutrition has the potential to improve patient outcomes such as less surgical site infection, improved wound healing, reduced mechanical ventilation times, shorter ICU stay, decreased hospital readmissions, and lower mortality.[28] The timing and duration of preoperative nutritional replacement is still unidentified.[14]

Box 2
Early extubation strategy across the entire perioperative pathway

Preoperative phase
  Nursing, anesthesia, and surgical preoperative assessment
  Cardiac prehabilitation including optimizing perioperative nutrition
  Carbohydrate preloading preoperatively in select patients

Intraoperative phase
  Reduced doses of opioids (fentanyl $\leq$20 μg/kg or equivalent) or the use of ultrashort-acting opioids
  Reserved use of short-acting benzodiazepines rather than long-acting benzodiazepines
  Lung-protective ventilation: low tidal volumes (6–8 mLkg−1 of predicted body weight) associated with higher positive end-expiratory pressure (PEEP), limitation of fraction of inspired oxygen (Fio$_2$)
  Recruitment maneuvers before weaning from cardiopulmonary bypass
  Multimodal analgesia

Postoperative phase
  Avoidance of postoperative hypothermia (<36°C)
  Monitoring and reversal of muscle paralysis
  Postoperative nurse-led weaning and extubation protocol with protective ventilation strategy
  Screening and active preemptive management of delirium

Cardiac prehabilitation includes aerobic exercise training, respiratory muscle training, smoking cessation, decreasing alcohol consumption, improving sleep patterns, weight control, optimization of medical comorbidities, and psychosocial assessment and education.[14] The primary goal of prehab is to reduce both the incidence and severity of postoperative complications.[29] A prehab course lasting between 6 and 8 weeks that is focused on the 3 key areas of preoperative physical exercise, nutritional care, and psychological support, seems to be a good compromise between feasibility and effectiveness[14] and may lead to the desired reductions in postoperative complications and hospital LOS.[15]

In noncardiac surgery it has been shown that oral administration of 25 to 50 g of carbohydrate preoperatively leads to a reduction in insulin resistance and perioperative hyperglycemia, hastens the return of gastrointestinal function, and improves patient satisfaction.[30] Studies have been carried out in cardiac surgery showing improvements in hemodynamic stability[31,32] with mixed results on the effects of insulin requirements intraoperatively.[33]

INTRAOPERATIVE

Reduced doses of opioids (fentanyl $\leq$20 μg/kg or equivalent), or the use of ultrashort-acting opioids, short-acting benzodiazepines, supplemented with propofol or etomidate, or volatile anesthesia[4] and additional doses of 1 to 3 mg/kg fentanyl up to a total dose of 10 to 20 mg/kg as needed, are the basis of enhanced recovery anesthesia.

Muscle paralysis should generally be maintained until separation from cardiopulmonary bypass. Patients receive an antifibrinolytic agent (eg, tranexamic acid or epsilon aminocaproic acid), insulin, as well as ionotropic and vasoactive medications as needed.[26] Some protocols avoid a second dose of benzodiazepine on pump due to increasing concern with postoperative cognitive dysfunction and delirium associated with benzodiazepines and reversal of paralytics after weaning from bypass.[26]

Ultrashort-acting opioids such as remifentanil have obvious favorable pharmacologic properties. A meta-analysis of remifentanil trials in cardiac surgery showed that remifentanil was associated with reduced time to extubation and length of hospital stay with no increase in risk of mortality when compared with use of fentanyl or sufentanil during general anesthesia.[34] The dose of fentanyl used in some of these trials has confounded the comparison in the literature. Lower dose fentanyl can also be used successfully. Longer acting opiate premedication, which was widely used historically has largely been superseded by short-acting hypnotics or no premedication.

ERAS Cardiac guidelines recommend management of patient and provider expectations, individualization of the dose and types of analgesics, consideration of the potential cardioprotective effects of opioids, and incorporating nonopiate approaches to pain management such as regional anesthesia.[14] Systematic reviews and meta-analyses have shown that the use of thoracic epidurals in patients undergoing coronary artery bypass graft surgery may reduce the risk of postoperative supraventricular arrhythmias and respiratory complications with no effects on the risk of mortality, myocardial infarction, or neurologic complications compared with general anesthesia alone.[35,36] Currently ERAS Cardiac has not recommended thoracic epidurals due to "additional studies needed to determine their true effectiveness and whether they should be applied to all patients or only a select few."[14]

Intraoperative ventilation strategies are important with high driving pressure resulting in more postoperative pulmonary complications.[37] The major components of protective ventilatory management include assist-controlled mechanical ventilation with low tidal volumes (6–8 mL/kg of predicted body weight) associated with higher positive end-expiratory pressure (PEEP), limitation of fraction of inspired oxygen (Fio_2), ventilation maintenance during cardiopulmonary bypass, and finally recruitment manoeuvers[38] before weaning from cardiopulmonary bypass in order to prevent atelectasis.[19] In protective ventilation during cardiac surgery, it is likely that a certain level of PEEP is necessary to reduce the risk of atelectasis due to low-volume ventilation. Several studies have demonstrated that PEEP reduces the incidence of postoperative atelectasis and improved respiratory function.[37,38] This may be problematic on occasions for surgical access when harvesting the internal thoracic artery, which may require disconnection from the ventilator and loss of PEEP.

Consensus on recruitment strategies for hypoxic cardiac surgical patients is still ongoing. Leme[39] suggested the use of an intensive (pressure-controlled ventilation plus positive end-expiratory pressure under a driving pressure of 15 cmH2O with PEEP fixed at 30 cmH2O for 3 cycles [60 seconds each]) alveolar recruitment strategy resulted in less severe pulmonary complications while in the hospital. These results have been criticized due to the study being unpowered and the possibility that the study patients already had underlying lung injury.[40] Recruitment at 40 cmH2O for 15 seconds performed before termination of cardiopulmonary bypass has been shown to be effective in reducing the incidence of atelectasis.[38,41] Overall, careful recruitment maneuvers with close monitoring of the hemodynamics of the patient may have benefit for some cardiac patients before chest closure.

Ventilation maintenance during bypass can prevent alveolar collapse, atelectasis, and therefore hypoxemia. There is some limited evidence that continuation of ventilation during cardiopulmonary bypass may be beneficial, although due to the technical limitations of this approach for surgery, it has not become mainstream practice.[38] Titration of Fio_2 is important, as high Fio_2 levels increase pulmonary oxygen toxicity, and hyperoxia can induce coronary vasospasm and a decrease in cerebral blood flow.[42] It is therefore recommended to limit Fio_2 in a range of values from 0.4 to 0.5[38] if clinically feasible.

On-table extubation postcardiac surgery in select patients requires standard enhanced recovery cardiac anesthesia techniques including the use of short-acting hypnotic drugs, reduced doses of opioids with a reduction of anesthesia at chest wiring with alveolar recruitment techniques, and initiation of spontaneous respiration. Patient selection is key for this group, and hemodynamic and respiratory function measures need to be matched intraoperatively and are a baseline for suitability. Studies have shown it to be safe in select patients,[16] but with no difference in length of ICU or hospital stay.[17] Postextubation ventilation was also a component of study protocols, where patients received noninvasive bilevel positive airway pressure ventilation via a face mask for 1 hour immediately after extubation at a pressure support of 10 to 15 cm H2O, PEEP of 5 cmH2O, and Fio_2 of 0.4. During the period of noninvasive ventilation, the pressure support was adapted to the patients' needs.[19]

POSTOPERATIVE

The application of enhanced recovery principles postoperatively including early intake of oral fluids and solids, ambulation, early mobilization, and removal of drains, all rely on discontinuation of ventilation and early extubation. Hence this is a pivotal point in the pathway. Most commonly patients are transferred to the ICU due to the low nurse-to-patient ratio and the physical concentration of skilled physicians, advanced practice providers, nurses, and therapists. It has been postulated that a mixed postsurgical ICU can act as a drag on time to extubation, as patients may be managed similar to long-term ventilated patients. Probst demonstrated the effectiveness of non-ICU

PACU-based care for earlier extubation and prompt discharge to a step-down unit without compromising patient safety.[19] It is essential to develop and implement efficient weaning and extubation protocols. The essence of such protocols is to define a phased approach to weaning of Fio_2, transfer from mandatory breathing to spontaneous supported breathing, cessation of sedation, and specific and nonrestrictive criteria for extubation. An effective protocol should have suggested progressive time points and be nurse-led.[43] Prompt physician or advanced practitioner consultation should be available when nurses have concerns about progressing through the protocol steps. If a patient fails any step of the protocol, then this step should be repeated after an appropriate intervention or pause. Contemporary postoperative ICU protocols usually include a protective ventilation strategy. The Probst study[19] specified a respiratory rate of 16 breaths per minute with a tidal volume of 8 mL/kg ideal body weight, although many contemporary protocols use lower volumes. It is important to ensure that any residual paralysis is reversed before the cessation of sedation at normothermia.

Finally delirium in the postoperative phase of cardiac surgical care can be a particularly problematic, affecting between 20% and 80% of patients.[44] Delirium increases complication rates, duration of mechanical ventilation, morbidity, and mortality and has been associated with long-term cognitive changes.[44,45] Published guidelines recommend screening patients routinely for known risk factors (frailty, genetics, lifestyle, underlying diseases, drug therapy, surgical trauma, anesthesia management [including the use of benzodiazepines], venous congestion, and pain management).[46] Nonpharmacologic strategies are recommended as first-line therapy such as early mobilization, pain management, minimization and targeted titration of sedation, avoidance of benzodiazepines and restraints, patient reorientation, cognitive stimulation, reduction of hearing and/or visual impairments, use of clocks/calendars, and promotion of normal sleep-wake circadian patterns.[14,46] Current guidelines recommend that nonbenzodiazepine sedatives (either propofol or dexmedetomidine) are preferable to benzodiazepine sedatives (either midazolam or lorazepam) because of improved short-term outcomes, such as ICU LOS, duration of mechanical ventilation, and delirium.[14,47]

SUMMARY

Early extubation has been demonstrated to be safe, effective, and feasible as part of an enhanced recovery protocol after cardiac surgery. It is an essential part of the pathway to enhance patient's recovery and mobilization. Continuous measurements of compliance with the extubation pathway is essential to ensure best practice and reduced variation.

DISCLOSURE

The authors have nothing to disclose.

REFERENCES

1. Ljungqvist O. The enhanced recovery after surgery in cardiac surgery revolution. JAMA Surg 2019;154(8):767.
2. Ljungqvist O, Scott M, Fearon KC. Enhanced recovery after surgery: a review. JAMA Surg 2017;152(3):292–8.
3. Engelman RM, Rousou JA, Flack JE 3rd, et al. Fast-track recovery of the coronary bypass patient. Ann Thorac Surg 1994;58(6):1742–6.

4. Myles PS, Daly DJ, Djaiani G, et al. A systematic review of the safety and effectiveness of fast-track cardiac anesthesia. Anesthesiology 2003;99(4):982–7.

5. Reyes A, Vega G, Blancas R, et al. Early vs conventional extubation after cardiac surgery with cardiopulmonary bypass. Chest 1997;112(1):193–201.

6. Engelman DT, Ben Ali W, Williams JB, et al. Guidelines for perioperative care in cardiac surgery: enhanced recovery after surgery society recommendations. JAMA Surg 2019;154(8):755–66.

7. Reddy SL, Grayson AD, Griffiths EM, et al. Logistic risk model for prolonged ventilation after adult cardiac surgery. Ann Thorac Surg 2007;84(2):528–36.

8. Wong WT, Lai VK, Chee YE, et al. Fast-track cardiac care for adult cardiac surgical patients. Cochrane Database Syst Rev 2016;9(9):CD003587.

9. Quasha AL, Loeber N, Feeley TW, et al. Postoperative respiratory care: a controlled trial of early and late extubation following coronary-artery bypass grafting. Anesthesiology 1980;52(2):135–41.

10. Mora CT, Dudek C, Torjman MC, et al. The effects of anesthetic technique on the hemodynamic response and recovery profile in coronary revascularization patients. Anesth Analg 1995;81(5):900–10.

11. Cheng DC, Karski J, Peniston C, et al. Early tracheal extubation after coronary artery bypass graft surgery reduces costs and improves resource usea prospective, randomized, controlled trial. Anesthesiology 1996;85(6):1300–10.

12. Zhu F, Lee A, Chee YE. Fast-track cardiac care for adult cardiac surgical patients. Cochrane Database Syst Rev 2012;(10):CD003587.

13. Wang W, Bagshaw SM, Norris CM, et al. Association between older age and outcome after cardiac surgery: a population-based cohort study. J Cardiothorac Surg 2014;9(1):177.

14. Gregory AJ, Grant MC, Manning MW, et al. Enhanced Recovery after Cardiac Surgery (ERAS cardiac) recommendations: an important first step-but there is much work to be done. J Cardiothorac Vasc Anesth 2020;34(1):39–47.

15. Marmelo F, Rocha V, Moreira-Gonçalves D. The impact of prehabilitation on postsurgical complications in patients undergoing non-urgent cardiovascular surgical intervention: systematic review and meta-analysis. Eur J Prev Cardiol 2018;25(4): 404–17.

16. Straka Z, Brucek P, Vanek T, et al. Routine immediate extubation for off-pump coronary artery bypass grafting without thoracic epidural analgesia. Ann Thorac Surg 2002;74(5):1544–7.

17. Montes FR, Sanchez SI, Giraldo JC, et al. The lack of benefit of tracheal extubation in the operating room after coronary artery bypass surgery. Anesth Analg 2000;91(4):776–80.

18. Ender J, Borger MA, Scholz M, et al. Cardiac surgery fast-track treatment in a postanesthetic care unitsix-month results of the leipzig fast-track concept. Anesthesiology 2008;109(1):61–6.

19. Probst S, Cech C, Haentschel D, et al. A specialized post anaesthetic care unit improves fast-track management in cardiac surgery: a prospective randomized trial. Crit Care 2014;18(4):468.

20. Vieillard-Baron A, Naeije R, Haddad F, et al. Diagnostic workup, etiologies and management of acute right ventricle failure : a state-of-the-art paper. Intensive Care Med 2018;44(6):774–90.

21. Hawkes CA, Dhileepan S, Foxcroft D. Early extubation for adult cardiac surgical patients. Cochrane Database Syst Rev 2003;(4):CD003587.

22. Blackwood B, Burns KE, Cardwell CR, et al. Protocolized versus non-protocolized weaning for reducing the duration of mechanical ventilation in critically ill adult patients. Cochrane Database Syst Rev 2010;(5):CD006904.

23. Kiessling AH, Huneke P, Reyher C, et al. Risk factor analysis for fast track protocol failure. J Cardiothorac Surg 2013;8(1):47.

24. Prabhakar S, Nanavati AJ. Enhanced recovery after surgery: if you are not implementing it, why not? Nutrition Issues in Gastroenterology, Series #151 2016;XL(4): 46–56.

25. Ramírez JM, Blasco JA, Roig JV, et al. Enhanced recovery in colorectal surgery: a multicentre study. BMC Surg 2011;11(1):9.

26. Fitch ZW, Debesa O, Ohkuma R, et al. A protocol-driven approach to early extubation after heart surgery. J Thorac Cardiovasc Surg 2014;147(4):1344–50.

27. van den Boom W, Schroeder RA, Manning MW, et al. Effect of A1C and glucose on postoperative mortality in noncardiac and cardiac surgeries. Diabetes Care 2018;41(4):782–8.

28. Stoppe C, Goetzenich A, Whitman G, et al. Role of nutrition support in adult cardiac surgery: a consensus statement from an international multidisciplinary expert group on nutrition in cardiac surgery. Crit Care 2017;21(1):131.

29. Arthur HM, Daniels C, McKelvie R, et al. Effect of a preoperative intervention on preoperative and postoperative outcomes in low-risk patients awaiting elective coronary artery bypass graft surgery: a randomized, controlled trial. Ann Intern Med 2000;133(4):253–62.

30. Bilku D, Dennison A, Hall T, et al. Role of preoperative carbohydrate loading: a systematic review. Ann R Coll Surg Engl 2014;96(1):15–22.

31. Breuer J-P, von Dossow V, von Heymann C, et al. Preoperative oral carbohydrate administration to ASA III-IV patients undergoing elective cardiac surgery. Anesth Analg 2006;103(5):1099–108.

32. Feguri GR, de Lima PRL, de Cerqueira Borges D, et al. Preoperative carbohydrate load and intraoperatively infused omega-3 polyunsaturated fatty acids positively impact nosocomial morbidity after coronary artery bypass grafting: a double-blind controlled randomized trial. Nutr J 2017;16(1):24.

33. Järvelä K, Maaranen P, Sisto T. Pre-operative oral carbohydrate treatment before coronary artery bypass surgery. Acta Anaesthesiol Scand 2008;52(6):793–7.

34. Greco M, Landoni G, Biondi-Zoccai G, et al. Remifentanil in cardiac surgery: a meta-analysis of randomized controlled trials. J Cardiothorac Vasc Anesth 2012;26(1):110–6.

35. Svircevic V, Passier MM, Nierich AP, et al. Epidural analgesia for cardiac surgery. Cochrane Database Syst Rev 2013;(6):CD006715.

36. Zhang S, Wu X, Guo H, et al. Thoracic epidural anesthesia improves outcomes in patients undergoing cardiac surgery: meta-analysis of randomized controlled trials. Eur J Med Res 2015;20(1):25.

37. Neto AS, Hemmes SN, Barbas CS, et al. Association between driving pressure and development of postoperative pulmonary complications in patients undergoing mechanical ventilation for general anaesthesia: a meta-analysis of individual patient data. Lancet Respir Med 2016;4(4):272–80.

38. Lellouche F, Delorme M, Bussieres J, et al. Perioperative ventilatory strategies in cardiac surgery. Best Pract Res Clin Anaesthesiol 2015;29(3):381–95.

39. Leme AC, Hajjar LA, Volpe MS, et al. Effect of intensive vs moderate alveolar recruitment strategies added to lung-protective ventilation on postoperative pulmonary complications: a randomized clinical trial. JAMA 2017;317(14):1422–32.

40. Patel JJ, Pfeifer K. Alveolar recruitment strategies after cardiac surgery. JAMA 2017;318(7):667–8.

41. Minkovich L, Djaiani G, Katznelson R, et al. Effects of alveolar recruitment on arterial oxygenation in patients after cardiac surgery: a prospective, randomized, controlled clinical trial. J Cardiothorac Vasc Anesth 2007;21(3):375–8.

42. McNulty PH, King N, Scott S, et al. Effects of supplemental oxygen administration on coronary blood flow in patients undergoing cardiac catheterization. Am J Physiol Heart Circ Physiol 2005;288(3):H1057–62.

43. Serena G, Corredor C, Fletcher N, et al. Implementation of a nurse-led protocol for early extubation after cardiac surgery: a pilot study. World J Crit Care Med 2019;8(3):28–35.

44. Ely EW, Shintani A, Truman B, et al. Delirium as a predictor of mortality in mechanically ventilated patients in the intensive care unit. JAMA 2004;291(14):1753–62.

45. Nomura Y, Nakano M, Bush B, et al. Observational study examining the association of baseline frailty and postcardiac surgery delirium and cognitive change. Anesth Analg 2019;129(2):507–14.

46. Baron R, Binder A, Biniek R, et al. Evidence and consensus based guideline for the management of delirium, analgesia, and sedation in intensive care medicine. Revision 2015 (DAS-Guideline 2015)–short version. GMS Med Sci 2015;13. https://doi.org/10.3205/000223.

47. Devlin JW, Skrobik Y, Gélinas C, et al. Executive summary: clinical practice guidelines for the prevention and management of pain, agitation/sedation, delirium, immobility, and sleep disruption in adult patients in the ICU. Crit Care Med 2018;46(9):1532–48.

48. Berry PD, Thomas SD, Mahon SP, et al. Myocardial ischaemia after coronary artery bypass grafting: early vs late extubation. Br J Anaesth 1998;80(1):20–5.

49. Engoren MC, Kraras C, Garzia F. Propofol-based versus fentanyl-isoflurane—Based anesthesia for cardiac surgery. J Cardiothorac Vasc Anesth 1998;12(2):177–81.

50. Zhu F, Gomersall CD, Ng SK, et al. A randomized controlled trial of adaptive support ventilation mode to wean patients after fast-track cardiac valvular surgery. Anesthesiology 2015;122(4):832–40.

51. Pettersson PH, Settergren G, Öwall A. Similar pain scores after early and late extubation in heart surgery with cardiopulmonary bypass. J Cardiothorac Vasc Anesth 2004;18(1):64–7.

52. Michalopoulos A, Nikolaides A, Antzaka C, et al. Change in anaesthesia practice and postoperative sedation shortens ICU and hospital length of stay following coronary artery bypass surgery. Respir Med 1998;92(8):1066–70.

53. Nicholson DJ, Kowalski SE, Hamilton GA, et al. Postoperative pulmonary function in coronary artery bypass graft surgery patients undergoing early tracheal extubation: a comparison between short-term mechanical ventilation and early extubation. J Cardiothorac Vasc Anesth 2002;16(1):27–31.

54. Salah M, Hosny H, Salah M, et al. Impact of immediate versus delayed tracheal extubation on length of ICU stay of cardiac surgical patients, a randomized trial. Heart Lung Vessel 2015;7(4):311.

55. Simeone F, Biagioli B, Scolletta S, et al. Optimization of mechanical ventilation support following cardiac surgery. J Cardiovasc Surg 2002;43(5):633–42.

56. Gruber P, Gomersall C, Leung P, et al. A randomized control trial comparing adaptive support ventilation with pressure-regulated volume control ventilation in weaning patients after cardiac surgery. Crit Care 2008;12(Suppl 2):P326.

Delirium Prevention in Postcardiac Surgical Critical Care

Rohan Sanjanwala, MD, MPH[a], Christian Stoppe, MD[b,c],
Ali Khoynezhad, MD, PhD, FHRS[d], Aileen Hill, MD[b],
Daniel T. Engelman, MD[e], Rakesh C. Arora, MD, PhD[a,f,*]

KEYWORDS

- Delirium • Enhanced recovery • Cardiac surgery • Intensive care unit
- Perioperative care

KEY POINTS

- Delirium is common after cardiac surgery, particularly in vulnerable older adults.
- The occurence of postoperative delirium is associated with worse short (in-hospital) and longer-term outcomes.
- Identifying patients who may be at risk prior to surgery is an important component of delirium prevention and management.
- The use of a systematic delirium screening tool, that encompasses the spectrum of delirium presentation should is an important component of an enhancing recovery protocol. Screening and identifying delirium at the earliest timepoint is essential to alert the perioperative team to search for the underlying etiology.
- Delirium management requires engagement of the entire interdisciplinary team.

INTRODUCTION

Delirium is an acute brain dysfunction, characterized by a transient, fluctuating course of inattention, impaired consciousness, and disordered cognition.[1] The syndrome can be difficult to diagnose and even more challenging to manage once it occurs given its

[a] Cardiac Sciences Program, St. Boniface Hospital, CR3015-369 Tache Avenue, Winnipeg, Manitoba R2H 2A6, Canada; [b] Department of Intensive Care Medicine, 3CARE—Cardiovascular Critical Care & Anesthesia Evaluation and Research, University Hospital RWTH Aachen, Pauwelsstraße 30, Aachen D-52074, Germany; [c] Department of Anesthesiology, Intensive Care Medicine and Pain Therapy, University Hospital Würzburg, Würzburg, Germany; [d] Department of Cardiothoracic Surgery, MemorialCare Long Beach Medical Center, 2801 Atlantic Avenue, Long Beach, CA 90806, USA; [e] Heart and Vascular Program, Baystate Health and University of Massachusetts Medical School–Baystate, 759 Chestnut Street, Springfield, MA 01199, USA; [f] Department of Surgery, Max Rady College of Medicine, University of Manitoba, Winnipeg, Manitoba, Canada
* Corresponding author. I.H. Asper Clinical Research Institute – St. Boniface Hospital, CR3015-369 Tache Avenue, Winnipeg, Manitoba R2H 2A6, Canada.
E-mail address: rakeshcarora@gmail.com

Crit Care Clin 36 (2020) 675–690
https://doi.org/10.1016/j.ccc.2020.06.001
criticalcare.theclinics.com
0749-0704/20/© 2020 Elsevier Inc. All rights reserved.

multifactorial cause and often subtle clinical presentation.[2] Disturbances of motor behavior are common presenting features of delirium representing clinically meaningful subtypes categorized as either hypoactive, hyperactive, or an overlap of both (ie, mixed). Patients with hyperactive delirium typically demonstrate features of restlessness and agitation and often experience hallucinations and delusions.[3] In contrast, patients with hypoactive delirium demonstrate features of lethargy, reduced motor activity, sluggishness, and abnormal drowsiness, which often remain unrecognized, taking a more insidious clinical course.[3]

There are numerous risk factors for delirium, predisposing individuals to and precipitating the syndrome. Delirium may resolve during hospitalization. However, patients experiencing delirium are at an increased risk of adverse events in both the short and the long term.[4] The goals of this review are to provide an overview of the key determinants of delirium and of the potential barriers to effective prevention and management in cardiac surgery patients. A practical approach for addressing new postoperative delirium involves identification of patient risk factors and adoption of strategies to prevent, and in lieu of prevention, to efficiently manage delirium to promote early enhanced recovery following cardiac surgery.[5]

HOW COMMON IS DELIRIUM AMONG POSTCARDIAC SURGERY PATIENTS?

There is a high prevalence of postoperative delirium because increasingly vulnerable patients (older, with advanced disease and multiple co-morbidities) are being offered cardiac surgery.[6] Although delirium is a common complication following cardiac surgery, there is wide discrepancy in reported incidence and prevalence, ranging from 8% to greater than 50% depending on the methodology of identification. In particular, the patients experiencing hypoactive delirium (accounting for >50% cases of delirium in a cardiac surgery intensive care unit [CS-ICU])[7,8] are often dismissed as "being sleepy" rather than being recognized as having an acute change in cognition. Furthermore, differing criteria for delirium diagnosis and screening tools, such as the frequency of screening, and administrator competency also influence delirium detection rates. However, when using a systematic screening tool, most contemporary estimates are that at least 1 in 5 patients following cardiac surgery experiences delirium.[8–11]

WHO GETS DELIRIOUS, AND WHY DOES IT HAPPEN AFTER CARDIAC SURGERY? THE RISK FACTORS OF DELIRIUM

Several factors, such as patients' baseline vulnerability (ie, frailty, hypertension, smoking, age, alcohol abuse, cognitive impairment), the complexity and duration of cardiac surgery, and severity of ICU stressors (eg, sedation and analgesia, duration of mechanical ventilation, ICU length of stay) strongly influence the incidence and risk of postcardiac surgery delirium[12] (**Fig. 1**). The assessment of risk, therefore, is an important initial step in the prevention of delirium.[8,13,14]

Preoperative Risk Factors: The Baseline Vulnerability

Advanced age is the most consistently observed predictor of delirium among cardiac surgery patients.[15] A metaanalysis of studies evaluating patients undergoing cardiac surgery demonstrated that every 1-year increase in age was associated with an 8% increase in the odds of a patient experiencing delirium.[16] Importantly, this risk is 3-fold higher for patients who are 65 years of age or older.[16–18] Furthermore, there is a sex difference in the risk of developing postoperative delirium, with multiple studies reporting that men are at increased risk.[12,19–23] In addition to these patient factors,

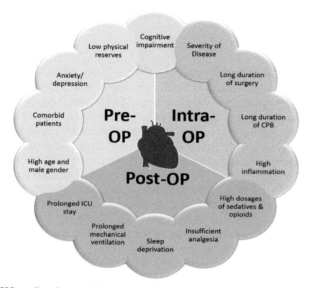

CPB cardiopulmonary bypass, Pre-Op preoperative, Intra-op intraoperative, Post-op postoperative.

Fig. 1. Risk factors for the development of delirium after cardiac surgery. Intra-OP, intraoperative; Post-OP, postoperative; Pre-OP, preoperative.

higher comorbid disease burden and severity of illness have both been independently associated with an increase in the risk of developing delirium following cardiac surgery.[12,20,24,25]

Frailty has been shown to increase the risk of delirium in the ICU by 3- to 8-fold among patients who underwent elective cardiac surgery.[8,11] Frailty encompasses the presence of low physiologic (ie, functional) and mental (both mood and cognitive) reserves that occur more commonly, although not exclusively, in older adult patients. In a study by Rudolph and colleagues,[26] standard testing of memory and executive functions was administered preoperatively to patients undergoing coronary artery bypass grafting (CABG) surgery. Poor preoperative performance on the neuropsychological battery (consisting of 5 executive function tests and 1 memory test) was independently associated with a greater risk of developing delirium after CABG.[26]

Behavioral factors, such as alcohol use and/or dependence and smoking, are associated with an increase in risk of postoperative delirium.[13,14] However, the association is not consistent across different studies and requires further validation. Last, neuropsychiatric disorders, including depression, anxiety, as well as the use of psychoactive medications, including antipsychotics and benzodiazepines (BZD), are associated with increased risk of postoperative delirium.[27,28]

Intraoperative Risk Factors

Intraoperative stressor events have been associated with an increased risk of postoperative delirium in the CS-ICU.[13] Inflammation and oxidative stress resulting from myocardial ischemia/reperfusion injury and emergency or urgent surgery are important precipitating factors.[4,19,29,30] In addition, intraaortic balloon pump support, valve surgery, and prolonged cardiopulmonary bypass (CPB) may also be associated with an increase in the risk of delirium; however, it is not clear if this is secondary to the use of CPB in and of itself or a surrogate for the severity of illness/cardiac disease.[24,31,32] Likewise, it is unclear whether off-pump coronary bypass is protective or carries equivalent risk.[33,34]

Postoperative Risk Factors

In 2018, the Society of Critical Care Medicine (SCCM) provided a detailed overview of ICU care–related factors that can contribute to the occurrence of new postoperative delirium.[35] Although a detailed review is beyond the scope of this review, management of postoperative pain and the appropriate selection of analgesia are important considerations.[35] The postoperative patients in the CS-ICU may experience pain at rest and during standard care procedures. A study evaluating pain among CABG patients using a self-reported pain scale demonstrated that severe pain at rest was reported in 49% of patients, severe pain when coughing in 78% of patients, and severe pain during movement in 62% of patients.[36] The severity and duration of postoperative pain, especially pain at rest, are reported to be a significant factor associated with an increase in the risk of delirium.[37–39] Although undertreatment of pain increases the risk of delirium, it is important to recognize that the excessive use of drugs used to alleviate pain, particularly opioids, is associated with higher risk of delirium.[37]

BZD agents are sedatives that are commonly used in the CS-ICU to alleviate the anxiety and discomfort associated with cardiac surgery and postoperative care (including mechanical ventilation, intubation, suction, chest tubes, and so forth). However, higher doses of BZD have been associated with increased risk of delirium.[40,41] Furthermore, BZD use is also associated with an increase in the duration of mechanical ventilation and ICU stay.[42] Prolonged mechanical ventilation (>24 hours) and duration of ICU stay, independently and in conjunction with BZD use, further compound the risk of delirium among cardiac surgery patients.[9] Last, sleep disturbances (especially sleep deprivation) are an important factor adding to the multitude of perioperative stressors that precipitate the risk of delirium.[4,29,40]

WHY DOES IT MATTER? THE SHORT- AND LONG-TERM IMPACT OF THE OCCURRENCE OF POSTOPERATIVE DELIRIUM FOLLOWING CARDIAC SURGERY

Delirium is recognized to be associated with a higher probability of adverse in-hospital and postdischarge outcomes, including death, morbidity, falls, cognitive decline, and loss of functional independence.[43–45] In addition, patients experiencing delirium are typically exposed to additional hospitalization-related stressors, including prolonged ICU stay, prolonged immobility, and higher risk of infections, resulting in an increase in the level of delirium, a higher deterioration in physiologic function, and decreased health-related quality of life following hospital discharge.[46,47]

The Impact of Delirium from the Patients' and Family Caregivers' Perspective

Postoperative delirium is now recognized to have long-term sequelae that extend beyond the patients' in-hospital stay. As such, patients experiencing delirium have an increased risk of death after discharge from the hospital.[48,49] A study evaluating patients undergoing a CABG procedure demonstrated an association between postoperative delirium and increased mortality at 6 months.[50] Other investigators have observed a sustained association with mortality for up to 10 years following hospital discharge.[10,51]

Delirium has also been independently associated with an increased risk of a decline in activities of daily living (ADL) when compared with a patient's prehospitalization status.[52–56] In a study of patients undergoing cardiac surgery, Rudolph and colleagues[8] observed postoperative delirium was associated with a functional decline at 1 and

12 months, independent of the patient's baseline status. In addition, postoperative delirium is associated with a significant decline in cognitive function. When examining cognitive function (using the Mini Mental Status examination), a prolonged episode of postoperative delirium has been associated with a decline in cognitive function at 1 year after cardiac surgery.[7,57] In addition, some patients never achieve baseline (ie, prehospitalization) status.[56] The persistent functional and cognitive impairment impedes ADL, resulting in a lower quality of life after hospital discharge.[44] Collectively, the neuropsychological, functional, and cognitive impairment associated with an ICU stay persisting following hospital discharge is termed the postintensive care unit syndrome (PICS).[58,59] Patients experiencing delirium are at increased risk of PICS following hospital discharge.[52,59,60]

Patients' experiences of delirium are diverse, with some patients having reported no memory of the event, and others having reported vivid recollection of the delirium. Fear and visual hallucinations are the most commonly recalled symptoms.[61] In addition, after hospital discharge, some patients experience anxiety, helplessness, disorientation, and delusions (change in reality, immersion in dramatic emotional scenes), which may significantly impact postoperative recovery.[56,62–64] There is a higher risk of long-term neuropsychological sequelae, such as depression, anxiety, and posttraumatic stress disorders, among patients experiencing delirium.[65,66] Koster and colleagues[56] evaluated the memories of delirium events among cardiac surgery patients at 1 year. They reported that patients described delirium as a fearful and an embarrassing event. Patients who remembered multiple traumatic episodes during their stay in the ICU following cardiac surgery were more likely to develop posttraumatic stress disorder–like symptoms.

More recently, it has been recognized that delirium-associated distress is also felt by family caregivers. The family caregiver's observations of patient's delirium symptoms (such as personality changes, inability to recognize family members), fear of such changes being permanent, as well as feelings of loss of control regarding appropriate care and safety, result in significant burden and stress when caring for delirious patients.[67] The family caregivers have reported feeling anxiety, fear, and depression, resulting in poor health and financial insecurities.[68,69] Additional studies are required, especially among cardiac surgery patients, to define a clear understanding and impact of delirium on the patients' family caregivers.

IDENTIFYING DELIRIUM IN CARDIAC SURGERY INTENSIVE CARE UNIT PATIENTS

The implementation and routine use of a validated delirium assessment tool are the key to prompt delirium detection in the immediate postoperative period. Numerous delirium screening tools can be applied based on the clinical setting.[29] Alertness or arousal should first be evaluated using a validated sedation-agitation scale, such as Richmond Agitation-Sedation Scale (RASS),[70] before assessing cognition for delirium. The Confusion Assessment Method for ICU and the Intensive Care Delirium Screening Checklist[71] are examples of commonly used delirium screening tools used in the ICU setting. In patients who are arousable to voice (RASS score ≥ 3; more alert), the systematic delirium screening tools have been reported to have 95% sensitivity and 89% specificity compared with a gold-standard psychiatric assessment.[72]

With adequate education and training, commonly perceived barriers, including intubated patients and screening tool complexity, can be addressed, allowing improved delirium detection. In a multicenter qualitative improvement initiative targeted toward improving delirium screening and detection, a multifaceted approach to educate nursing staff was implemented. Through education and teaching with monthly staff meetings and one-on-one teaching with experts, compliance of more than 84% was achieved. This approach facilitated efficient utilization of a delirium screening tool with increased frequency of assessment.[73]

IT TAKES A TEAM! A MULTICOMPONENT APPROACH TO DELIRIUM MANAGEMENT

A multicomponent approach, targeting risk factors of delirium, is the most effective and consistent strategy for prevention of delirium.[74–78] Multiple studies have demonstrated its effectiveness in reducing the incidence of delirium and improvement in other clinical outcomes, including preventing falls, reducing length of stay, and hospital readmissions.[79] Several research studies and practice guidelines have encouraged implementation strategies to prevent delirium in cardiac and noncardiac surgical as well as medical ICU patients.[80] The most widely disseminated approaches include the ICU liberation bundle,[81] the Hospital Elder Life Program,[74] and others,[82,83] which are multicomponent intervention strategies with demonstrated effectiveness in preventing delirium and functional decline.[84,85] The interventions included are described in **Box 1**. Finally, the use of a dedicated clinical pathway that incorporates a multicomponent strategy is essential to facilitate early enhanced recovery following cardiac surgery.

For the cardiac surgery patient, establishing baseline preoperative vulnerability through appropriate screening (eg, a risk assessment tool[86]) for patient risk factors for delirium should be initiated in the preoperative setting if possible and should involve an assessment of cognition (eg, the Mini mental status examination,[87] Montreal Cognitive Assessment,[88] or Mini-Cog[89]), assessment of baseline frailty (using

---

Box 1
Delirium prevention intervention

1. Early mobilization
   - Prompt removal of mechanical ventilation, drips, and other immobilizing equipment
   - Get out of bed and early physiotherapy initiation

2. Reorientation
   - Orient to time, place, person; frequent reorientation to reason for hospitalization
   - Include family caregivers

3. Sleep hygiene promotion
   - Increase daytime activities; maintain sleep-wake cycle
   - Avoid caffeine and sleep medications
   - Provide sleep aids, for example, ear plugs, sleeping masks

4. Meet daily requirements for hydration and macronutrients
   - Early recognition of dehydration; encourage greater than 1.2 L/d of fluid intake
   - Early initiation of oral feeds and maintanance of protein caloric daily requirements

5. Provide visual and hearing adaptations
   - Provide glasses, lenses
   - Provide portable amplifying devices

6. Therapeutic activities
   - Cognitive stimulation activities, such as availing language-friendly reading materials: newspapers, magazines

7. Reduce use and dosage of "deliriogenic" medication
   - Reduce the use of deliriogenic medications, such as BZD, opioids, anticholinergics
   - Simultaneously ensure adequate pain management

From Inouye SK, Bogardus ST, Baker DI, et al. The Hospital Elder Life Program: a model of care to prevent cognitive and functional decline in older hospitalized patients. Hospital Elder Life Program. J Am Geriatr Soc. 2000;48(12):1697–706; with permission.

screening tools such as the Clinical Frailty Scale or other more comprehensive tools),[90] mood disorders (anxiety, neuropsychiatric impairment such as depression), and assessment of hazardous substance or alcohol abuse. In addition, preoperative delineation of a strategy for postoperative pain management and setting goals for postoperative mobilization with the patient and caregivers set the stage for enhanced postoperative recovery.

Delirium Management

The main aspects of managing delirium include preventing delirium, minimizing the duration, and managing the severity of delirium in the postoperative period.[91] Delirium can be addressed with nonpharmacologic and pharmacologic interventions.

Analgesia and Sedation in the Postoperative Cardiac Surgery Patient

An optimal use of analgesia is necessary to achieve a balance between adequate pain control and excessive use of analgesic medications, to avoid precipitating the risk of delirium. This balance can be achieved through targeting pain control to the lowest effective dose using a validated pain scale, that is, Visual Analogue Scale[92] for verbal or Critical Care Pain Observation Tool or Behavioral Pain Scale[93] for nonverbal patients. In addition, applying a multimodal opioid-sparing approach (including regional analgesia nerve blocks) to optimize pain management and avoiding excess use of sedating or opioid drugs can improve patient comfort and potentially reduce the risk of postcardiac surgery delirium.

A relatively small percentage of patients with a prolonged ICU stay following cardiac surgery may require prolonged sedation.[94,95] In most other cases, the goal is for the patient to be calm and cooperative and to reduce postprocedural discomfort.[96,97] Data from large trials, such as the SEDCOM,[98] MENDS,[99] and DEXCOM[100] studies, demonstrated that using dexmedetomidine as a sedative agent was associated with less delirium compared with other agents, including BZDs, propofol, and opiates. However, although seminal, these studies were conducted in noncardiac surgical settings.[101–103]

Several smaller studies have shown an association between the use of dexmedetomidine for sedation and reduced incidence, onset, and duration of delirium in postcardiac surgery patients compared with the use of propofol sedation.[96,100,104] A recent randomized trial involving 121 cardiac surgery patients studied dexmedetomidine and intravenous acetaminophen for the prevention of postoperative delirium following cardiac surgery (DEXACET study).[105] The study compared sedation with dexmedetomidine versus propofol with and without the concurrent use of acetaminophen. The investigators observed a reduction in the occurrence of postoperative delirium following cardiac surgery with dexmedetomidine.[106] In agreement with these findings, the SCCM have recommended the use of non-BZDs, such as dexmedetomidine and propofol, for sedation in mechanically ventilated cardiac surgery patients with a goal to reduce the time of mechanical ventilation, facilitate mobilization, and reduce the risk of delirium.[35] Furthermore, a more recent concept, eCASH, providing a personalized, patient-centered approach to sedation, has been proposed to reduce the risk of delirium.[107]

Does an "Ounce of Prevention" Work?

Numerous psychopharmacologic agents have been proposed for the management of delirium.[108,109] Randomized studies were reviewed for haloperidol,[103,110] atypical antipsychoticziprasidone,[110] olanzapine,[111,112] and the use of a hydroxy-methylglutaryl-coenzyme A reductase (HMG-CoA reductase) inhibitor (ie, statins).[113] At this time, there is no evidence demonstrating the benefits of using these agents to reduce the duration of delirium, mechanical ventilation, length of ICU stay, and mortality. The lack of apparent effectiveness of any one agent is likely due to the multifactorial nature of delirium and underlying systemic end-organ dysfunction, likely making the use of a single pharmacologic agent or intervention ineffective in reducing the incidence of delirium or modifying delirium-related clinical outcomes.[114,115]

Similarly for the cardiac surgery patient, systematic review and metaanalysis of 13 randomized controlled trials did not demonstrate a reduction in postoperative delirium nor a reduction in mortality or ICU or hospital length of stay with the use of prophylactic neuroactive medications, such as rivastigmine or risperidone, following cardiac surgery.[116–118] As such, the 2018 SCCM Pain, Agitation, Delirium, Immobility, and Sleep disturbance Guidelines have recommended against the routine use of medications (such as haloperidol, dexmedetomidine, statins, or ketamine)[35,119–121] for either the prevention or the treatment of new delirium. There is an exception for the management of patients who experience significant distress secondary to symptoms of delirium or may be physically harmful to themselves or others.

Nonpharmacologic Delirium Management

The nonpharmacologic management of delirium in the CS-ICU primarily focuses on providing perioperative orientation and early mobilization after surgery. A multicomponent reorientation approach should be used, including visual cues or daily reminders of time, place, and reason for hospitalization. Sleep preservation should be facilitated through reduced ICU-related disturbances (eg, noise, high-intensity lighting, avoiding patient care during night hours). The early use of sensory assistive devices (hearing aids, eyeglasses) and early mobilization (both passive and active) may also reduce the incidence and duration of delirium.[122,123]

Extensive adaptation and sustainability of such approaches, however, require considerable resource commitment, effective delirium champions, and most importantly, long-term multidisciplinary support. Furthermore, the effectiveness and usability of these multicomponent approaches will require validation in different health care systems as well as in the cardiac surgical setting to ensure real-world effectiveness.

CALL FOR ACTION/FUTURE WORK

Health care professionals caring for cardiac surgical patients should perform a preoperative assessment of delirium risk factors. This preoperative assessment should include assessments of frailty, baseline assessment of cognition, sensory defects (ie, poor vision or hearing), mood disorders, severe illness, and presence of infection. However, despite extensive research, there is a further need to elucidate the potential mechanisms resulting in delirium and large multicenter studies to confirm perioperative modifiable risk factors that are associated with postoperative delirium. Furthermore, targeting modifiable risk factors through interventions, such as providing prehabilitation (nutrition, exercise, and mental health optimization strategies) to decrease patient vulnerability in the preoperative window, or considering minimizing surgery-related inflammatory responses (through minimally invasive cardiac surgical approaches), requires additional study.

SUMMARY

Delirium is the most common neurologic complication following cardiac surgery. Identification of patient and care factors as well as the use of a systematic delirium screening approach is essential to the care of the contemporary cardiac surgery patient. Importantly, although the acute symptoms of delirium may resolve during the hospital stay, patients who develop delirium are at a significantly higher risk of adverse events following hospital discharge that directly affects ADL and quality of life. Therefore, heath care provider teams need to develop a patient-centered delirium prevention/management plan. Early diagnosis of delirium will facilitate implementing effective management strategies that may reduce the duration of delirium as well as mitigate the associated adverse short- and long-term outcomes. Nonetheless, additional inquiry is necessary to elucidate complete pathogenesis, risk factors, and the impact of delirium for cardiac surgery patients.

FUNDING AND CONFLICTS OF INTEREST

The authors have not received any funding for this article. R.C. Arora has received an unrestricted educational grant from Pfizer Canada Inc and has received honoraria from Abbott Nutrition and Edwards Lifesciences that are unrelated to the current article. D.T. Engelman consults for Edwards Lifesciences.

REFERENCES

1. Association AP. Diagnostic and statistical manual of mental disorders (DSM-5®). American Psychiatric Pub; 2013.
2. Brown CH. Delirium in the cardiac surgical ICU. Curr Opin Anaesthesiol 2014; 27(2):117–22. Available at: http://proxycheck.lib.umanitoba.ca/libraries/online/proxy.php?http://ovidsp.ovid.com/ovidweb.cgi?T=JS&CSC=Y&NEWS=N&PAGE=fulltext&D=medl&AN=24514034.
3. Lipowski ZJ. Transient cognitive disorders (delirium, acute confusional states) in the elderly. Am J Psychiatry 1983;140(11):1426–36.
4. Hayhurst CJ, Pandharipande PP, Hughes CG. Intensive care unit delirium: a review of diagnosis, prevention, and treatment. Anesthesiology 2016;125(6): 1229–41.
5. Engelman DT, Ben Ali W, Williams JB, et al. Guidelines for perioperative care in cardiac surgery: enhanced recovery after surgery society recommendations. JAMA Surg 2019;154(8):755–66.
6. Goldfarb M, Bendayan M, Rudski LG, et al. Cost of cardiac surgery in frail compared with nonfrail older adults. Can J Cardiol 2017;33(8):1020–6.
7. Saczynski JS, Marcantonio ER, Quach L, et al. Cognitive trajectories after postoperative delirium. N Engl J Med 2012;367(1):30–9.
8. Rudolph JL, Inouye SK, Jones RN, et al. Delirium: an independent predictor of functional decline after cardiac surgery. J Am Geriatr Soc 2010;58(4):643–9.
9. Pandharipande PP. Delirium in the cardiovascular ICU: exploring modifiable risk factors (vol 41, pg 405, 2013). Crit Care Med 2013;41(4):E41.
10. Gottesman RF, Grega MA, Bailey MM, et al. Delirium after coronary artery bypass graft surgery and late mortality. Ann Neurol 2010;67(3):338–44.
11. Brown CH 4th, Max L, Laflam A, et al. The association between preoperative frailty and postoperative delirium after cardiac surgery. Anesth Analg 2016; 123(2):430–5.
12. Norkiene I, Ringaitiene D, Misiuriene I, et al. Incidence and precipitating factors of delirium after coronary artery bypass grafting. Scand Cardiovasc J 2007; 41(3):180–5.
13. Zaal IJ, Devlin JW, Peelen LM, et al. A systematic review of risk factors for delirium in the ICU. Crit Care Med 2015;43(1):40–7.

14. Huai J, Ye X. A meta-analysis of critically ill patients reveals several potential risk factors for delirium. Gen Hosp Psychiatry 2014;36(5):488–96.
15. Kotfis K, Szylinska A, Listewnik M, et al. Early delirium after cardiac surgery: an analysis of incidence and risk factors in elderly (≥65 years) and very elderly (≥80 years) patients. Clin Interv Aging 2018;13:1061–70. Available at: http://proxycheck.lib.umanitoba.ca/libraries/online/proxy.php?http://ovidsp.ovid.com/ovidweb.cgi?T=JS&CSC=Y&NEWS=N&PAGE=fulltext&D=medl&AN= 29881262 https://primo-pmtna01.hosted.exlibrisgroup.com/primo-explore/openurl?institution=UMB&vid=umb_services_p.
16. Lin Y, Chen J, Wang Z. Meta-analysis of factors which influence delirium following cardiac surgery. J Card Surg 2012;27(4):481–92.
17. Bohner H, Hummel TC, Habel U, et al. Predicting delirium after vascular surgery: a model based on pre- and intraoperative data. Ann Surg 2003;238(1):149–56.
18. Bryson GL, Wyand A, Wozny D, et al. A prospective cohort study evaluating associations among delirium, postoperative cognitive dysfunction, and apolipoprotein E genotype following open aortic repair. Can J Anaesth 2011;58(3): 246–55.
19. Afonso A, Scurlock C, Reich D, et al. Predictive model for postoperative delirium in cardiac surgical patients. Semin Cardiothorac Vasc Anesth 2010;14(3):212–7.
20. Oldroyd C, Scholz AFM, Hinchliffe RJ, et al. A systematic review and meta-analysis of factors for delirium in vascular surgical patients. J Vasc Surg 2017; 66(4):1269–79.e9.
21. Chang Y-L, Tsai Y, Lin P, et al. Prevalence and risk factors for postoperative delirium in a cardiovascular intensive care unit. Am J Crit Care 2008;17(6): 567–75.
22. Burkhart CS, Dell-Kuster S, Gamberini M, et al. Modifiable and nonmodifiable risk factors for postoperative delirium after cardiac surgery with cardiopulmonary bypass. J Cardiothorac Vasc Anesth 2010;24(4):555–9.
23. Andrejaitiene J, Sirvinskas E. Early post-cardiac surgery delirium risk factors. Perfusion 2012;27(2):105–12.
24. Bakker RC, Osse RJ, Tulen JHM, et al. Preoperative and operative predictors of delirium after cardiac surgery in elderly patients. Eur J Cardiothorac Surg 2011; 41(3):544–9.
25. Guenther U, Theuerkauf N, Frommann I, et al. Predisposing and precipitating factors of delirium after cardiac surgery: a prospective observational cohort study. Ann Surg 2013;257(6):1160–7.
26. Rudolph JL, Jones RN, Grande LJ, et al. Impaired executive function is associated with delirium after coronary artery bypass graft surgery. J Am Geriatr Soc 2006;54(6):937–41.
27. Kim H, Chung S, Joo YH, et al. The major risk factors for delirium in a clinical setting. Neuropsychiatr Dis Treat 2016;12:1787–93. Available at: https://www.ncbi.nlm.nih.gov/pubmed/27499625.
28. Al-Qadheeb NS, O'Connor HH, White AC, et al. Antipsychotic prescribing patterns, and the factors and outcomes associated with their use, among patients requiring prolonged mechanical ventilation in the long-term acute care hospital setting. Ann Pharmacother 2013;47(2):181–8.
29. Inouye SK, Westendorp RGJ, Saczynski JS. Delirium in elderly people. Lancet 2014;383(9920):911–22.
30. Arenson BG, Macdonald L a, Grocott HP, et al. Effect of intensive care unit environment on in-hospital delirium after cardiac surgery. J Thorac Cardiovasc Surg 2013;146:172–8.

31. Osse RJ, Fekkes D, Tulen JHM, et al. High preoperative plasma neopterin predicts delirium after cardiac surgery in older adults. J Am Geriatr Soc 2012;60(4): 661–8.
32. Rolfson DB, McElhaney JE, Rockwood K, et al. Incidence and risk factors for delirium and other adverse outcomes in older adults after coronary artery bypass graft surgery. Can J Cardiol 1999;15(7):771–6.
33. Bucerius J, Gummert JF, Borger MA, et al. Predictors of delirium after cardiac surgery delirium: effect of beating-heart (off-pump) surgery. J Thorac Cardiovasc Surg 2004;127(1):57–64.
34. Liu Y-H, Wang D-X, Li L-H, et al. The effects of cardiopulmonary bypass on the number of cerebral microemboli and the incidence of cognitive dysfunction after coronary artery bypass graft surgery. Anesth Analg 2009;109(4):1013–22.
35. Devlin JW, Skrobik Y, Gelinas C, et al. Clinical practice guidelines for the prevention and management of pain, agitation/sedation, delirium, immobility, and sleep disruption in adult patients in the ICU. Crit Care Med 2018;46(9):e825–73.
36. Milgrom LB, Brooks JA, Qi R, et al. Pain levels experienced with activities after cardiac surgery. Am J Crit Care 2004;13(2):116–25.
37. Vaurio LE, Sands LP, Wang Y, et al. Postoperative delirium: the importance of pain and pain management. Anesth Analg 2006;102(4):1267–73.
38. Kumar AK, Jayant A, Arya VK, et al. Delirium after cardiac surgery: a pilot study from a single tertiary referral center. Ann Card Anaesth 2017;20(1):76–82. Available at: https://www.ncbi.nlm.nih.gov/pubmed/28074801.
39. Smulter N, Lingehall HC, Gustafson Y, et al. Delirium after cardiac surgery: incidence and risk factors. Interact Cardiovasc Thorac Surg 2013;17(5):790–6.
40. Kamdar BB, Niessen T, Colantuoni E, et al. Delirium transitions in the medical ICU: exploring the role of sleep quality and other factors. Crit Care Med 2015;43(1): 135–41. Available at: http://uml.idm.oclc.org/login?url=http://search.ebscohost.com/login.aspx?direct=true&db=c8h&AN=103863846&site=ehost-live.
41. Pandharipande PP, Shintani A, Peterson J, et al. Lorazepam is an independent risk factor for transitioning to delirium in intensive care unit patients. Anesthesiology 2006;104(1):21–6.
42. Jarvela K, Porkkala H, Karlsson S, et al. Postoperative delirium in cardiac surgery patients. J Cardiothorac Vasc Anesth 2018;32(4):1597–602.
43. Crocker E, Beggs T, Hassan A, et al. Long-term effects of postoperative delirium in patients undergoing cardiac operation: a systematic review. Ann Thorac Surg 2016;102(4):1391–9.
44. Patel N, Minhas JS, Chung EML. Risk factors associated with cognitive decline after cardiac surgery: a systematic review. Cardiovasc Psychiatry Neurol 2015; 2015:370612. Available at: http://www.hindawi.com/journals/cpn/%5Cnhttp://ovidsp.ovid.com/ovidweb.cgi?T=JS&PAGE=reference&D=emed13&NEWS=N&AN=2015445631.
45. Newman MF, Grocott HP, Mathew JP, et al. Report of the substudy assessing the impact of neurocognitive function on quality of life 5 years after cardiac surgery. Stroke 2001;32(12):2874–9.
46. Widyastuti Y, Stenseth R, Wahba A, et al. Length of intensive care unit stay following cardiac surgery: is it impossible to find a universal prediction model? Interact Cardiovasc Thorac Surg 2012;15(5):825–32.
47. Schelling G, Richter M, Roozendaal B, et al. Exposure to high stress in the intensive care unit may have negative effects on health-related quality-of-life outcomes after cardiac surgery. Crit Care Med 2003;31(7):1971–80.

48. Diwell RA, Davis DH, Vickerstaff V, et al. Key components of the delirium syndrome and mortality: greater impact of acute change and disorganised thinking in a prospective cohort study. BMC Geriatr 2018;18(1):1–8.

49. Moskowitz EE, Overbey DM, Jones TS, et al. Post-operative delirium is associated with increased 5-year mortality. Am J Surg 2017;214(6):1036–8.

50. Koster S, Hensens AG, Schuurmans MJ, et al. Consequences of delirium after cardiac operations. Ann Thorac Surg 2012;93(3):705–11.

51. Pisani MA, Kong SYJ, Kasl SV, et al. Days of delirium are associated with 1-year mortality in an older intensive care unit population. Am J Respir Crit Care Med 2009;180(11):1092–7.

52. Brummel NE, Jackson JC, Pandharipande PP, et al. Delirium in the ICU and subsequent long-term disability among survivors of mechanical ventilation. Crit Care Med 2014;42(2):369–77.

53. Huff T, Khan B. Functional performance outcomes after ICU delirium. In: C50 critical care: delirium and sedation in the ICU. American Thoracic Society; 2016. p. A5273.

54. Altman MT, Knauert MP, Murphy TE, et al. Association of intensive care unit delirium with sleep disturbance and functional disability after critical illness: an observational cohort study. Ann Intensive Care 2018;8(1):63.

55. Rengel KF, Hayhurst CJ, Pandharipande PP, et al. Long-term cognitive and functional impairments after critical illness. Anesth Analg 2019;128(4):772–80.

56. Koster S, Hensens AG, van der Palen J. The long-term cognitive and functional outcomes of postoperative delirium after cardiac surgery. Ann Thorac Surg 2009;87(5):1469–74. Available at: https://www.scopus.com/inward/record.uri?eid=2-s2.0-64649084172&doi=10.1016%2Fj.athoracsur.2009.02.080&partnerID=40&md5=d72e4daeb28aae2278d101e2f035f7d5.

57. Rothenhäusler HB, Grieser B, Nollert G, et al. Psychiatric and psychosocial outcome of cardiac surgery with cardiopulmonary bypass: a prospective 12-month follow-up study. Gen Hosp Psychiatry 2005;27(1):18–28.

58. Rawal G, Yadav S, Kumar R. Post-intensive care syndrome: an overview. J Transl Int Med 2017;5(2):90–2.

59. Needham DM, Davidson J, Cohen H, et al. Improving long-term outcomes after discharge from intensive care unit: report from a stakeholders' conference. Crit Care Med 2012;40(2):502–9.

60. Griffiths J, Hatch RA, Bishop J, et al. An exploration of social and economic outcome and associated health-related quality of life after critical illness in general intensive care unit survivors: a 12-month follow-up study. Crit Care 2013;17(3):R100.

61. Grover S, Ghosh A, Ghormode D. Experience in delirium: is it distressing? J Neuropsychiatry Clin Neurosci 2015;27(2):139–46. Available at: http://psychiatryonline.org/doi/10.1176/appi.neuropsych.13110329.

62. Andersson EM, Hallberg IR, Norberg A, et al. The meaning of acute confusional state from the perspective of elderly patients. Int J Geriatr Psychiatry 2002;17(7):652–63.

63. Lingehall HC, Smulter NS, Lindahl E, et al. Preoperative cognitive performance and postoperative delirium are independently associated with future dementia in older people who have undergone cardiac surgery: a longitudinal cohort study. Crit Care Med 2017;45(8):1295–303.

64. Duppils GS, Wikblad K. Patients' experiences of being delirious. J Clin Nurs 2007;16(5):810–8.

65. Ackerman MG, Shapiro PA. Psychological effects of invasive cardiac surgery and cardiac transplantation. In: Alvarenga ME, Byrne D, editors. Handbook of Psychocardiology. Singapore: Springer Singapore; 2016. p. 567–84.

66. Wolters AE, Peelen LM, Welling MC, et al. Long-term mental health problems after delirium in the ICU. Crit Care Med 2016;44(10):1808–13.

67. Schmitt EM, Gallagher J, Albuquerque A, et al. Perspectives on the delirium experience and its burden: common themes among older patients, their family caregivers, and nurses. Gerontologist 2017;59(2):327–37.

68. Partridge JSL, Martin FC, Harari D, et al. The delirium experience: what is the effect on patients, relatives and staff and what can be done to modify this? Int J Geriatr Psychiatry 2013;28(8):804–12.

69. Breitbart W, Gibson C, Tremblay A. The delirium experience: delirium recall and delirium-related distress in hospitalized patients with cancer, their spouses/caregivers, and their nurses. Psychosomatics 2002;43(3):183–94.

70. Ely EW, Truman B, Shintani A, et al. Monitoring sedation status over time in ICU patients: reliability and validity of the Richmond Agitation-Sedation Scale (RASS). JAMA 2003;289(22):2983–91.

71. Bergeron N, Dubois M-JJ, Dumont M, et al. Intensive care delirium screening checklist: evaluation of a new screening tool. Intensive Care Med 2001;27(5):859–64.

72. Inouye SK, van Dyck CH, Alessi CA, et al. Clarifying confusion: the confusion assessment method. A new method for detection of delirium. Ann Intern Med 1990;113(12):941–8.

73. Pun BT, Gordon SM, Peterson JF, et al. Large-scale implementation of sedation and delirium monitoring in the intensive care unit: a report from two medical centers. Crit Care Med 2005;33(6):1199–205.

74. Inouye SK, Bogardus ST, Baker DI, et al. The Hospital Elder Life Program: a model of care to prevent cognitive and functional decline in older hospitalized patients. Hospital Elder Life Program. J Am Geriatr Soc 2000;48(12):1697–706.

75. O'Mahony R, Murthy L, Akunne A, et al. Synopsis of the National Institute for Health and Clinical Excellence guideline for prevention of delirium. Ann Intern Med 2011;154(11):746–51.

76. Inouye SK. Delirium in older persons. N Engl J Med 2006;354(11):1157–65.

77. Wei LA, Fearing MA, Sternberg EJ, et al. The confusion assessment method: a systematic review of current usage. J Am Geriatr Soc 2008;56(5):823–30.

78. Inouye SK, Robinson T, Blaum C, et al. American Geriatrics Society abstracted clinical practice guideline for postoperative delirium in older adults. J Am Geriatr Soc 2015;63(1):142–50.

79. Smith CD, Grami P. Feasibility and effectiveness of a delirium prevention bundle in critically ill patients. Am J Crit Care 2016;26(1):19–27.

80. Hshieh TT, Yue J, Oh E, et al. Effectiveness of multicomponent nonpharmacological delirium interventions: a meta-analysis. JAMA Intern Med 2015;175(4):512–20.

81. Marra A, Ely EW, Pandharipande PP, et al. The ABCDEF bundle in critical care. Crit Care Clin 2017;33(2):225–43.

82. Young J, Murthy L, Westby M, et al. Diagnosis, prevention, and management of delirium: summary of NICE guidance. BMJ 2010;341:c3704.

83. Samuel M. Postoperative delirium in older adults: best practice statement from the American Geriatrics Society. J Am Coll Surg 2015;220:136–49.

84. Rizzo JA, Bogardus STJ, Leo-Summers L, et al. Multicomponent targeted intervention to prevent delirium in hospitalized older patients: what is the economic value? Med Care 2001;39(7):740–52.

85. Leslie DL, Zhang Y, Bogardus ST, et al. Consequences of preventing delirium in hospitalized older adults on nursing home costs. J Am Geriatr Soc 2005;53(3):405–9.

86. Ministry of Health New South Wales. Delirium screen for older adults. 2014. p. 23–4. Available at: https://www.aci.health.nsw.gov.au/__data/assets/pdf_file/0010/286156/NSW_HEALTH_Delirium_Screen_for_Older_Adults_-_240714.pdf. Accessed July 11, 2020.

87. Heun R, Papassotiropoulos A, Jennssen F. The validity of psychometric instruments for detection of dementia in the elderly general population. Int J Geriatr Psychiatry 1998;13(6):368–80.

88. Nasreddine Z, Phillips N. The Montreal Cognitive Assessment, MoCA: a brief screening tool for mild cognitive impairment. J Am Geriatr Soc 2005;53(4):695–9.

89. Borson S, Scanlan J, Brush M, et al. The mini-cog: a cognitive "vital signs" measure for dementia screening in multi-lingual elderly. Int J Geriatr Psychiatry 2000;15(11):1021–7.

90. Donald GW, Ghaffarian AA, Isaac F, et al. Preoperative frailty assessment predicts loss of independence after vascular surgery. J Vasc Surg 2018;68(5):1382–9.

91. Devlin JW, Fong JJ, Schumaker G, et al. Use of a validated delirium assessment tool improves the ability of physicians to identify delirium in medical intensive care unit patients. Crit Care Med 2007;35(12):2721–4 [quiz: 2725].

92. van Dijk JFM, van Wijck AJM, Kappen TH, et al. Postoperative pain assessment based on numeric ratings is not the same for patients and professionals: a cross-sectional study. Int J Nurs Stud 2012;49(1):65–71.

93. Rijkenberg S, Stilma W, Bosman RJ, et al. Pain measurement in mechanically ventilated patients after cardiac surgery: comparison of the Behavioral Pain Scale (BPS) and the Critical-Care Pain Observation Tool (CPOT). J Cardiothorac Vasc Anesth 2017;31(4):1227–34.

94. Manji RA, Arora RC, Singal RK, et al. Long-term outcome and predictors of noninstitutionalized survival subsequent to prolonged intensive care unit stay after cardiac surgical procedures. Ann Thorac Surg 2016;101(1):56–63 [discussion: 63].

95. Muller Moran HR, Maguire D, Maguire D, et al. Association of earlier extubation and postoperative delirium after coronary artery bypass grafting. J Thorac Cardiovasc Surg 2019. [Epub ahead of print].

96. Priye S, Jagannath S, Singh D, et al. Dexmedetomidine as an adjunct in postoperative analgesia following cardiac surgery: a randomized, double-blind study. Saudi J Anaesth 2015;9(4):353–8.

97. Manji RA, Arora RC, Singal RK, et al. Early rehospitalization after prolonged intensive care unit stay post cardiac surgery: outcomes and modifiable risk factors. J Am Heart Assoc 2017;6(2):e004072.

98. Dasta JF, Kane-Gill SL, Pencina M, et al. A cost-minimization analysis of dexmedetomidine compared with midazolam for long-term sedation in the intensive care unit. Crit Care Med 2010;38(2):497–503.

99. Pandharipande PP, Pun BT, Herr DL, et al. Effect of sedation with dexmedetomidine vs lorazepam on acute brain dysfunction in mechanically ventilated patients: the MENDS randomized controlled trial. JAMA 2007;298(22):2644–53.

100. Shehabi Y, Grant P, Wolfenden H, et al. Prevalence of delirium with dexmedeto-midine compared with morphine based therapy after cardiac surgery: a ran-domized controlled trial (DEXmedetomidine COmpared to Morphine-DEXCOM Study). Anesthesiology 2009;111(5):1075–84.

101. Wang W, Li H-L, Wang D-X, et al. Haloperidol prophylaxis decreases delirium incidence in elderly patients after noncardiac surgery: a randomized controlled trial*. Crit Care Med 2012;40(3):731–9.

102. Al-Qadheeb NS, Balk EM, Fraser GL, et al. Randomized ICU trials do not demonstrate an association between interventions that reduce delirium duration and short-term mortality: a systematic review and meta-analysis. Crit Care Med 2014;42(6):1442–54.

103. Page VJ, Ely EW, Gates S, et al. Effect of intravenous haloperidol on the duration of delirium and coma in critically ill patients (Hope-ICU): a randomised, double-blind, placebo-controlled trial. Lancet Respir Med 2013;1(7):515–23.

104. Djaiani G, Silverton N, Fedorko L, et al. Dexmedetomidine versus propofol seda-tion reduces delirium after cardiac surgery: a randomized controlled trial. Anes-thesiology 2016;124(2):362–8.

105. Shankar P, Mueller A, Packiasabapathy S, et al. Dexmedetomidine and intrave-nous acetaminophen for the prevention of postoperative delirium following car-diac surgery (DEXACET trial): protocol for a prospective randomized controlled trial. Trials 2018;19(1):326.

106. Lin YY, He B, Chen J, et al. Can dexmedetomidine be a safe and efficacious sedative agent in post-cardiac surgery patients? A meta-analysis. Crit Care 2012;16(5):R169. Available at: http://proxycheck.lib.umanitoba.ca/libraries/online/proxy.php?http://ovidsp.ovid.com/ovidweb.cgi?T=JS&CSC=Y&NEWS=N&PAGE=fulltext&D=med7&AN=23016926.

107. Vincent J-L, Shehabi Y, Walsh TS, et al. Comfort and patient-centred care without excessive sedation: the eCASH concept. Intensive Care Med 2016;42(6):962–71.

108. Fok MC, Sepehry AA, Frisch L, et al. Do antipsychotics prevent postoperative delirium? A systematic review and meta-analysis. Int J Geriatr Psychiatry 2015;30(4):333–44.

109. Siddiqi N, Harrison JK, Clegg A, et al. Interventions for preventing delirium in hospitalised non-ICU patients. Cochrane Database Syst Rev 2016;(3):CD005563.

110. Girard TD, Pandharipande PP, Carson SS, et al. Feasibility, efficacy, and safety of antipsychotics for intensive care unit delirium: the MIND randomized, placebo-controlled trial. Crit Care Med 2010;38(2):428–37.

111. Devlin JW, Roberts RJ, Fong JJ, et al. Efficacy and safety of quetiapine in crit-ically ill patients with delirium: a prospective, multicenter, randomized, double-blind, placebo-controlled pilot study. Crit Care Med 2010;38(2):419–27.

112. Skrobik YK, Bergeron N, Dumont M, et al. Olanzapine vs haloperidol: treating delirium in a critical care setting. Intensive Care Med 2004;30(3):444–9.

113. Needham DM, Colantuoni E, Dinglas VD, et al. Rosuvastatin versus placebo for delirium in intensive care and subsequent cognitive impairment in patients with sepsis-associated acute respiratory distress syndrome: an ancillary study to a randomised controlled trial. Lancet Respir Med 2016;4(3):203–12.

114. Pauley E, Lishmanov A, Schumann S, et al. Delirium is a robust predictor of morbidity and mortality among critically ill patients treated in the cardiac inten-sive care unit. Am Heart J 2015;170(1):79–86.e1.

115. Maldonado JR. Pathoetiological model of delirium: a comprehensive understanding of the neurobiology of delirium and an evidence-based approach to prevention and treatment. Crit Care Clin 2008;24(4):789–856, ix.
116. Mu JL, Lee A, Joynt GM. Pharmacologic agents for the prevention and treatment of delirium in patients undergoing cardiac surgery: systematic review and metaanalysis. Crit Care Med 2015;43(1):194–204.
117. Serafim RB, Bozza FA, Soares M, do Brasil PEAA, Tura BR, Ely EW, et al. Pharmacologic prevention and treatment of delirium in intensive care patients: a systematic review. J Crit Care 2015;30(4):799–807.
118. Neufeld KJ, Yue J, Robinson TN, et al. Antipsychotic medication for prevention and treatment of delirium in hospitalized adults: a systematic review and meta-analysis. J Am Geriatr Soc 2016;64(4):705–14.
119. Prakanrattana U, Prapaitrakool S. Efficacy of risperidone for prevention of postoperative delirium in cardiac surgery. Anaesth Intensive Care 2007;35(5):714–9.
120. Su X, Meng Z-T, Wu X-H, et al. Dexmedetomidine for prevention of delirium in elderly patients after non-cardiac surgery: a randomised, double-blind, placebo-controlled trial. Lancet 2016;388(10054):1893–902.
121. van den Boogaard M, Slooter AJC, Bruggemann RJM, et al. Effect of haloperidol on survival among critically ill adults with a high risk of delirium: the REDUCE randomized clinical trial. JAMA 2018;319(7):680–90.
122. Vidan MT, Sanchez E, Alonso M, et al. An intervention integrated into daily clinical practice reduces the incidence of delirium during hospitalization in elderly patients. J Am Geriatr Soc 2009;57(11):2029–36.
123. Inouye SK, Bogardus STJ, Charpentier PA, et al. A multicomponent intervention to prevent delirium in hospitalized older patients. N Engl J Med 1999;340(9): 669–76.

Prevention of Acute Kidney Injury

Mira Küllmar, MD[a], Alexander Zarbock, MD[a,*], Daniel T. Engelman, MD[b],
Subhasis Chatterjee, MD[c,d], Nana-Maria Wagner, MD[a]

KEYWORDS

- Acute kidney injury (AKI) • Cardiac surgery • KDIGO bundles • Renal biomarkers
- Prevention of acute kidney injury (AKI)

KEY POINTS

- Cardiac surgery–associated acute kidney injury (CSA-AKI) is a common complication of cardiac surgery and independently associated with worse outcome.
- Risk identification and prevention of CSA-AKI play a crucial role in improving patient outcomes after cardiac surgery.
- Implementation of the Kidney Disease: Improving Global Outcomes bundles in high-risk patients has been demonstrated to be an effective strategy to decrease the incidence of CSA-AKI.
- Remote ischemic preconditioning in high-risk patients may be an effective preventive management strategy.

INTRODUCTION

Cardiac surgery–associated acute kidney injury (CSA-AKI) is one of the major complications after cardiac surgery and independently associated with worse short-term and long-term outcomes.[1,2] Depending on the specific criteria used, up to 42% of cardiac surgery patients undergoing cardiopulmonary bypass (CPB) suffer from CSA-AKI postoperatively, doubling hospital costs.[1,3–5] In 1% to 5% of these patients, renal replacement therapy (RRT) is required with its associated decreased survial.[6] Besides RRT as a supportive measure, therapeutic options are limited, highlighting the importance of risk identification, prevention, and early recognition of CSA-AKI in daily clinical practice. Based on current evidence, this review provides an overview of the "what, why, who, when, and if" of CSA-AKI, with a focus on

[a] Department of Anesthesiology, Intensive Care and Pain Medicine, University of Münster, Albert-Schweitzer-Campus 1, Building A1, Münster 48149, Germany; [b] Heart and Vascular Program, Baystate Health and University of Massachusetts Medical School–Baystate, 759 Chestnut Street, Springfield, MA 01199, USA; [c] Department of Surgery, Baylor College of Medicine, One Baylor Plaza, MS: BCM 390, Houston, TX 77030, USA; [d] Division of Cardiovascular Surgery, Texas Heart Institute, Houston, TX, USA
* Corresponding author.
E-mail address: zarbock@uni-muenster.de

Crit Care Clin 36 (2020) 691–704
https://doi.org/10.1016/j.ccc.2020.07.002
0749-0704/20/© 2020 Elsevier Inc. All rights reserved.

criticalcare.theclinics.com

risk identification and preventive measures to improve patient outcomes after cardiac surgery.

WHAT? DEFINITION OF ACUTE KIDNEY INJURY

Acute kidney injury (AKI), including CSA-AKI, is defined by the Kidney Disease: Improving Global Outcomes (KDIGO) criteria as an increase in serum creatinine (SCr) by greater than or equal to 0.3 mg/dL within 48 hours or to greater than or equal to 1.5-times to 1.9-times baseline values within 7 days and/or a urine output (UO) less than or equal to 0.5 mL/kg/h for at least 6 hours and differentiates into 2 stages of severity (**Fig. 1**).[7] The most recent KDIGO definition and criteria for diagnosis and staging of AKI were developed over many years. After a long period without standardized definition, the risk, injury, failure, loss, and end-stage kidney disease (RIFLE) criteria were formulated in 2004 and defined AKI through elevation in SCr and/or decline in UO.[8] In 2007, the more specified Acute Kidney Injury Network (AKIN) criteria extended the RIFLE criteria by defining AKI as an increase in SCr by greater than or equal to 0.3 mg/dL within 48 hours.[9] Since 2012, the KDIGO criteria were merged with the RIFLE and the AKIN criteria and were shown to be more sensitive for AKI detection.[10] Together with the adapted criteria for AKI definition, the formerly used term, *acute renal failure*, was replaced by the term, *acute kidney injury*, and includes not only loss of kidney function based on damage but also injury without loss of function. Even this so-called subclinical AKI—clinically silent due to the preserved organ function and thus undetectable by the KDIGO criteria—has been demonstrated to be

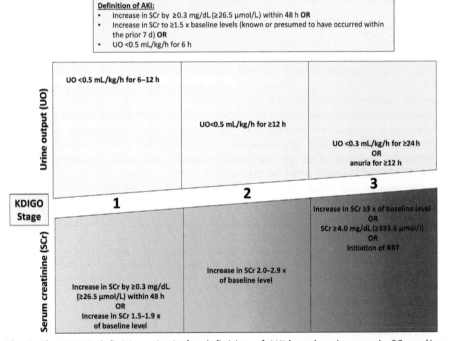

Fig. 1. The KDIGO definition criteria for definition of AKI based on increase in SCr and/or decrease in UO. The KDIGO criteria can be used for diagnosis and staging CSA-AKI. (*Data from* KDIGO Board Members. Kidney international supplements. Mar 2012;2(1):3.)

associated with worse outcome[11] and further emphasizes the characteristics of AKI as a syndrome along a continuum.[12]

WHY? PATHOGENESIS OF CARDIAC SURGERY–ASSOCIATED ACUTE KIDNEY INJURY

The pathogenesis of CSA-AKI is complex, multifactorial, and still poorly understood. A few major pathophysiologic mechanisms, however, have been identified.[13]

Hemodynamics, Inflammation, and Hemolysis

The use of CPB is associated with decreased and nonpulsatile renal blood flow, hemodilution, and hypothermia. Renal autoregulation is impaired, resulting in renal hypoperfusion and a decrease in glomerular filtration rate. Low cardiac output perioperatively contributes to renal hypoperfusion and increased risk of CSA-AKI.[14] In addition, low cardiac output induces activation of the sympathetic nervous and renin-angiotensin systems and increases vasopressin release, leading to vasoconstriction and renal hypoperfusion.[15] In congestive heart failure, the associated increased central venous pressure and venous congestion are additional risk factors for the development of AKI.[16,17] The use of CPB, surgical trauma, and the concomitant systemic inflammatory response results in increased proinflammatory cytokine levels and complement activation, further contributing to CSA-AKI.[18,19] Perioperatively occurring ischemia-reperfusion injury can further promote CSA-AKI by inducing a burst in oxygen species and activation of renal inflammatory pathways that facilitate tubular epithelial cell damage.[20] Low hemoglobin levels, red blood cell transfusion, and hemolysis during CPB result in reduced oxygen supply and iron release constituting additional risk factors for the development of CSA-AKI.[21,22] Finally, renal blood flow can be endangered by surgical manipulation and embolization during CPB cannulation and cross-clamping, making the exact culprits of CPB associated CSA-AKI particularly difficult to identify.[13] Nonetheless, several studies have not detected a benefit of off-pump cardiac surgery in relation to long-term renal function and the requirement for RRT.[23,24]

Nephrotoxic Agents

Before and after cardiac surgery, patient exposure to nephrotoxic agents, such as antibiotics (aminogylcosides[25] and vancomycin[26]); nonsteroidal anti-inflammatory drugs,[27] including aspirin[28]; angiotensin-converting enzyme inhibitors; and angiotensin-receptor blockers,[29] often is unavoidable. Intravenous radiocontrast agents commonly are used for perioperative diagnostic purposes, such as coronary angiography or computer tomography. Contrast agent–induced AKI is a well-known complication after administration of radiocontrast agents, depending on dose and time of administration, hydration status, and age.[30]

Genetics

Genetic polymorphisms have been shown to correlate with an increased risk for CSA-AKI[31,32] and 2 new loci recently were identified.[33] Despite these interesting approaches regarding risk identification and prevention, clear evidence is still lacking and further research is required.

WHO? RISK STRATIFICATION AND PREDICTION

Risk factors for CSA-AKI can be categorized as preoperative, intraoperative, and postoperative and as patient-related and procedure-related risk factors (**Table 1**). Because there currently is no curative therapy for CSA-AKI, the Acute Disease Quality Initiative (ADQI) group recommends continuous intraoperative and postoperative

Table 1
Risk factors for cardiac surgery–associated acute kidney injury

Preoperative Risk Factors	Intraoperative Risk Factors	Postoperative Risk Factors
• Higher age	• Type of procedure	• Nephrotoxic agents
• Female sex	• CPB	• Sepsis
• Preexisting renal dysfunction/	• Duration of CPB	• Cardiogenic shock
chronic kidney disease	• Cross-clamp time	• Low cardiac output
• Chronic obstructive	• Hemodilution	• Hypotension
pulmonary disease	• Transfusion of	
• Insulin-dependent	red blood cells	
diabetes mellitus	• Embolism	
• Heart failure		
• Low cardiac output		
• Coronary heart disease		
• Peripheral vascular disease		
• Intra-aortic balloon pump		
• Emergency surgery		
• Previous cardiac surgery		
• Nephrotoxic agents		

patient re-evaluation for risk and preventative strategy implementation.[34] Preoperative risk factors are of particular importance in predicting CSA-AKI and mostly are patient-related and typically nonmodifiable. These include age, female gender, preexisting chronic kidney disease, and comorbidities, such as chronic obstructive pulmonary disease, insulin-dependent diabetes mellitus, peripheral and coronary artery disease, hypertension, congestive heart failure and decreased left ventricular ejection fraction (<35%), need for intra-aortic balloon pump therapy, and emergency or previous cardiac surgery.[34,35] In contrast, intraoperative and postoperative risk factors mostly are procedure-related and potentially addressable within preventive strategies. For example, valve surgery (with or without coronary artery bypass graft) is associated with a higher risk for CSA-AKI than coronary artery bypass graft alone.[35] Further intraoperative risk factors are cross-clamp time, duration of CPB, and type of surgical procedure.[36] Postoperative exposure to nephrotoxic agents, conditions of hypovolemia and hypotension, or development of sepsis or cardiogenic shock (associated with renal vasoconstriction) also are consistent with an increased risk for CSA-AKI.[34] Based on these risk factors, several risk-prediction scores have been proposed as clinical tools for the identification of patients at high risk. Only a few of them have been validated externally.[6,35,37,38] Most of these risk scores aim to identify severe CSA-AKI requiring RRT, such as the Simplified Predictive Renal Index[39], the Metha Score[6] and the Cleveland Score.[35] Recently, Birnie and colleagues[40] postulated "the all stage AKI score" as the first score to identify all stages of CSA-AKI. Further promising approaches additionally integrate novel biomarkers into risk prediction models for CSA-AKI.[41,42] Although there are no guidelines for the implementation of existing risk-prediction scores, their preoperative use as well as a continued intraoperative and postoperative assessment is recommended by the ADQI group for patients undergoing cardiac surgery.[34]

WHEN? CARDIAC SURGERY–ASSOCIATED ACUTE KIDNEY INJURY—DIAGNOSIS AND EARLY RECOGNITION

CSA-AKI is diagnosed according to the KDIGO definition criteria based on elevated SCr and/or decrease in UO (see **Fig. 1**).[7] With respect to subclinical AKI, these 2

AKI-defining functional parameters have important limitations. Because the kidneys have a notable functional reserve, an increase in SCr level does not become significant before 50% of the renal glomerular filtration capacity is impaired. Thus, elevations in SCr indicate advanced renal dysfunction but do not detect AKI at an early stage. SCr can be affected by a broad range of factors (drugs, fluids administered, hemodilution, and reduced muscle mass).[43] UO is a functional marker with low sensitivity and specificity because oliguria may occur due to various reasons (eg, sepsis, shock, and obstruction) or it might be a physiologic response to hypovolemia. To detect AKI prior to loss of function, early renal biomarkers are required[44] and several have been proposed to predict CSA-AKI.[45] The most extensively investigated biomarkers are neutrophil gelatinase–associated lipocalin (NGAL), tissue inhibitor of metalloproteinases-2 (TIMP-2), and insulinlike growth factor binding protein 7 (IGFBP7). TIMP-2 and IGFBP7 are proteins involved in the G_1 cell-cycle arrest of tubular epithelial cells.[46,47] Both of them were demonstrated to predict CSA-AKI.[48] NGAL is released by injured renal tubular epithelial cells in the absence of functional AKI in adults and particularly in children.[49,50] This predictive value is limited, however, to patients with preoperative unimpaired kidney function.[50,51] NGAL was postulated as a troponin-like biomarker for early detection of AKI in patients with increased risk.[52] New approaches have proposed NGAL measurements during the perioperative period to guide clinical management and implement early preventive strategies.[53] The investigators generated an NGAL-based injury score for patients undergoing cardiac surgery, the CSA-NGAL score.[53] Despite these promising data, NGAL has not yet been established in clinical practice, due to a lack of cutoff values, variability in results, and limitations in available NGAL assays.[49]

Multiplication of the values of biomarkers TIMP-2 and IGFBP7 (ie, [TIMP-2] × [IGFBP7], respectively), has been shown to be superior to other biomarkers in predicting AKI.[46,54,55] The need for RRT, renal recovery after AKI, and mortality in patients after cardiac surgery were shown to be predicted by elevations of [TIMP-2] × [IGFBP7].[56,57] Several studies have demonstrated an association of [TIMP-2] × [IGFBP7] and development of CSA-AKI 4 hours after CPB[57–59] or the association of moderate and severe CSA-AKI with bimodal elevations of [TIMP-2] × [IGFBP7] (intraoperatively and 6 hours after CPB).[60] Some trials have not been able to confirm these results in low risk patients.[61] Other investigators, however, have been able to utilize the routine measurement of [TIMP-2] × [IGFBP7] to guide therapeutic interventions in all cardiac surgery patients resulting in a significant decrease in stage 2/3 AKI following cardiac surgery.[62] The ADQI group suggests detection of renal biomarkers only in high-risk patients in the presence of clinical risk factors.[34] The Enhanced Recovery After Cardiac Surgery (ERACS) Society [Guidelines] suggest routine early detection of kidney stress (using biomarkers) and interventions to avoid AKI after cardiac surgery.[63]

If...Prevention OF CARDIAC SURGERY–ASSOCIATED ACUTE KIDNEY INJURY

A variety of pharmacologic and nonpharmacologic approaches to prevent CSA-AKI have been proposed. Most of these strategies, however, currently lack evidence to effectively reduce CSA-AKI.

Pharmacologic Strategies

Statins were demonstrated to exert protective effects by preserving endothelial function, ameliorating inflammation, and increasing nitric oxide bioavailability, thus supporting a potential role of statins in the protection from CSA-AKI.[64] A retrospective study suggested the perioperative use of statins to reduce the risk of postoperative CSA-AKI.[65] These results could not be confirmed, however, in recently published meta-analyses.[66,67] Previous data suggested fenoldopam, a selective dopamine receptor agonist, reduces CSA-AKI.[68] In a larger multicenter, randomized, placebo-controlled trial, however, fenoldopam was not effective in CSA-AKI prevention but was associated with hypotension.[69] Numerous other approaches (eg, with levosimendan, N-acetylcysteine, sodium bicarbonate, or erythropoetin) also failed to clearly demonstrate preventive effects on CSA-AKI.[34] Diuretics commonly are administered in the setting of cardiac surgery to prevent fluid overload and venous congestion and to increase renal blood flow. There is no evidence, however, of any preventive effects utilizing diuretics on CSA-AKI, and the KDIGO guidelines do not recommend diuretics as a preventive measure.[7] Intraoperatively administered volatile anesthetics were shown to be protective against CSA-AKI.[70,71]

Fluid Management

Perioperative fluid management plays a pivotal role in CSA-AKI prevention. It is a balancing act between avoiding hypovolemia or hypervolemia with both renal hypoperfusion and fluid overload associated with CSA-AKI and worse outcome.[72] The type of fluids used also might have an impact on renal function and is controversial. A meta-analysis of 21 studies with 6253 patients demonstrated that high-chloride fluids are associated with a significantly increased risk for AKI.[73] In contrast, a large multicenter, cluster-randomized, double-crossover trial in 2278 patients requiring crystalloid fluid therapy was unable to confirm these results because the use of buffered crystalloid solutions compared with saline did not reduce the risk of AKI.[74] This trial was criticized, however, for several limitations (eg, limited fluid doses and inclusion of patients with low disease severity).[75] A recently published cluster-randomized, multiple-crossover trial among 7942 critically ill patients indicated that the use of balanced crystalloids resulted in lower rates of RRT or persistent renal dysfunction within 30 days,[76] which currently is recommended.[34] Additional large randomized trials are needed to specifically investigate whether the results of fluid regimes applied to the critically ill extend to prevention of CSA-AKI.

Kidney Disease: Improving Global Outcomes Bundles

The KDIGO group proposed the "KDIGO bundle of care" in their guideline strategies for prevention of AKI (**Fig. 2**).[7] These bundles incorporate optimization of volume status and perfusion pressure, consideration of invasive hemodynamic monitoring, avoidance of hyperglycemia and nephrotoxic agents, and consideration of alternatives to radiocontrast media as well as close monitoring of SCr and UO.[7] Data from 33,330 noncardiac surgical patients demonstrated the significant association between short periods (<5 minutes) of intraoperative hypotension (mean arterial blood pressure of <55 mm Hg) and the development of AKI,[77] supporting hemodynamic optimization as a central component of CSA-AKI prevention. Glycemic control was studied in a prospective, randomized controlled trial with 1548 patients and demonstrated intensive insulin therapy (target blood glucose ≤ 110 mg/dL) to significantly reduce the incidence of AKI in critically ill patients.[78] Subsequent studies suggested that conventional (target blood glucose <200 mg/dL)[79] and moderate (target blood glucose 127–179 mg/dL)[80] glucose management is superior to tight glycemic control. The postoperative implementation of the KDIGO bundles in patients at high risk for CSA-AKI identified by the biomarkers [TIMP-2] × [IGFBP7] recently was demonstrated to reduce the frequency and severity of CSA-AKI compared with standard care.[81] This single-center, randomized controlled trial with 276 patients undergoing cardiac

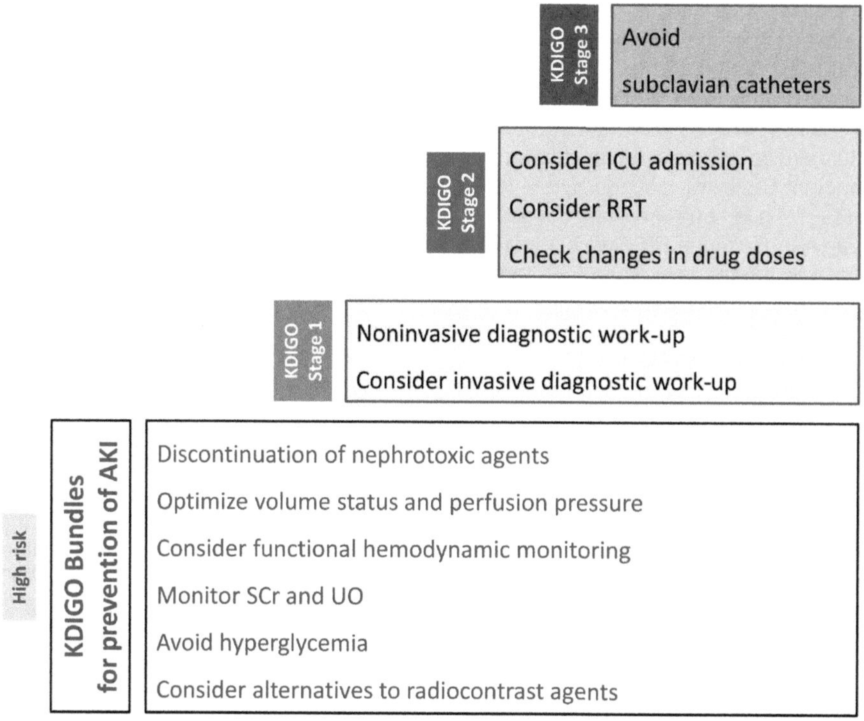

Fig. 2. The KDIGO bundles of care for AKI. To prevent AKI the KDIGO guidelines recommend the implementation of the KDIGO bundles in high- risk patients. ICU, intensive care unit. (*From* KDIGO Board Members. Section 2: AKI Definitions. Kidney international supplements. Mar 2012;2(1):2; with permission.)

surgery with CPB was the first to demonstrate that the implementation of the KDIGO bundles is effective in preventing CSA-AKI. One of the crucial questions is the adherence of intensivists to the KDIGO bundles in daily clinical routine. A recently performed multicenter, multinational, randomized controlled trial investigated the compliance rate of adherence to the KDIGO bundles in high-risk patients after cardiac surgery (NCT03244514) with results currently pending for publication.

Remote Ischemic Preconditioning

Remote ischemic preconditioning (RIPC) may be performed preoperatively and includes several brief episodes of ischemia and reperfusion to a remote tissue (eg, the upper arm) before the actual injury occurs. The definitive mechanism is unclear. RIPC is suggested to attenuate renal injury by exploiting cellular defense mechanisms.[82] RIPC is postulated to induce immunomodulatory pathways similar to those occurring after ischemia/reperfusion injury, which then result in natural defense mechanisms, such as transient cell-cycle arrest. Data indicating the efficiency of RIPC are controversial. Smaller randomized controlled trials demonstrated a reduced incidence for CSA-AKI after RIPC was performed.[58,83] In contrast, 2 large multicenter, randomized controlled trials could not demonstrate a benefit of RIPC for prevention of CSA-AKI.[84,85] These controversial results are hardly comparable, however, due to differing endpoints, heterogeneous patient populations, different definitions of AKI, and the use of propofol. Propofol has been shown to impair the efficiency of RIPC.[86]

A current trial investigates the effect of different anesthetic regimes on the renoprotective effect of RIPC in high-risk patients undergoing cardiac surgery (DRKS00014989). Additionally, a meta-analysis of 30 randomized controlled trials demonstrated evidence for the preventive effect of RIPC on CSA-AKI.[87] This conclusion is supported by recently published data of a randomized controlled trial including 130 cardiac surgery patients who received RIPC or Sham-RIPC.[88] The primary endpoint CSA-AKI, defined by the KDIGO criteria, was reduced in patients receiving RIPC.[88] Thus, current data suggest RIPC as a potential preventive measure for CSA-AKI. Because RIPC is a noninvasive intervention with little risk of side effects, it may be worth considering RIPC as part of preventive strategies in high-risk patients for CSA-AKI in clinical routine.

How...Clinical MANAGEMENT

When severe CSA-AKI postoperatively occurs, initiation of RRT is the only therapeutic option to support renal function. Besides the intensity, the modalities, duration, and timing of RRT initiation primarily affect patient outcome. The KDIGO guidelines recommend the immediate initiation of RRT in cases of life-threatening complications (eg, hyperkalemia or metabolic acidosis).[7] In the absence of such complications, the timing of RRT remains unclear. Several large randomized controlled trials investigated early versus delayed initiation of RRT and demonstrated controversial results.[89–91] Due to different definitions of early versus late initiation of RRT and differences in the definition criteria of AKI used, these trials are of only limited comparability. Only 1 of these trials performed a biomarker-guided approach by identifying high-risk patients for AKI prior to inclusion.[89] Data from this trial demonstrated reduced mortality in patients receiving early (KDIGO stage 2) RRT[89] but further evidence is required. Although RRT is an invasive measure, which might cause severe complications, the CSA-AKI underlying pathophysiology supports consideration of early RRT initiation to avoid further harm to the kidneys. In this regard, a recently completed large multinational, randomized controlled trial soon may provide new insights (NCT02568722).

SUMMARY

CSA-AKI is a common and severe complication in patients undergoing cardiac surgery and an independent risk factor for worse outcomes. In severe CSA-AKI, RRT is the only available therapeutic intervention, although it solely constitutes a supportive measure. Therefore, perioperative risk identification, prevention, and early diagnosis play a pivotal role to improve care. Risk assessment should be regularly re-evaluated during the perioperative period and implementation of new biomarkers may be helpful to identify patients at an increased risk for CSA-AKI. In high-risk patients, implementation of the KDIGO bundles may reduce the incidence of CSA-AKI while evidence supporting most preventive approaches remains poor.

ACKNOWLEDGMENTS

This work was supported by the German Research Foundation (ZA428/14-1, KFO 342/1, ZA 428/18-1, ZA 428/10-1).

DISCLOSURE

M. Küllmar and N-M. Wagner declare no conflicts of interest. A. Zarbock received fees from Astute Medical, BioMerieux, Braun, Baxter, Fresenius, AM Pharma, Amomed,

AM Pharma, Ratiopharm, and Astellas and funding from Astute Medical, Astellas, Fresenius, Baxter, German Research Foundation, GIF, and BMBF. D. Engelman consults for Edwards Lifesciences.

REFERENCES

1. Machado MN, Nakazone MA, Maia LN. Prognostic value of acute kidney injury after cardiac surgery according to kidney disease: improving global outcomes definition and staging (KDIGO) criteria. PLoS One 2014;9(5):e98028.
2. Hobson CE, Yavas S, Segal MS, et al. Acute kidney injury is associated with increased long-term mortality after cardiothoracic surgery. Circulation 2009; 119(18):2444–53.
3. Fuhrman DY, Kellum JA. Epidemiology and pathophysiology of cardiac surgery-associated acute kidney injury. Curr Opin Anaesthesiol 2017;30(1):60–5.
4. Hu J, Chen R, Liu S, et al. Global incidence and outcomes of adult patients with acute kidney injury after cardiac surgery: a systematic review and meta-analysis. J Cardiothorac Vasc Anesth 2016;30(1):82–9.
5. Xie X, Wan X, Ji X, et al. Reassessment of acute kidney injury after cardiac surgery: a retrospective study. Intern Med 2017;56(3):275–82.
6. Mehta RH, Grab JD, O'Brien SM, et al. Bedside tool for predicting the risk of postoperative dialysis in patients undergoing cardiac surgery. Circulation 2006; 114(21):2208–16 [quiz: 2208].
7. oard members. Kidney Int supplements 2012;2(1):3.
8. Bellomo R, Ronco C, Kellum JA, et al. Acute Dialysis Quality Initiative w. Acute renal failure - definition, outcome measures, animal models, fluid therapy and information technology needs: the Second International Consensus Conference of the Acute Dialysis Quality Initiative (ADQI) Group. Crit Care 2004;8(4):R204–12.
9. Mehta RL, Kellum JA, Shah SV, et al. Acute Kidney Injury Network: report of an initiative to improve outcomes in acute kidney injury. Crit Care 2007;11(2):R31.
10. Luo X, Jiang L, Du B, et al. A comparison of different diagnostic criteria of acute kidney injury in critically ill patients. Crit Care 2014;18(4):R144.
11. Ronco C, Kellum JA, Haase M. Subclinical AKI is still AKI. Crit Care 2012; 16(3):313.
12. Lameire N, Biesen WV, Vanholder R. Acute kidney injury. Lancet 2008;372(9653): 1863–5.
13. Bellomo R, Auriemma S, Fabbri A, et al. The pathophysiology of cardiac surgery-associated acute kidney injury (CSA-AKI). Int J Artif Organs 2008;31(2):166–78.
14. Hudson C, Hudson J, Swaminathan M, et al. Emerging concepts in acute kidney injury following cardiac surgery. Semin Cardiothorac Vasc Anesth 2008;12(4): 320–30.
15. McFarlane SI, Winer N, Sowers JR. Role of the natriuretic peptide system in cardiorenal protection. Arch Intern Med 2003;163(22):2696–704.
16. Afsar B, Ortiz A, Covic A, et al. Focus on renal congestion in heart failure. Clin Kidney J 2016;9(1):39–47.
17. Gambardella I, Gaudino M, Ronco C, et al. Congestive kidney failure in cardiac surgery: the relationship between central venous pressure and acute kidney injury. Interact Cardiovasc Thorac Surg 2016;23(5):800–5.
18. Zhang WR, Garg AX, Coca SG, et al. Plasma IL-6 and IL-10 concentrations predict AKI and long-term mortality in adults after cardiac surgery. J Am Soc Nephrol 2015;26(12):3123–32.

19. Laffey JG, Boylan JF, Cheng DC. The systemic inflammatory response to cardiac surgery: implications for the anesthesiologist. Anesthesiology 2002;97(1):215–52.

20. Haase M, Bellomo R, Haase-Fielitz A. Novel biomarkers, oxidative stress, and the role of labile iron toxicity in cardiopulmonary bypass-associated acute kidney injury. J Am Coll Cardiol 2010;55(19):2024–33.

21. Vermeulen Windsant IC, de Wit NC, Sertorio JT, et al. Hemolysis during cardiac surgery is associated with increased intravascular nitric oxide consumption and perioperative kidney and intestinal tissue damage. Front Physiol 2014;5:340.

22. Haase M, Bellomo R, Story D, et al. Effect of mean arterial pressure, haemoglobin and blood transfusion during cardiopulmonary bypass on post-operative acute kidney injury. Nephrol Dial Transplant 2012;27(1):153–60.

23. Garg AX, Devereaux PJ, Yusuf S, et al. Kidney function after off-pump or on-pump coronary artery bypass graft surgery: a randomized clinical trial. JAMA 2014;311(21):2191–8.

24. Lamy A, Devereaux PJ, Prabhakaran D, et al. Five-year outcomes after off-pump or on-pump coronary-artery bypass grafting. N Engl J Med 2016;375(24): 2359–68.

25. Pagkalis S, Mantadakis E, Mavros MN, et al. Pharmacological considerations for the proper clinical use of aminoglycosides. Drugs 2011;71(17):2277–94.

26. Cappelletty D, Jablonski A, Jung R. Risk factors for acute kidney injury in adult patients receiving vancomycin. Clin Drug Investig 2014;34(3):189–93.

27. Ungprasert P, Cheungpasitporn W, Crowson CS, et al. Individual non-steroidal anti-inflammatory drugs and risk of acute kidney injury: a systematic review and meta-analysis of observational studies. Eur J Intern Med 2015;26(4):285–91.

28. Aboul-Hassan SS, Stankowski T, Marczak J, et al. The use of preoperative aspirin in cardiac surgery: a systematic review and meta-analysis. J Card Surg 2017; 32(12):758–74.

29. Yacoub R, Patel N, Lohr JW, et al. Acute kidney injury and death associated with renin angiotensin system blockade in cardiothoracic surgery: a meta-analysis of observational studies. Am J Kidney Dis 2013;62(6):1077–86.

30. Morcos R, Kucharik M, Bansal P, et al. Contrast-induced acute kidney injury: review and practical update. Clin Med Insights Cardiol 2019;13. 1179546819878680.

31. Isbir SC, Tekeli A, Ergen A, et al. Genetic polymorphisms contribute to acute kidney injury after coronary artery bypass grafting. Heart Surg Forum 2007;10(6): E439–44.

32. Gaudino M, Di Castelnuovo A, Zamparelli R, et al. Genetic control of postoperative systemic inflammatory reaction and pulmonary and renal complications after coronary artery surgery. J Thorac Cardiovasc Surg 2003;126(4):1107–12.

33. Stafford-Smith M, Li YJ, Mathew JP, et al. Genome-wide association study of acute kidney injury after coronary bypass graft surgery identifies susceptibility loci. Kidney Int 2015;88(4):823–32.

34. Nadim MK, Forni LG, Bihorac A, et al. Cardiac and vascular surgery-associated acute kidney injury: the 20th international consensus conference of the ADQI (Acute Disease Quality Initiative) Group. J Am Heart Assoc 2018;7(11):e008834.

35. Thakar CV, Arrigain S, Worley S, et al. A clinical score to predict acute renal failure after cardiac surgery. J Am Soc Nephrol 2005;16(1):162–8.

36. Yi Q, Li K, Jian Z, et al. Risk factors for acute kidney injury after cardiovascular surgery: evidence from 2,157 cases and 49,777 controls - a meta-analysis. Cardiorenal Med 2016;6(3):237–50.

37. Jorge-Monjas P, Bustamante-Munguira J, Lorenzo M, et al. Predicting cardiac surgery-associated acute kidney injury: the CRATE score. J Crit Care 2016; 31(1):130–8.

38. Pannu N, Graham M, Klarenbach S, et al. A new model to predict acute kidney injury requiring renal replacement therapy after cardiac surgery. CMAJ 2016; 188(15):1076–83.

39. Wijeysundera DN, Karkouti K, Dupuis JY, et al. Derivation and validation of a simplified predictive index for renal replacement therapy after cardiac surgery. JAMA 2007;297(16):1801–9.

40. Birnie K, Verheyden V, Pagano D, et al. Predictive models for kidney disease: improving global outcomes (KDIGO) defined acute kidney injury in UK cardiac surgery. Crit Care 2014;18(6):606.

41. Parikh CR, Devarajan P, Zappitelli M, et al. Postoperative biomarkers predict acute kidney injury and poor outcomes after pediatric cardiac surgery. J Am Soc Nephrol 2011;22(9):1737–47.

42. Albert C, Haase M, Albert A, et al. Urinary biomarkers may complement the Cleveland score for prediction of adverse kidney events after cardiac surgery: a pilot study. Ann Lab Med 2020;40(2):131–41.

43. Samra M, Abcar AC. False estimates of elevated creatinine. Perm J 2012; 16(2):51–2.

44. Chawla LS, Bellomo R, Bihorac A, et al. Acute kidney disease and renal recovery: consensus report of the Acute Disease Quality Initiative (ADQI) 16 Workgroup. Nat Rev Nephrol 2017;13(4):241–57.

45. Mayer T, Bolliger D, Scholz M, et al. Urine biomarkers of tubular renal cell damage for the prediction of acute kidney injury after cardiac surgery—a pilot study. J Cardiothorac Vasc Anesth 2017;31(6):2072–9.

46. Kashani K, Al-Khafaji A, Ardiles T, et al. Discovery and validation of cell cycle arrest biomarkers in human acute kidney injury. Crit Care 2013;17(1):R25.

47. Vanmassenhove J, Vanholder R, Nagler E, et al. Urinary and serum biomarkers for the diagnosis of acute kidney injury: an in-depth review of the literature. Nephrol Dial Transplant 2013;28(2):254–73.

48. Vandenberghe W, De Loor J, Hoste EA. Diagnosis of cardiac surgery-associated acute kidney injury from functional to damage biomarkers. Curr Opin Anaesthesiol 2017;30(1):66–75.

49. Haase-Fielitz A, Haase M, Devarajan P. Neutrophil gelatinase-associated lipocalin as a biomarker of acute kidney injury: a critical evaluation of current status. Ann Clin Biochem 2014;51(Pt 3):335–51.

50. Zhou F, Luo Q, Wang L, et al. Diagnostic value of neutrophil gelatinase-associated lipocalin for early diagnosis of cardiac surgery-associated acute kidney injury: a meta-analysis. Eur J Cardiothorac Surg 2016;49(3):746–55.

51. McIlroy DR, Wagener G, Lee HT. Neutrophil gelatinase-associated lipocalin and acute kidney injury after cardiac surgery: the effect of baseline renal function on diagnostic performance. Clin J Am Soc Nephrol 2010;5(2):211–9.

52. Devarajan P. Review: neutrophil gelatinase-associated lipocalin: a troponin-like biomarker for human acute kidney injury. Nephrology (Carlton) 2010;15(4): 419–28.

53. de Geus HR, Ronco C, Haase M, et al. The cardiac surgery-associated neutrophil gelatinase-associated lipocalin (CSA-NGAL) score: a potential tool to monitor acute tubular damage. J Thorac Cardiovasc Surg 2016;151(6):1476–81.

54. Su LJ, Li YM, Kellum JA, et al. Predictive value of cell cycle arrest biomarkers for cardiac surgery-associated acute kidney injury: a meta-analysis. Br J Anaesth 2018;121(2):350–7.

55. Wang Y, Zou Z, Jin J, et al. Urinary TIMP-2 and IGFBP7 for the prediction of acute kidney injury following cardiac surgery. BMC Nephrol 2017;18(1):177.

56. Jia HM, Huang LF, Zheng Y, et al. Prognostic value of cell cycle arrest biomarkers in patients at high risk for acute kidney injury: a systematic review and meta-analysis. Nephrology (Carlton) 2017;22(11):831–7.

57. Meersch M, Schmidt C, Van Aken H, et al. Urinary TIMP-2 and IGFBP7 as early biomarkers of acute kidney injury and renal recovery following cardiac surgery. PLoS One 2014;9(3):e93460.

58. Zarbock A, Schmidt C, Van Aken H, et al. Effect of remote ischemic preconditioning on kidney injury among high-risk patients undergoing cardiac surgery: a randomized clinical trial. JAMA 2015;313(21):2133–41.

59. Pilarczyk K, Edayadiyil-Dudasova M, Wendt D, et al. Urinary [TIMP-2]*[IGFBP7] for early prediction of acute kidney injury after coronary artery bypass surgery. Ann Intensive Care 2015;5(1):50.

60. Cummings JJ, Shaw AD, Shi J, et al. Intraoperative prediction of cardiac surgery-associated acute kidney injury using urinary biomarkers of cell cycle arrest. J Thorac Cardiovasc Surg 2019;157(4):1545–53.e5.

61. Wetz AJ, Richardt EM, Wand S, et al. Quantification of urinary TIMP-2 and IGFBP-7: an adequate diagnostic test to predict acute kidney injury after cardiac surgery? Crit Care 2015;19:3.

62. Engelman DT, Crisafi C, Germain M, et al. Utilizing urinary biomarkers to reduce acute kidney injury following cardiac surgery. J Thorac Cardiovasc Surg 2019.

63. Engelman DT, Ali WB, Williams JB, et al. Guidelines for perioperative care in cardiac surgery: enhanced recovery after surgery society recommendations. JAMA Surg 2019;154(8):755–66.

64. Galyfos G, Sianou A, Filis K. Pleiotropic effects of statins in the perioperative setting. Ann Card Anaesth 2017;20(Supplement):S43–8.

65. Layton JB, Kshirsagar AV, Simpson RJ Jr, et al. Effect of statin use on acute kidney injury risk following coronary artery bypass grafting. Am J Cardiol 2013; 111(6):823–8.

66. Putzu A, de Carvalho ESC, de Almeida JP, et al. Perioperative statin therapy in cardiac and non-cardiac surgery: a systematic review and meta-analysis of randomized controlled trials. Ann Intensive Care 2018;8(1):95.

67. He SJ, Liu Q, Li HQ, et al. Role of statins in preventing cardiac surgery-associated acute kidney injury: an updated meta-analysis of randomized controlled trials. Ther Clin Risk Manag 2018;14:475–82.

68. Zangrillo A, Biondi-Zoccai GG, Frati E, et al. Fenoldopam and acute renal failure in cardiac surgery: a meta-analysis of randomized placebo-controlled trials. J Cardiothorac Vasc Anesth 2012;26(3):407–13.

69. Bove T, Zangrillo A, Guarracino F, et al. Effect of fenoldopam on use of renal replacement therapy among patients with acute kidney injury after cardiac surgery: a randomized clinical trial. JAMA 2014;312(21):2244–53.

70. Yoo YC, Shim JK, Song Y, et al. Anesthetics influence the incidence of acute kidney injury following valvular heart surgery. Kidney Int 2014;86(2):414–22.

71. Cai J, Xu R, Yu X, et al. Volatile anesthetics in preventing acute kidney injury after cardiac surgery: a systematic review and meta-analysis. J Thorac Cardiovasc Surg 2014;148(6):3127–36.

72. Haase-Fielitz A, Haase M, Bellomo R, et al. Perioperative hemodynamic instability and fluid overload are associated with increasing acute kidney injury severity and worse outcome after cardiac surgery. Blood Purif 2017;43(4):298–308.

73. Krajewski ML, Raghunathan K, Paluszkiewicz SM, et al. Meta-analysis of high-versus low-chloride content in perioperative and critical care fluid resuscitation. Br J Surg 2015;102(1):24–36.

74. Young P, Bailey M, Beasley R, et al. Effect of a buffered crystalloid solution vs saline on acute kidney injury among patients in the intensive care unit: the SPLIT randomized clinical trial. JAMA 2015;314(16):1701–10.

75. Joannidis M, Forni LG. Acute kidney injury: buffered crystalloids or saline in the ICU–a SPLIT decision. Nat Rev Nephrol 2016;12(1):6–8.

76. Semler MW, Self WH, Wanderer JP, et al. Balanced crystalloids versus saline in critically ill adults. N Engl J Med 2018;378(9):829–39.

77. Walsh M, Devereaux PJ, Garg AX, et al. Relationship between intraoperative mean arterial pressure and clinical outcomes after noncardiac surgery: toward an empirical definition of hypotension. Anesthesiology 2013;119(3):507–15.

78. van den Berghe G, Wouters P, Weekers F, et al. Intensive insulin therapy in critically ill patients. N Engl J Med 2001;345(19):1359–67.

79. Gandhi GY, Nuttall GA, Abel MD, et al. Intensive intraoperative insulin therapy versus conventional glucose management during cardiac surgery: a randomized trial. Ann Intern Med 2007;146(4):233–43.

80. Bhamidipati CM, LaPar DJ, Stukenborg GJ, et al. Superiority of moderate control of hyperglycemia to tight control in patients undergoing coronary artery bypass grafting. J Thorac Cardiovasc Surg 2011;141(2):543–51.

81. Meersch M, Schmidt C, Hoffmeier A, et al. Prevention of cardiac surgery-associated AKI by implementing the KDIGO guidelines in high risk patients identified by biomarkers: the PrevAKI randomized controlled trial. Intensive Care Med 2017;43(11):1551–61.

82. Jaeschke H. Mechanisms of Liver Injury. II. Mechanisms of neutrophil-induced liver cell injury during hepatic ischemia-reperfusion and other acute inflammatory conditions. Am J Physiol Gastrointest Liver Physiol 2006;290(6):G1083–8.

83. Zimmerman RF, Ezeanuna PU, Kane JC, et al. Ischemic preconditioning at a remote site prevents acute kidney injury in patients following cardiac surgery. Kidney Int 2011;80(8):861–7.

84. Meybohm P, Bein B, Brosteanu O, et al. A multicenter trial of remote ischemic preconditioning for heart surgery. N Engl J Med 2015;373(15):1397–407.

85. Hausenloy DJ, Candilio L, Evans R, et al. Remote ischemic preconditioning and outcomes of cardiac surgery. N Engl J Med 2015;373(15):1408–17.

86. Kottenberg E, Thielmann M, Bergmann L, et al. Protection by remote ischemic preconditioning during coronary artery bypass graft surgery with isoflurane but not propofol - a clinical trial. Acta Anaesthesiol Scand 2012;56(1):30–8.

87. Hu J, Liu S, Jia P, et al. Protection of remote ischemic preconditioning against acute kidney injury: a systematic review and meta-analysis. Crit Care 2016;20(1):111.

88. Zhou H, Yang L, Wang G, et al. Remote ischemic preconditioning prevents postoperative acute kidney injury after open total aortic arch replacement: a double-blind, randomized, sham-controlled trial. Anesth Analg 2019;129(1):287–93.

89. Zarbock A, Kellum JA, Schmidt C, et al. Effect of early vs delayed initiation of renal replacement therapy on mortality in critically ill patients with acute

kidney injury: the ELAIN randomized clinical trial. JAMA 2016;315(20):2190–9.

90. Gaudry S, Hajage D, Dreyfuss D. Initiation of renal-replacement therapy in the intensive care unit. N Engl J Med 2016;375(19):1901–2.

91. Barbar SD, Clere-Jehl R, Bourredjem A, et al. Timing of renal-replacement therapy in patients with acute kidney injury and sepsis. N Engl J Med 2018;379(15):1431–42.

Section 2: New Developments in Cardiopulmonary Resuscitation

Preface

Implications of Cardiac Arrest and Resuscitation for Critical Care Medicine

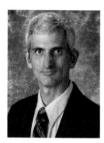

Clifton W. Callaway, MD, PhD
Editor

Cardiopulmonary resuscitation (CPR) has a history spanning hundreds of years. Modern attempts to restore function and to promote recovery for people who appeared to be dead developed directly from the artificial breathing techniques pioneered by European humane societies that were devoted to the rescue of drowned persons in the eighteenth century. Development of electrical defibrillation in the early twentieth century and rediscovery of chest compressions to sustain blood flow in the mid-twentieth century resulted in the CPR that we practice today.

Developments in CPR stimulated many practices that define critical care medicine. These include artificial airways, artificial breathing, circulatory support, electrical therapy for the heart, and pharmacologic support of the cardiovascular system. Over time, we learned how to support other organ systems and refined the interventions used originally for "people who appeared dead." Combined with the huge advances in perioperative medicine and anesthesia during the twentieth century, multiple organ support resulted in critical care medicine as a practice to support people through situations that would otherwise progress to death. Modern practice focuses on earlier intervention, preventing progression, and optimizing the chances for patients to heal.

In the first 2 decades of the twenty-first century, critical care medicine has refined CPR. Technical advances in airway management and cardiopulmonary support provide more options for restoring oxygen delivery. Experience has demonstrated that vasopressor drugs have both positive and negative effects. Cardiology has identified many of the root causes of sudden cardiovascular collapse and developed approaches to support freshly injured hearts. Finally, practitioners of CPR have recognized that we must individualize resuscitation therapies for different patients based on their underlying disease process.

Crit Care Clin 36 (2020) xix–xx
https://doi.org/10.1016/j.ccc.2020.07.011
0749-0704/20/© 2020 Published by Elsevier Inc.

In this issue of *Critical Care Clinics*, the authors describe the current status of CPR and resuscitation. Randomized clinical trials that required decades to develop and complete have provided higher-quality evidence about airway management, pharmacotherapy, and mechanical cardiovascular support. The epidemiology of cardiac arrest has also evolved. Respiratory failure is more common in the hospital, and respiratory failure from opioid overdose became a major public health problem. Two articles in this issue explore how resuscitation may change for these patients.

These clinical overviews represent a snapshot in a long history of advances in resuscitation. It is important to recognize how CPR and resuscitation do not only benefit "people who appeared dead." CPR and resuscitation advances inform care for all patients who may require critical care or organ support. We can hope that as we continue to push the envelope of support for these most severe patients, new knowledge will benefit and allow recovery for all people who would otherwise progress to death.

Clifton W. Callaway, MD, PhD
University of Pittsburgh School of Medicine
University of Pittsburgh
400A Iroquois
3600 Forbes Avenue
Pittsburgh, PA 15260, USA

E-mail address:
callawaycw@upmc.edu

Optimal Airway Management in Cardiac Arrest

Jestin N. Carlson, MD, MS[a],*, Henry E. Wang, MD, MS[b]

KEYWORDS

- Cardiopulmonary arrest • Airway management • Intubation (intratracheal)
- Supraglottic airway • Bag-valve mask

KEY POINTS

- Bag-valve mask ventilation is associated with improved outcomes compared with endotracheal intubation in retrospectives studies; however, prospective trials are inconclusive.
- When performing bag-valve mask ventilation, utilize a 2-hand technique to improve the seal and ventilation.
- Two large randomized controlled trials in the prehospital setting suggest that supraglottic airways are at least as effective as endotracheal intubation in out-of-hospital cardiac arrest.
- Endotracheal intubation should not be prioritized during the first 15 minutes of the resuscitation for in-hospital cardiac arrest over other interventions (eg, high-quality chest compressions).
- Hyperventilation may have a negative impact on patients and providers should avoid hyperventilation in patients with cardiac arrest.

INTRODUCTION

Airway management is a key component in the resuscitation of critically ill patients. Although historically airway management was the initial step in resuscitation (airway-breathing-circulation), a better understanding of the potential pitfalls associated with airway management at the expense of other aspects of resuscitation (eg, circulation) has helped to refine understanding of the role of airway management in cardiac arrest. Several recent studies have helped to further advance knowledge of how to optimally manage the airway during cardiac arrest.

Financial support and sponsorship: J.N. Carlson and H.E. Wang are supported by UH2-HL125163 from the National Heart, Lung, and Blood Institute (NHLBI) for the Pragmatic Airway Resuscitation Trial.
Conflicts of interest: J.N. Carlson and H.E. Wang are investigators of the Pragmatic Airway Resuscitation Trial.
a Department of Emergency Medicine, Saint Vincent Hospital, Allegheny Health Network, 232 West 25th Street, Erie, PA 16544, USA; b Department of Emergency Medicine, The University of Texas Health Science Center at Houston, 64312 Fannin Street, JJL 434, Houston, TX 77030, USA
* Corresponding author.
E-mail address: jcarlson@ahn-emp.com

Although several recent trials have been published, most data come from retrospective analyses. In addition, multiple endpoints in these studies include return of spontaneous circulation (ROSC), survival to hospital admission, 72-hour survival, survival to hospital discharge, and favorable neurologic status at discharge. As such, the interpretation of these observational studies and their subsequent results requires understanding of the limitations of this methodology.

BAG-VALVE MASK VENTILATION

Multiple methods of managing the airway exist, ranging from bag-valve mask ventilation (BVM) to supraglottic airways (SGAs) to endotracheal intubation (ETI). Although ETI often is considered the gold standard for airway management, recent studies question the benefit of ETI in patients in cardiac arrest. Previous work in the prehospital setting reveals frequent and prolonged breaks in chest compressions for ETI.[1] In addition, intubation is a complex skill with more than 100 subtasks and requires significant initial training and ongoing skill practice to maintain proficiency.[2] Given the complexity of ETI and potential detrimental effects of interrupting chest compressions, some experts advocate for less invasive strategies, such as BVM. A previous systematic review suggested that patient outcomes were improved when providers used BVM rather than advanced airway management strategies (SGA or ETI).[3] This review has a major limitation in that the majority of the data came from a single, retrospective study.[4]

CARDIAC ARREST AIRWAY MANAGEMENT TRIAL

Given the equipoise regarding BVM-only in cardiac arrest, a group in France and Belgium conducted the Cardiac Arrest Airway Management (CAAM) trial.[5] The CAAM trial was a noninferiority, prospective randomized clinical trial comparing BVM and ETI placed by prehospital physicians in adult out-of-hospital cardiac arrest (OHCA). The primary outcome was favorable neurologic function at 28 days. A total of 2043 patients were enrolled, 1020 randomly assigned to BVM and 1023 randomly assigned to ETI. Favorable neurologic function at 28 days was similar between BVM (4.3%) and ETI (4.2%) (difference 0.11%; 1-sided 97.5% CI [−1.64% to infinity]). Complications occurred more frequently, however, in the BVM group, including higher rates of ventilation failure (BVM 6.7%; ETI 2.1%) and regurgitation of gastric contents (BVM 15.2%; ETI 7.5%). Given these results, the investigators were unable to conclude noninferiority of BVM relative to ETI.

BAG-VALVE MASK PERFORMANCE

One key challenge with BVM is ensuring an adequate seal around the face, especially in patients who are edentulous or who have facial trauma or facial hair. Although the traditional E-C technique is taught, where by the third, fourth, and fifth digits of a provider's hand form an E shape to lift the mandible while the thumb and index finger form a C shape around the mask, this technique can be challenging. The other hand then squeezes the bag to deliver the ventilations. The E-C technique is a 1-person technique, although 2-person techniques are preferable because they help ensure a more adequate seal and provide larger tidal volumes.[6] When 2 providers are available, 1 provider may seal the mask by using the E-C approach with each hand while the other squeezes the bag to deliver the ventilations. In an alternative 2-person technique, the provider places the thenar eminence and thumb of each hand on the mask and the second through fifth digits grasp the mandible to help lift the jaw.

Both 2-handed techniques provide similar tidal volumes.[6] Finally, a positive end-expiratory pressure (PEEP) valve may be attached to the reservoir port of the bag to help maintain PEEP and to allow for better oxygenation and ventilation while performing BVM ventilations. Adequate oxygenation and ventilation with a BVM require a good face mask seal, which may be difficult in patients with facial trauma, facial hair, or anatomic anomalies or in those who are edentulous.[7]

SUPRAGLOTTIC AIRWAYS

SGAs, including the King LT (Ambu, Copenhagen, Denmark) and i-gel (Intersurgical, Wokingham, Berkshire, United Kingdom), have been suggested as primary airway management strategy in cardiac arrest because they can successfully be placed rapidly and potentially reduce interrupts in chest compressions.[8,9] These benefits have led some investigators to believe that SGAs may be associated with improved outcomes in cardiac arrest; however, previous retrospective studies found associations between SGAs use and improved patient outcomes compared with ETI in OHCA.[10,11] In a meta-analysis by Benoit and colleagues,[11] examining 10 retrospective studies with a total of 34,533 ETI patients and 41,116 SGA patients, outcomes were improved with SGA for ROSC (odds ratio [OR] 1.28; 95% CI, −1.05–1.55), survival to hospital admission (OR 1.34; 95% CI, 1.03–1.75), and neurologically intact survival (OR 1.33; 95% CI, 1.09–1.61). These retrospective studies suffered from confounding by indication, a form of bias whereby the type of intervention that a patient receives is related to measurable or unmeasurable reasons that are direct influences on outcome. For example, a patient who the provider believes has a better chance of survival (eg, a witnessed OHCA where the patient was shocked once and regains ROSC) may receive ETI whereas another patient (a patient with an unwitnessed arrest found in asystole) may receive an SGA. The only way to overcome this bias is by performing a randomized controlled trial (RCT). Two recent RCTs were published comparing SGAs and ETI in OHCA.

PRAGMATIC AIRWAY RESUSCITATION TRIAL

The Pragmatic Airway Resuscitation Trial (PART) was a prospective, multicenter, cluster-randomized, crossover trial comparing 72-hour survival in adult OHCA patients treated with either laryngeal tube (LT) (King LT) or ETI placed by emergency medical services (EMS) providers.[12,13] The primary outcomes was survival at 72 hours. A total of 3004 patients were enrolled, 1505 randomly assigned to LT and 1499 randomly assigned to ETI. Survival at 72 hours was higher in the LT (18.3%) than ETI (15.4%) group (adjusted difference 3.6%; 95% CI, 0.3%–6.8%). Similar results were seen in secondary outcomes (ROSC, survival to hospital discharge, and favorable neurologic status at discharge). One important element of PART was the first-attempt success rate of the airway strategies: 51% for ETI compared with 90.6% for LT. These results were consistent in a subsequent post hoc bayesian analysis of these data.[14]

AIRWAYS-2

A second multicenter RCT, Airways-2, compared favorable functional outcome at either hospital discharge or 30-days between adult OHCA patients treated with either paramedic placed i-gel or ETI.[15] Airways-2 enrolled a total of 9296 patients; 4886 i-gel and 4410 ETI. Patients treated with the i-gel had similar rates of favorable function outcome (i-gel 6.4%; ETI 6.8%; adjusted risk difference (RD) −0.6%; 95% CI, −1.6%–0.4%). In the per protocol analysis, however, patients treated with the i-gel had better functional status (i-gel 3.9%; ETI 2.6%; adjusted RD 1.4%; 95% CI, 0.5%–2.2%).

Although these studies focus on cardiac arrest in the out-of-hospital setting, several themes are present. Previous retrospective analyses found an association between ETI and improved outcomes.[10,11] This was not noted in either of the 2 large RCTs or in a subsequent meta-analysis of these RCTs.[16] Both in the primary analysis of PART, a subsequent bayesian, and the per protocol analysis of Airways-2, however, SGA use was associated with improved patient outcomes.[13–15] Although only a single trial has demonstrated superiority of SGA over ETI in OHCA, both trials suggest that there is no clear benefit of ETI over SGA and providers should feel comfortable utilizing either strategy in OHCA patients as long as that strategy does not interfere with other aspects of the resuscitation.

ENDOTRACHEAL INTUBATION

ETI long has been considered the preferred airway management strategy in cardiac arrest although there are several questions surrounding the timing of ETI, ideal technique, importance of procedural success, and training issues surrounding proficiency and skill maintenance with ETI.

Andersen and colleagues[17] performed a retrospective, propensity-matched study examining the impact of ETI and timing of ETI during in-hospital cardiac arrest patients utilizing a large database. They identified 108,079 adult patients who suffered an in-hospital cardiac arrest and compared outcomes between those who received ETI within the first 15 minutes of the resuscitation and those who had not received ETI by that same time interval. Outcomes were worse for patients who were intubated within the first 15 minutes, including survival (16.3% vs 19.4%, respectively; risk ratio [RR] 0.84; 95% CI, 0.81–0.87; $P < .001$), ROSC (57.8% vs 59.3%, respectively; RR 0.97; 95% CI, 0.96–0.99; $P < .001$), and good functional outcome (10.6% vs 13.6%, respectively; RR 0.78; 95% CI, 0.75–0.81; $P < .001$). Results were similar after adjusting for all prespecified subgroups (initial rhythm [shockable vs nonshockable], timing of the matching, illness category, preceding respiratory insufficiency and location within the hospital). These results suggest that early intubation is not associated with improved outcomes and may detract from other resuscitative efforts (eg, chest compressions). Although this analysis is limited by its retrospective design, it suggests the potential harms of early ETI.

Additional work in the prehospital setting has identified discordant findings. Izawa and colleagues[18] performed a time-dependent propensity matched retrospective analysis of a large cardiac arrest database comparing patients with advanced airway management. Izawa and colleagues examined the impact of advanced airway management (ETI or SGA) on survival at 1 month or to hospital discharge within 1 month and patients with advanced airways were matched to those without based on time intervals throughout the resuscitation. The analysis was divided based on initial rhythms; shockable (ventricular fibrillation and ventricular tachycardia; n = 16,114 patients) and nonshockable (pulseless electrical activity and asystole; n = 236,042 patients). Overall, advanced airway management was not associated with improved outcomes in patients with shockable rhythms (adjusted RR [ARR] 1; 95% CI, 0.93–1.07) but was associated with improved outcomes in the nonshockable cohort (ARR 1.27; 1.2–1.35).[18] These data suggest that the impact of advanced airway management on patient outcomes may be more dependent on the initial rhythm (and potentially the underlying etiology of the cardiac arrest) and less on when they are placed during the resuscitation. Additional research is needed in this area to better understanding the ideal timing of airway management strategies in cardiac arrest.

FIRST-ATTEMPT SUCCESS

ETI is a complicated procedure and previous work has shown complications when attempted during cardiac arrest.[19,20] The number of complications increases with the number of attempts required to secure the airway, highlighting the importance of first-attempt success.[21] Using a national EMS database, Jarvis and colleagues[22] identified that 4 attempts were required to obtain a success plateau of 91.5% (95% CI, 91.2%–91.9%) with a first-attempt success of 71.4% (95% CI, 70.9%–71.9%). Although these numbers come from paramedics in the prehospital setting, similar first-pass success rates are seen in emergency physicians (70%) based on large prospective study enrolling 3360 cardiac arrest patients in Japan.[23] Not only have multiple attempts been associated with complications, new data suggest that first-attempt success may be associated with improved outcomes. In a retrospective analysis of OHCA cases, first-attempt success was associated with increased ROSC and 72-hour survival highlighting the importance of maximizing first-attempt success.(Lupton In Press).

INTUBATION SKILL DEVELOPMENT AND MAINTENANCE

Emergent ETI is challenging in due to the undifferentiated nature of the patients, the unique pathology of critically ill patients, and the limited preparation time and resources available in acute settings and in patients with cardiac arrest. Frequent practice may be needed to ensure proficiency with this critical skill, especially in patients in cardiac arrest.[24] ETI in the prehospital setting has been noted to be infrequent with the median annual number of ETIs per year approximately 1; however, until recently, the frequency of ETI in others settings was unknown.[25]

A recent study by Carlson and colleagues[26] examined the frequency of ETI in US emergency department (EDs) using a large database of 135 EDs over 6 years, including 2108 emergency physicians and 53,904 ETIs. The investigators found that ETI performance at the provider level varies widely in any given year (minimum 0 and maximum 109 ETIs) with a median of 10 (interquartile range 5–17) ETIs per year.[26] ETI also is performed infrequently by some ED providers, with approximately 1 in 4 providers performing few than 5 ETIs per year.[26] These numbers represent ETI for all conditions. ETI in the ED is performed less frequently for cardiac arrest. Data from the National Emergency Airway Registry by Brown and colleagues[27] report that only 7% of all ED intubations are performed for cardiac arrest. Extrapolating the data from Brown and colleagues[27] and Carlson and colleagues,[26] if the median number of ETIs per year for practicing emergency physicians is 10 and only 7% of ED ETIs are for patients in cardiac arrest, then many emergency physicians will perform less than 1 ETI for cardiac arrest annually. Recent work has suggested that, given the complexities of ETI in cardiac arrest, more than 240 ETIs attempts may be needed to attain a first-attempt success rate over 90%.[28] Providers may require ongoing training and practice to maintain proficiency with ETI in cardiac arrest as clinical practice alone may not provide enough opportunities to maintain this critical skill.

ADJUNCTS FOR INTUBATION
Video Laryngoscopy

Given the complexities with direct laryngoscopy (DL), several studies examined the utility of video laryngoscopy (VL) in patients in cardiac arrest. VL offers several potential advantages over DL, including improved glottis views and more rapid learning curve.

Emergency department video laryngoscopy

Okamoto and colleagues[23] examined the first-attempt success rates between VL and DL in a prospectively collected database of ED providers in Japan. The investigators identified 3360 patients in cardiac arrest who underwent ETI and identified higher first-attempt success rates in the VL group compared with the DL group (78% vs 70%, respectively; unadjusted OR 1.61 [95% CI, 1.26–2.06]; $P<.001$). These results were consistent after adjusting for multiple potential confounders and within-ED clustering and in a propensity score–matched analysis. Although the provider experience ranged greatly in Okamato study, VL also was associated with improved first-attempt success in novice providers along when performing ETI on ED patients in cardiac arrest (VL 91.8% vs DL 55.9%; $P<.001$).[29]

In-hospital video laryngoscopy

VL produces similar results when used during in-hospital cardiac arrest. Lee and colleagues[30] performed a prospective, observational study comparing first-attempt success in DL and VL. They report data on 229 patients, with 121 DL and with 108 VL. First-attempt success was higher with VL compared with DL (71.9% vs 52.8%, respectively; $P = .003$). In their multivariate model, predicted difficult airway, operator experience, and use of VL were independently associated with first-attempt success.

Prehospital Video laryngoscopy

Although VL is associated with improved odds of first attempt in multiple ED and in-hospital studies, results in the prehospital setting are mixed.[31] A systematic review, including 8 studies, suggested improvement in first-attempt success with VL in "nonphysician providers with less experience with DL" but no improvement in the performance of experienced physicians.[31] A recent prospective, randomized trial comparing intubation outcomes between DL and VL in adult patients in the out-of-hospital setting has added to this body of evidence.[32] Ducharme and colleagues[32] enrolled 82 patients; with 42 DL and with 40 VL with a majority in cardiac arrest (76/82; 92.6%). Overall, first-attempt success was similar between DL and VL (28/42, 66.7%, vs 25/40, 62.5%, respectively; $P = .69$) Overall success and glottic view as measured by Cormack-Lehane and percentage of glottis opening also were similar between groups.

Gum elastic bougie

Multiple airway adjuncts have been advocated to help improve first-attempt success. One commonly advocated is the gum elastic bougie (or bougie). Previously, the majority of work examining the utility of the bougie relied on retrospective data or data extrapolated from the operating room.[33,34] The recently published Bougie use in Emergency Airway Management (BEAM) trial, by Driver and colleagues,[35] was a randomized clinical trial comparing first-attempt success between bougie-facilitated intubation and intubation with a styletted endotracheal tube. This was performed in a single large urban ED and enrolled all patients greater than or equal to 18 years old undergoing ETI in the ED. Their primary outcome was first-attempt success in patients with at least 1 difficult airway characteristic (large tongue, obesity, facial trauma, and so forth). A total of 757 patients were enrolled, 381 bougie and 376 stylets. For patients with at least 1 difficult airway characteristic, first-attempt success was higher in the bougie group (96% vs 82%, respectively; absolute between-group difference, 14% [95% CI, 8%–20%]). First-attempt success also was higher in the bougie when examining all patients (98% vs 87%, respectively; absolute difference, 11% [95% CI, 7% to 14%]). Other outcomes, including duration of first intubation attempt and hypoxemia, were similar between the bougie and stylet.

Although the BEAM study suggests the bougie results in improved first-attempt success, it is important to remember that the study was performed at a single center where the providers routinely use the bougie.[35] As such, the stylet arm was a common technique in this population of providers. Despite this potential for significant benefits, the bougie is used infrequently for ED intubations (approximately 5%).[27] The results of the BEAM study suggest that the bougie may have a role during primary ETI and not simply reserved as a backup device when traditional ETI is unsuccessful. Given the lower rate of first-attempt success in patients in cardiac arrest; the association between improved first-attempt success and patient outcomes and the improved first-attempt success seen with the bougie in BEAM, providers should consider utilizing the bougie as a first-line device to help facilitate intubation in patients in cardiac arrest.

Hyperventilation

Although much attention has been paid to the device used to secure the airway in patients in cardiac arrest, the ventilation strategies employed after a device is placed also are important. Previous work suggests that hyperventilation in cardiac arrest patients occurs frequently and may have a negative impact on patient outcomes.[36] Hyperventilation is believed to worsen outcomes in myriad different ways, specifically with regards to neurologic outcomes. Hyperventilation increases intrathoracic pressure thereby decreasing mean arterial pressure and increasing jugular venous pressure—both resulting in decreased perfusion to the central nervous system.[37] Hyperventilation also decreases $Paco_2$ that also results in decreased central nervous system perfusion through vasoconstriction.[37]

Many of the theoretically detrimental effects of hyperventilation are believed to have a direct impact on the brain at a time when it is particularly sensitive to injury during and after cardiac arrest. Although large scale trials evaluating hyperventilation in cardiac arrest are lacking, the Excellence in Prehospital Care Study by Spaite and colleagues[38] suggested the potentially beneficial effect of controlled ventilations in patients with severe traumatic brain injury; a population where the brain also is sensitive to the effects of hyperventilation. The EPIC study reports on a before/after state-wide implementation of practice guidelines directing care in patients with traumatic brain injury, including prevention and correction of hyperventilation. Their outcome included survival to hospital discharge (primary) and survival to hospital admission (secondary). During the study period (January 1, 2007, to June 30, 2015), more than 20,000 patients were enrolled from 130 EMS agencies. Although the overall survival to hospital discharge did not differ (adjusted OR [aOR] 1.06; 95% CI, 0.93–1.21), survival was improved in the severely injured and intubated subgroup as measured by 2 different markers of severity (injury severity score 16–24: aOR, 3.28; 95% CI, 1.19–11.34, and regional severity score–head 3–4: aOR, 3.14; 95% CI, 1.65–5.98).[38]

Although previous, small studies suggest that hyperventilation occurs frequently and is associated with worse neurologic outcomes, recent studies question these findings.[36,39,40] In a retrospective analysis of 337 OHCA cases, Vissers and colleagues[39] did not find any association between ventilation rate and patient outcomes (ROSC, survival to hospital discharge, and 1 year neurologically intact survival). In a prospective, observational study of 47 pediatric patients with cardiac arrest in pediatric intensive care units, although hyperventilation was common, increased ventilation rate was associated with improved patient outcomes, including ROSC, survival to hospital discharge, and survival with favorable neurologic outcome in their unadjusted models as well as models adjusting for location of arrest and time of day/day of week.[40]

Given the potential risks of hyperventilation, various approaches have been advocated to control ventilation, including focused training, higher compression-to-ventilation ratios, metronome-guided ventilations, feedback devices, and ventilators.[41] One promising approach is compression-adjusted ventilation whereby ventilations are given based on a specified number of chest compressions (eg, 1 breath per every 12 chest compression). In a simulated model of cardiac arrest conducted by Nikolla and colleagues, emergency medical technicians and firefighters with basic life support training were advised to perform either standard ventilations or compression-adjusted ventilations.[42] The number of ventilations per minute were higher at all time intervals for standard ventilations compared with compression-adjusted ventilations. In addition, hyperventilation (defined as ventilation rates as >10 breaths/minute) occurred 64% of the time in the standard ventilation group compared with 1% of the time in the compression-adjusted ventilation group.[42]

SUMMARY

Airway management is a cornerstone in the resuscitation of critically ill patients, including those in cardiac arrest. Multiple recent trials have helped to better shape understanding of how the airway is managed during cardiac arrest. ETI, once considered the gold standard for airway management in cardiac arrest, is associated with worsened patient outcomes if performed early during in-hospital arrests.[17] Several large, recent prospective randomized trials compare alternatives to ETI, including BVM and SGAs.[5,13,15] These studies suggest that SGAs are at least as effective as ETI and may result in improved outcomes, with lower complication rates in select populations.[13,15] If a decision is made to perform ETI, providers should consider the use of VL, which is associated with improved outcomes in several setting.[23,30] Despite these advances, ETI in cardiac arrest is infrequent at the provider level, and providers should look for additional opportunities to train with and practice this critical skill. There are theoretic risks to hyperventilation and efforts should be made to maintain specific ventilation rates.

REFERENCES

1. Wang HE, Simeone SJ, Weaver MD, et al. Interruptions in cardiopulmonary resuscitation from paramedic endotracheal intubation. Ann Emerg Med 2009;54(5): 645–52.e1.

2. Wang HE, Kupas DF, Greenwood MJ, et al. An algorithmic approach to prehospital airway management. Prehosp Emerg Care 2005;9(2):145–55.

3. Fouche PF, Simpson PM, Bendall J, et al. Airways in out-of-hospital cardiac arrest: systematic review and meta-analysis. Prehosp Emerg Care 2014;18(2): 244–56.

4. Hasegawa K, Hiraide A, Chang Y, et al. Association of prehospital advanced airway management with neurologic outcome and survival in patients with out-of-hospital cardiac arrest. JAMA 2013;309(3):257–66.

5. Jabre P, Penaloza A, Pinero D, et al. Effect of bag-mask ventilation vs endotracheal intubation during cardiopulmonary resuscitation on neurological outcome after out-of-hospital cardiorespiratory arrest: a randomized clinical trial. JAMA 2018;319(8):779–87.

6. Otten D, Liao MM, Wolken R, et al. Comparison of bag-valve-mask hand-sealing techniques in a simulated model. Ann Emerg Med 2014;63(1):6–12.e13.

7. Campbell TP, Stewart RD, Kaplan RM, et al. Oxygen enrichment of bag-valve-mask units during positive-pressure ventilation: a comparison of various techniques. Ann Emerg Med 1988;17(3):232–5.

8. Guyette F, Greenwood MJ, Neubecker D, et al. Alternative airway in the prehospital setting (resource document to NAEMSP position statement). Prehosp Emerg Care 2007;11(1):56–61.

9. Beauchamp G, Phrampus P, Guyette FX. Simulated rescue airway use by laypersons with scripted telephonic instruction. Resuscitation 2009;80(8):925–9.

10. Wang HE, Szydlo D, Stouffer JA, et al. Endotracheal intubation versus supraglottic airway insertion in out-of-hospital cardiac arrest. Resuscitation 2012;83(9): 1061–6.

11. Benoit JL, Gerecht RB, Steuerwald MT, et al. Endotracheal intubation versus supraglottic airway placement in out-of-hospital cardiac arrest: a meta-analysis. Resuscitation 2015;93:20–6.

12. Wang HE, Prince DK, Stephens SW, et al. Design and implementation of the resuscitation outcomes consortium pragmatic airway resuscitation trial (PART). Resuscitation 2016;101:57–64.

13. Wang HE, Schmicker RH, Daya MR, et al. Effect of a strategy of initial laryngeal tube insertion vs endotracheal intubation on 72-hour survival in adults with out-of-hospital cardiac arrest: a randomized clinical trial. JAMA 2018;320(8):769–78.

14. Wang HE, Humbert A, Nichol G, et al. Bayesian analysis of the pragmatic airway resuscitation trial. Ann Emerg Med 2019;74(6):809–17.

15. Benger JR, Kirby K, Black S, et al. Effect of a strategy of a supraglottic airway device vs tracheal intubation during out-of-hospital cardiac arrest on functional outcome: the AIRWAYS-2 randomized clinical trial. JAMA 2018;320(8):779–91.

16. White L, Melhuish T, Holyoak R, et al. Advanced airway management in out of hospital cardiac arrest: a systematic review and meta-analysis. Am J Emerg Med 2018;36(12):2298–306.

17. Andersen LW, Granfeldt A, Callaway CW, et al. Association between tracheal intubation during adult in-hospital cardiac arrest and survival. JAMA 2017;317(5): 494–506.

18. Izawa J, Komukai S, Gibo K, et al. Pre-hospital advanced airway management for adults with out-of-hospital cardiac arrest: nationwide cohort study. BMJ 2019;364: l430.

19. Mort TC. The incidence and risk factors for cardiac arrest during emergency tracheal intubation: a justification for incorporating the ASA Guidelines in the remote location. J Clin Anesth 2004;16(7):508–16.

20. Mort TC. Emergency tracheal intubation: complications associated with repeated laryngoscopic attempts. Anesth Analg 2004;99(2):607–13, table of contents.

21. Sakles JC, Chiu S, Mosier J, et al. The importance of first pass success when performing orotracheal intubation in the emergency department. Acad Emerg Med 2013;20(1):71–8.

22. Jarvis JL, Barton D, Wang H. Defining the plateau point: when are further attempts futile in out-of-hospital advanced airway management? Resuscitation 2018;130:57–60.

23. Okamoto H, Goto T, Wong ZSY, et al. Comparison of video laryngoscopy versus direct laryngoscopy for intubation in emergency department patients with cardiac arrest: a multicentre study. Resuscitation 2019;136:70–7.

24. Kerrey BT, Wang H. Intubation by emergency physicians: how often is enough? Ann Emerg Med 2019;74(6):795–6.

25. Wang HE, Yealy DM. How many attempts are required to accomplish out-of-hospital endotracheal intubation. Acad Emerg Med 2006;13(4):372–7.

26. Carlson JN, Zocchi M, Marsh K, et al. Procedural experience with intubation: results from a national emergency medicine group. Ann Emerg Med 2019;74(6):786–94.

27. Brown CA 3rd, Bair AE, Pallin DJ, et al. Techniques, success, and adverse events of emergency department adult intubations. Ann Emerg Med 2015;65(4):363–70.e1.

28. Kim SY, Park SO, Kim JW, et al. How much experience do rescuers require to achieve successful tracheal intubation during cardiopulmonary resuscitation? Resuscitation 2018;133:187–92.

29. Park SO, Kim JW, Na JH, et al. Video laryngoscopy improves the first-attempt success in endotracheal intubation during cardiopulmonary resuscitation among novice physicians. Resuscitation. 2015;89:188–94.

30. Lee DH, Han M, An JY, et al. Video laryngoscopy versus direct laryngoscopy for tracheal intubation during in-hospital cardiopulmonary resuscitation. Resuscitation 2015;89:195–9.

31. Savino PB, Reichelderfer S, Mercer MP, et al. Direct versus video laryngoscopy for prehospital intubation: a systematic review and meta-analysis. Acad Emerg Med 2017;24(8):1018–26.

32. Ducharme S, Kramer B, Gelbart D, et al. A pilot, prospective, randomized trial of video versus direct laryngoscopy for paramedic endotracheal intubation. Resuscitation 2017;114:121–6.

33. Driver B, Dodd K, Klein LR, et al. The bougie and first-pass success in the emergency department. Ann Emerg Med 2017;70(4):473–8.e1.

34. Tandon N, McCarthy M, Forehand B, et al. Comparison of intubation modalities in a simulated cardiac arrest with uninterrupted chest compressions. Emerg Med J 2013;31(10):799–802.

35. Driver BE, Prekker ME, Klein LR, et al. Effect of use of a bougie vs endotracheal tube and stylet on first-attempt intubation success among patients with difficult airways undergoing emergency intubation: a randomized clinical trial. JAMA 2018;319(21):2179–89.

36. Aufderheide TP, Lurie KG. Death by hyperventilation: a common and life-threatening problem during cardiopulmonary resuscitation. Crit Care Med 2004;32(9 Suppl):S345–51.

37. Gaither JB, Spaite DW, Bobrow BJ, et al. Balancing the potential risks and benefits of out-of-hospital intubation in traumatic brain injury: the intubation/hyperventilation effect. Ann Emerg Med 2012;60(6):732–6.

38. Spaite DW, Bobrow BJ, Keim SM, et al. Association of statewide implementation of the prehospital traumatic brain injury treatment guidelines with patient survival following traumatic brain injury: the excellence in prehospital injury care (EPIC) Study. JAMA Surg 2019;154(7):e191152.

39. Vissers G, Duchatelet C, Huybrechts SA, et al. The effect of ventilation rate on outcome in adults receiving cardiopulmonary resuscitation. Resuscitation 2019;138:243–9.

40. Sutton RM, Reeder RW, Landis WP, et al. Ventilation rates and pediatric in-hospital cardiac arrest survival outcomes. Crit Care Med 2019;47(11):1627–36.

41. Nikolla D, Lewandowski T, Carlson J. Mitigating hyperventilation during cardiopulmonary resuscitation. Am J Emerg Med 2016;34(3):643–6.

42. Nikolla DA, Kramer BJ, Carlson JN. A cross-over trial comparing conventional to compression-adjusted ventilations with metronome-guided compressions. Prehosp Disaster Med 2019;34(2):220–3.

Role of Vasopressors in Cardiac Arrest

Laurie J. Morrison, MD, MSc, FRCPC[a,b]

KEYWORDS

- Cardiac arrest • Sudden cardiac death • Resuscitation • Vasopressors

KEY POINTS

- Epinephrine has been used routinely in cardiac arrest for decades without strong scientific evidence.
- Recent clinical trials and studies indicate that any beneficial effects of epinephrine are small, and there is some risk of restoring cardiac activity in patients who are not able to recover functionally.
- Clinical trials do not support any superiority of higher doses of epinephrine or of alternative drugs such as vasopressin.
- Routine use of epinephrine in cardiac arrest has weak supporting evidence, and use of this drug must be tested in efficacy trials that control for other important factors in resuscitation.

INTRODUCTION

Epinephrine has been administered for decades in efforts to restore circulation during cardiac arrest. The original use of this drug was prompted by its ability to promote return of spontaneous circulation (ROSC) in animals. Subsequent clinical experience confirmed that ROSC is more likely after epinephrine administration. However, there are fewer data about more patient-focused outcomes. Moreover, evidence has accumulated that quality of cardiopulmonary resuscitation (CPR) and peri-CPR clinical care have large effects on patient outcome. However, CPR and periarrest or postarrest care were largely ignored in early clinical testing of vasopressor drugs. This article points out that it is unlikely that there is a role for vasopressors or drugs of any kind given routinely to all adult cardiac arrests where high-quality CPR is performed and postarrest care is guideline compliant. It is likely that the usefulness of vasopressors is under-researched and there is much to be learned by well-designed efficacy studies that control for important resuscitation variables.

[a] Rescu, Li Ka Shing Knowledge Institute, St Michael's Hospital, 30 Bond Street, Toronto, ON M5B 1W8, Canada; [b] Division of Emergency Medicine, Department of Medicine, Faculty of Medicine, University of Toronto, Toronto, ON, Canada
E-mail address: Laurie.Morrison@unityhealth.to

Crit Care Clin 36 (2020) 715–721
https://doi.org/10.1016/j.ccc.2020.07.009
0749-0704/20/© 2020 Elsevier Inc. All rights reserved.

REVIEW OF EVIDENCE

Successful cardiac arrest resuscitation both in hospital and out of hospital depends on timely high-quality CPR and early defibrillation when indicated, and anything that takes the focus away from these important interventions is likely to have a negative impact on outcomes. This point was summarized nicely by Perkins and Deakin[5] (the Paramedic2 investigators) because the number of patients who would need to be treated to prevent 1 death after cardiac arrest was 112 with epinephrine compared with 11 for early recognition of cardiac arrest, 15 for bystander CPR, and only 5 for early defibrillation.

A novel and courageous randomized trial by Olasveengen and colleagues[1] in Norway compared drugs versus no drugs in the management of out-of-hospital cardiac arrest (OHCA). The Norwegian paramedics randomized all adult OHCA to intravenous (IV) or no IV such that only the IV arm received drugs. The team and paramedics services performing the study were the first to measure CPR metrics and are known internationally for the quality and timeliness of CPR. This trial was no exception. CPR quality was high in both cohorts. The survival to hospital discharge rate was consistent across both cohorts as 9.2% (no IV) versus 10.5% (IV). Thus, the lack of any benefit to the IV arm suggests that drug administration is not additive or effective in OHCA when patients are given the drug late and their CPR quality metrics are optimized.

This finding is consistent with the 3-phase model first proposed by Weisfeldt and Becker[2] in 2002. The 3-phase model (**Fig. 1**) suggests that, after 10 minutes of resuscitation, the survival rate is poor, and this is attributed to tissue injury from whole-body ischemia circulating metabolic factors during cell reperfusion that cause additional injury. The investigators question whether this injury is irreversible or whether therapeutic approaches fail to correct important factors in this phase. As an example, vasopressors given late without blood flow generated by optimized CPR metrics may have extensive tissue injury and organ dysfunction and may not generate a response similar to what is seen in the experimental laboratory tests. This premise was partially tested with in-hospital cardiac arrests, where time to drug interval is faster (median time to first dose was 3 minutes, interquartile range of 1–5 minutes). Donnino and colleagues[3] showed a stepwise decrease in survival with 3-minute incremental increases in time to drug; adjusted odds ratio (OR) 1.0 for 1 to 3 minutes as the reference group;

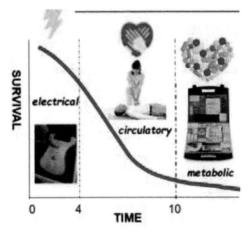

Fig. 1. Three-phase model of survival after cardiac arrest. (*Adapted from* Weisfeldt and Becker Jama 2002.)

0.91 (95% confidence interval [CI], 0.82–1.00; $P = .055$) for 4 to 6 minutes; 0.74 (95% CI, 0.63–0.88; $P<.001$) for 7 to 9 minutes; and 0.63 (95% CI, 0.52–0.76; $P<.001$) for more than 9 minutes. The same relationship was found with time to drug and ROSC, survival at 24 hours, and favorable neurologic status (Cerebral Performance Score of 1 or 2). CPR quality metrics were not reported.

A post hoc analysis of the Norwegian randomized trial data to compare randomized patients who received epinephrine in the intervention arm was unable to show a significant difference in survival to hospital discharge with epinephrine; adjusted for confounders (OR, 0.52; 95% CI, 0.29, 0.92). Similar findings were seen for survival with good neurologic outcome.[4] The survival rate in the no-IV group was 13% and in the epinephrine arm was 7%. As in the primary trial, CPR metrics in both cohorts were rigorously optimized and similar in both groups (**Table 1**).

There are 2 placebo controlled randomized trials (1 in the United Kingdom and 1 in Australia) that showed similar findings when 1 mg of epinephrine was given by protocol every 3 to 5 minutes in adult OHCA.[5,6] Both showed increased rates of ROSC in the epinephrine cohort. Survival at 30 days and at 3 months was significantly higher with epinephrine compared with placebo in the UK trial but the trial was neutral for good neurologic outcome at 30 days. The rate for those surviving with a poor neurologic outcome at 30 days was higher in the epinephrine arm. The survival rate overall in both groups was disappointingly low at 3.2% versus 2.4%. The quality of CPR provided was not optimized prior to the trial nor measured by protocol across all randomized patients in either trial. The time to drug administration was long, with a median of 21 minutes and a range from 16 to 27 minutes in both arms.[5] This time interval for drug administration is comparable with other trials. The Amiodarone Lidocaine Placebo controlled randomized trial reported similar time intervals in North American emergency medical services (EMS) systems.[7]

In both of these trials, the quality of postarrest care was not measured or prescribed as part of the routine care. The postarrest care is challenging to control given the number of institutions and treating physicians involved in the destination hospitals, but not impossible. The Targeted Temperature Management (TTM) trial investigators achieved this consistency in guideline-compliant postarrest care, with in-hospital survival in both arms of the trial of approximately 50% where 20% of patients recruited presented initially with pulseless electrical activity (PEA) or asystole.[8] When postarrest care is not controlled well in the trial, the in-hospital survival rate can be unpredictable or low. In the UK trial, the survival to hospital discharge for patients admitted to hospital was 13.5% for epinephrine and 29% for placebo. In the Australian

Table 1				
Cardiopulmonary resuscitation metric				
CPR Metric	**Measure**	**No Intravenous** **N = 433**	**Intravenous** **N = 418**	**P** **Value**
CPR rate	Mean rate per minute (95% CI)	116 (115, 117)	117 (116, 119)	.12
Hands-off ratio	Median (range)	0.14 (0.01–0.59)	0.15 (0.02–0.89)	.16
Compressions	Mean number per minute (95% CI)	94 (93, 96)	—	—
Ventilations	Mean number per minute (95% CI)	11 (10, 11)	11 (11, 11)	.48
Preshock pause	Median in seconds (range)	11 (1–74)	12 (1–82)	.58

Data from Olasveengen TM, Wik L, Sunde K, et al. Outcome when adrenaline (epinephrine) was actually given vs. not given - post hoc analysis of a randomized clinical trial. Resuscitation 2012;83(3):327-32. Olasveengen TM et al Jama 2009 Vol 302 p 2222-2229 abstracted from Table 1 of this source.

trial, the in-hospital survival for those who survived long enough to be admitted to hospital was 15.9% for epinephrine and 14.7% for placebo.

The UK and Australian OHCA trials recruited dissimilar cohorts in terms of initial rhythm; however, both showed an advantage for restoring circulation with epinephrine. The UK trial recruited 50% PEA or asystole, whereas the Australian trial recruited 20% PEA or asystole. A prespecified subgroup analysis comparing outcomes for shockable versus nonshockable rhythms in the Australian trial suggested a magnitude of effect in favor of epinephrine for the cohort with an initial nonshockable rhythm. OR for ROSC was 2.4 (95% CI, 1.2, 4.5) versus 6.9 (95% CI, 2.6, 18.4) and for admitted to hospital it was 2.2 (95% CI, 1.2, 4.1) versus 2.5 (95% CI,1.3, 4.8).[6] This trial was stopped prematurely secondary to ethical concerns in the press and the involvement of local politicians. As a result, the subgroup sample size is too small to compare for the primary outcome of survival to hospital discharge. In the UK trial, a significant difference in the effect of epinephrine based on initial rhythm and favoring the 2 nonshockable rhythms was observed with ROSC, survival to hospital discharge, and survival at 3 months. A meta-analysis completed in 2019 reported a cumulative OR for survival to hospital discharge in the nonshockable cohort of patients randomized to receive epinephrine of 1% (34 out of 3,302) compared with placebo with 0.4% (13 out of 3,317; relative risk 2.56; 95% CI, 1.37, 4.8). When converted to absolute risk difference, this translated to 6 more patients with a nonshockable rhythm surviving to hospital discharge when given epinephrine compared with those given placebo. This significant difference was not observed in the shockable cohort. The effect of epinephrine seemed to be more pronounced in the nonshockable cohort versus the shockable cohort (*P* value for the interaction was <.01 for ROSC and .04 for survival to hospital discharge) (**Fig. 2**).[9]

As a result of this meta-analysis, the International Liaison Committee on Resuscitation (ILCOR) Advanced Life Support Task Force published a consensus on science (https://www.ilcor.org/) suggesting there was sufficient evidence to recommend epinephrine during cardiac arrest with low to moderate certainty and to recommend epinephrine as soon as feasible during adult cardiac arrest in any setting where the initial rhythm is nonshockable with a very low certainty of evidence. In patients with an initial shockable rhythm, the task force suggested epinephrine be considered if defibrillation attempts are unsuccessful, again with very low certainty of evidence.

Vasopressin alone or in combination with epinephrine was evaluated by randomized trials that date from 1997 until 2011. Every trial was neutral for benefit or harm in cardiac arrest. The same issues identified for the epinephrine versus placebo studies are applicable here: lack of CPR metrics, given late in the resuscitation without protocolized postarrest care. The task force weighed the risk of making the algorithm complex and decided to err on the side of simplicity. Thus the task force suggested against the use of any other vasopressor in cardiac arrest based on a weak recommendation and very low certainty of evidence. A search of (https://www.clinicaltrials.gov/) identified 2 randomized trials comparing vasopressin with or without a steroid in cardiac arrest that are actively recruiting: 1 in Asia and another in Europe.

High-dose epinephrine was evaluated by randomized trials that also predated the emphasis on CPR metrics and postarrest care in communities where the survival rate was low. The 6 articles that address this comparison date from 1992 to 1998. A systematic review published in 2014 reported a cumulative event rate of survival to discharge of 77 in 2779 with standard-dose epinephrine cohort and 78 in 2859 for the higher-dose epinephrine cohort.[10] The meta-analysis was indeterminate for the

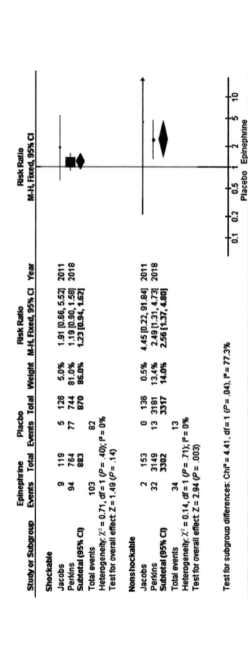

Fig. 2. Survival to hospital discharge stratified by initial rhythm. Pooled estimates for controlled trials of epinephrine compared with placebo stratified by initial rhythm. Pooled estimates for ROSC stratified by shockable and nonshockable rhythms. Horizontal lines indicate 95% confidence intervals (CIs) of the estimate. The studies are ordered by year of publication within each analysis. df, degrees of freedom; M-H, Mantel-Haenszel analysis. (*Adapted from* Holmberg MJ, Issa MS, Moskowitz A, et al. Vasopressors during adult cardiac arrest: A systematic review and meta-analysis. Resuscitation 2019;139:106-21; with permission.)

critical outcomes of survival to discharge and neurologic function at discharge. Standard-dose epinephrine had lower rates of ROSC (RR, 2.80; 95% CI, 1.78, 4.41; P<.00001) and survival to hospital admission (RR, 1.95; 95% CI, 1.34–2.84; P = .0004) compared with higher-dose epinephrine. ILCOR summarized these trials and some observational data in 2015 to derive a consensus that high-dose epinephrine should not be used. This recommendation will not be revisited unless there are new randomized trials on dosage.

The lack of evidence for the use of epinephrine in cardiac arrest is profound for a drug that is used every day in resuscitations all over the world. Given its legacy of use, the Norwegian, UK, and Australian investigator teams had tremendous courage to randomize patients to placebo. This was admirable as it enabled the science and refined the treatment recommendations based on more evidence than prior versions. However, the certainty of evidence is at best moderate, most recommendations are weak, and there is still community equipoise for how to use epinephrine in cardiac arrests.

An experimental study conducted at the University of Pennsylvania by Sutton and colleagues[11] suggested the approach to cardiac arrest should move away from guideline-based medicine to a guided approach based on physiologic metrics. Cardiac arrest resuscitation needs to move to patient-specific care. When a patient arrests in the intensive care unit, with various invasive measures at the bedside, this presents an opportunity to directly and indirectly measure blood flow and brain oxygenation in order to identify who is a vasopressor responder, to guide the timing and the dosage of epinephrine, and to adjust the quality of the CPR. Together with optimized postarrest care, there is the opportunity to measure efficacy under well-controlled circumstances rather than continuing to conduct pragmatic trials routinely giving the drug without focusing on other interventions that are known to improve survival with a low number needed to treat. Teasing out which patients will benefit from epinephrine using a bedside metric translatable to the prehospital environment, and at what dose, and given at what time are the questions for future trials.

SUMMARY

The current interpretation of the evidence by ILCOR may be too generous. Epinephrine is effective at improving clinical outcomes of ROSC, admission to hospital, discharge from hospital, alive at 30 days, and alive at 3 months in patients who are treated by EMS services, with low survival rates after OHCA and unmeasured CPR metrics that routinely give the drug at least 20 minutes after arrest and patients are transported to hospitals where the quality and consistency of evidence-based postarrest care is unknown. However, the downside of generic use of the drug in these pragmatic or nonoptimized settings is that the proportion of patients surviving with a poor neurologic function at 30 days may be higher with epinephrine. In contrast, in settings where the quality of CPR and postarrest care are optimized, the additive effect of epinephrine may not be significant, as was seen in the Norwegian trial. This same evidence could argue against the routine use of epinephrine.

Alternatively, perhaps the detrimental effects of epinephrine on neurologic function are not present for in-hospital cardiac arrest or out-of-hospital patients with good CPR sustained throughout the resuscitation. In these settings, perhaps early drug administration of a small dose of epinephrine will start the heart and encourage ROSC. More courage is needed to take on these important scientific questions and advance the evidence for vasopressor drugs through well-designed efficacy trials.

ACKNOWLEDGMENTS

Dr Morrison currently holds peer reviewed operating grants from the Canadian Institute of Health Research evaluating the the use of epinephrine and naloxone in cardiac arrest.

REFERENCES

1. Olasveengen TM, Sunde K, Brunborg C, et al. Intravenous drug administration during out-of-hospital cardiac arrest: a randomized trial. JAMA 2009;302(20): 2222–9.
2. Weisfeldt ML, Becker LB. Resuscitation after cardiac arrest: a 3-phase time-sensitive model. JAMA 2002;288(23):3035–8.
3. Donnino MW, Salciccioli JD, Howell MD, et al. Time to administration of epinephrine and outcome after in-hospital cardiac arrest with non-shockable rhythms: retrospective analysis of large in-hospital data registry. BMJ 2014;348:g3028.
4. Olasveengen TM, Wik L, Sunde K, et al. Outcome when adrenaline (epinephrine) was actually given vs. not given - post hoc analysis of a randomized clinical trial. Resuscitation 2012;83(3):327–32.
5. Perkins GD, Ji C, Deakin CD, et al. A randomized trial of epinephrine in out-of-hospital cardiac arrest. N Engl J Med 2018;379(8):711–21.
6. Jacobs IG, Finn JC, Jelinek GA, et al. Effect of adrenaline on survival in out-of-hospital cardiac arrest: a randomised double-blind placebo-controlled trial. Resuscitation 2011;82(9):1138–43.
7. Kudenchuk PJ, Brown SP, Daya M, et al. Amiodarone, lidocaine, or placebo in out-of-hospital cardiac arrest. N Engl J Med 2016;374(18):1711–22.
8. Nielsen N, Wetterslev J, Cronberg T, et al. Targeted temperature management at 33 degrees C versus 36 degrees C after cardiac arrest. N Engl J Med 2013; 369(23):2197–206.
9. Holmberg MJ, Issa MS, Moskowitz A, et al. Vasopressors during adult cardiac arrest: a systematic review and meta-analysis. Resuscitation 2019;139:106–21.
10. Lin S, Callaway CW, Shah PS, et al. Adrenaline for out-of-hospital cardiac arrest resuscitation: a systematic review and meta-analysis of randomized controlled trials. Resuscitation 2014;85(6):732–40.
11. Sutton RM, Friess SH, Naim MY, et al. Patient-centric blood pressure-targeted cardiopulmonary resuscitation improves survival from cardiac arrest. Am J Respir Crit Care Med 2014;190(11):1255–62.

Current Work in Extracorporeal Cardiopulmonary Resuscitation

Scott T. Youngquist, MD, MS[a,*], Joseph L. Tonna, MD[a,b],
Jason A. Bartos, MD, PhD[c,d], Michael Austin Johnson, MD, PhD[a],
Guillaume L. Hoareau, PhD[a], Alice Hutin, MD, PhD[e],
Lionel Lamhaut, MD, PhD[e]

KEYWORDS

- Extracorporeal pulmonary resuscitation • Extracorporeal membrane oxygenation
- Cardiac arrest

KEY POINTS

- ECPR holds tremendous promise as a rescue therapy for refractory cardiac arrest. The last decade has seen a rapid rise in programs to treat out-of-hospital cardiac arrest patients.
- As time from collapse to cannulation is one of the most important prognostic factors for neurologic survival, logistical hurdles remain an important consideration of the approach.
- Areas of active research include the optimal location of cannulation (prehospital vs hospital), the training required to achieve proficiency, the optimal initial ECMO settings, and adjunctive critical care.

INTRODUCTION

For over 50 years, cardiopulmonary resuscitation (CPR) has consisted primarily of 2 treatments: rhythmically compressing the patient's chest to circulate blood and rapidly defibrillating those with a shockable rhythm (ie, ventricular fibrillation or pulseless ventricular tachycardia). Despite process and system improvements, these 2 therapies have led to only modest increases in survival in out-of-hospital cardiac arrest (OHCA) in recent years.[1–6] However, even when good CPR and early defibrillation are available, for most cardiac arrest victims, the results are the same: death or severe disability after 80% to 90% of resuscitation attempts. The highest cardiac arrest

[a] Division of Emergency Medicine, University of Utah School of Medicine, 30 North 1900 East, Room 1C26 SOM, Salt Lake City, UT 84132, USA; [b] Division of Cardiothoracic Surgery, University of Utah, Salt Lake City, UT, USA; [c] Cardiovascular Division, University of Minnesota, 420 Delaware Street SE, MMC 508 Mayo, 8508A, Minneapolis, MN 55455, USA; [d] Center for Resuscitation Medicine, Minneapolis, MN, USA; [e] SAMU de Paris, Necker Hospital, 149 Rue de Sevres, Paris 75015, France
* Corresponding author. 30 North 1900 East, Room 1C26 SOM, Salt Lake City, UT 84132.
E-mail address: scott.youngquist@utah.edu

Crit Care Clin 36 (2020) 723–735
https://doi.org/10.1016/j.ccc.2020.07.004
0749-0704/20/© 2020 Elsevier Inc. All rights reserved.

survival is achieved by a category of patients with a bystander-witnessed arrest and an initial shockable rhythm (31%), although overall survival to discharge in the United States for all comers is only 8%.[7]

Closed chest compressions are often insufficient to stop the march of global ischemia. Estimates of blood flow achieved by chest compressions under laboratory conditions are 15% to 25% of native flow.[8,9] Moreover, in a dog model of cardiac arrest, when CPR was delayed for as little as 6 minutes after arrest, the blood flow to the brain during chest compressions was below the ischemic threshold needed to maintain cerebral metabolism.[10] CPR is also often the author of its own therapeutic demise: rib and sternal fractures from CPR lead to loss of chest wall integrity and a decline in CPR efficacy as the thoracic recoil contribution to blood flow is diminished or lost. Hypoxic vasoconstriction of pulmonary arteries and the loss of arterial vasomotor tone as adrenergic tachyphylaxis sets in can further reduce effective blood flow. The sum of these physiologic limitations is a rapid decrease in the probability of survival over time, as demonstrated in large observational cohorts that account for resuscitation duration.[11,12] CPR is thus, in most cases, an insufficient and time-limited treatment for cardiac arrest with a narrow therapeutic window. Ultimately, the objective of CPR is not only to obtain return of spontaneous circulation (ROSC) but also to provide sufficient organ perfusion, especially to the brain, to preserve function until circulation can be durably restored. The main patient-oriented endpoint is not ROSC but neurologically intact survival.

Mechanical circulatory support has been used for decades for the temporary perioperative support of patients undergoing cardiothoracic surgery, and, more recently, for the treatment of severe chronic heart failure with advances in device technology. One of these technologies, extracorporeal membrane oxygenation (ECMO), has become a paradigm-changing intervention that can be implemented on an emergency basis following recent reductions in relative cost along with design improvements, coupled with new, cross-disciplinary collaborations.[13] ECMO offers an appealing rescue (or second-line) therapy for select patients who do not respond to initial CPR attempts, because it produces physiologic (and even supraphysiologic) levels of blood flow, organ perfusion, and oxygen delivery. Extracorporeal cardiopulmonary resuscitation (ECPR) is the term used to denote the deployment of ECMO in the treatment of cardiac arrest. ECMO works by withdrawing venous blood from the central circulation via a percutaneous cannula, passing it through a pump and an oxygenator, and then returning oxygenated blood under pressure to the distal aorta through a return cannula (**Fig. 1**). ECPR can provide full cardiopulmonary support (replacing the function of the heart and lungs) without the physical trauma of prolonged external chest compressions. In theory, initiation of ECPR terminates ongoing ischemia and provides adequate end-organ perfusion, which allows time to evaluate and treat the underlying cause of cardiac arrest. Coronary artery disease accounts for approximately 80% of cases of refractory cardiac arrest in which the presenting rhythm is shockable.[14,15] Often in refractory cases, coronary occlusion is proximal and affects multiple vessels.[16] In this scenario, ECPR takes over the work of the arrested heart to perfuse vital organs until coronary revascularization, and, ultimately, native cardiac output can be restored. Conceptually, however, ECPR could be used to treat any reversible cause of cardiac arrest, such as pulmonary embolism, overdose, and hypothermia.

In addition to refractory cardiac arrest, approximately 18% of patients who obtain ROSC with standard ACLS will ultimately rearrest,[17] and approximately 50% will exhibit hypotension in the postarrest period.[18] Both of these events portend a worse outcome despite achievement of sustained ROSC. Moreover, patients who experience ROSC at any time, even if they subsequently become unstable, exhibit a level

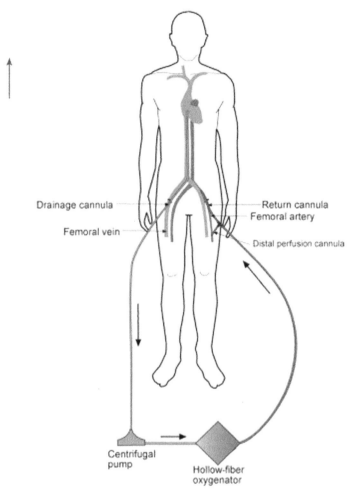

Fig. 1. ECMO diagram. (*From* Sidebotham A, McGeorge A, McGuinness S, et al. Extracorporeal Membrane Oxygenation for Treating Severe Cardiac and Respiratory Failure in Adults: Part 2 – Technical Considerations. Journal of Cardiothoracic and Vascular Anesthesia. 2010;24(1): p.164-172; with permission. (Figure 1 in original).)

of physiologic responsiveness that indicates survivability.[15,19,20] Thus, ECPR and ECMO may also be considered as support for patients who have achieved ROSC but are hemodynamically unstable. However, this post-ROSC ECMO remains to be studied and compared with ECPR.

CURRENT EVIDENCE SUGGESTING EXTRACORPOREAL PULMONARY RESUSCITATION IMPROVES SURVIVAL AND STRENGTH OF EVIDENCE

Most, but not all, case series of ECPR demonstrate higher survival than matched controls when accounting for duration of CPR.[21–25] These observational studies of ECPR demonstrate a wide range of survival from 10% to 45%,[20,22,26–28] suggesting that patient selection is an important determinant of outcome. However, variations in technique and critical care remain understudied. In larger meta-analyses, improved survival is associated with ECPR compared with conventional CPR among patients with in-hospital cardiac arrest (IHCA).[29,30] A recent large registry study of IHCA in the United States demonstrated highly selective use of ECPR. Even after multivariate case-mix adjustment, patients who received ECPR remained profoundly different than non-ECPR treated patients in terms of clinical characteristics such as age and pre-existing comorbidities (Tonna, private communication, 2019). In 2 propensity-matched studies of ECPR, most patients could not be matched because of their char-acteristic differences.[22,31]

Duration of CPR prior to ROSC is inversely associated with survival for conventional CPR,[32,33] so the observed survival advantage for IHCA ECPR, compared to OHCA, may reflect shorter durations of CPR until ECMO initiation. Indeed, shorter durations of CPR before ECMO initiation, and the correlate of lower markers of ischemia (such as lactate), are associated with improved survival for both in-hospital and OHCA among patients treated with ECPR.[34–36]

Randomized trials to overcome this selection bias have been completed or are un-derway in the Czech Republic, France, and in the United States.

SELECTED PROGRAM DEVELOPMENT AROUND THE WORLD
United States

The first cases of ECPR use were published in the 1970s[37] and by 2012, the first description of an emergency department-based program in the United States was published from San Diego,[38] followed soon by others.[13] Registry reports from the Extracorporeal Life Support Organization (ELSO) in 2020 demonstrated that 430 cen-ters had reported cases of ECPR use in adults, although many of these were restricted to inpatient arrest. By 2016, 37 programs throughout the United States reported per-forming ECPR in the emergency department, but only one-third used formal criteria and protocols to identify and treat these patients with ECPR.[39] The University of Min-nesota and the Minnesota Resuscitation Consortium have developed one of the most successful and high-volume coronary catheterization laboratory (CCL)-based ECPR programs for refractory OHCA in the United States.[15,36] Their work represents the largest series of OHCA ECPR cases at a single institution in North America and has had an influence on the development of programs at other institutions. Based on their encouraging results, the creators of the program have undertaken an ambitious proj-ect to bring a specialized, CCL-equipped ambulance carrying a highly trained team to rendezvous with ambulance units transporting refractory cardiac arrest patients to community hospitals.

France

In France, basic life support (BLS) for OHCA is managed by fire squadron members until a mobile intensive care unit (ICU) with a physician arrives to deliver advanced life support (ALS). Although ECPR has been available at receiving hospitals in Paris for some time, because of the difficulties of negotiating Paris traffic, prehospital imple-mentation of ECPR was developed in Paris as recently as 2011 – and more recently in other cities – in an attempt to decrease time to cannulation and restoration of blood flow for cases of refractory cardiac arrest. Early efforts did not use strict selection criteria, nor had care protocols been firmly established, and the results were mixed. Since that time, rigorous patient selection criteria and aggressive, protocol-driven pa-tient management have been implemented to better standardize the approach. Some studies in Paris have reported improved outcomes when compared with standard therapy,[40] although more recent nationwide reports have suggested equivalent outcomes compared with conventional CPR.[41] These more recent reports are concerning; equivalent outcomes in the ECPR patient group and a select patient cohort with a favorable probability of survival with conventional CPR, raise the question of whether outcomes would be worse in the ECPR cohort if selection bias were removed. Admittedly, selection criteria, while generally biasing outcomes toward higher survival, may be more than offset by resuscitation time bias.[42] Such competing bias means selected patients start off with a high chance of survival based on favorable clinical and arrest characteristics, but after failing to regain a pulse following a generally prolonged period of resuscitation they have a revised probability of survival that is substantially lower. It should be noted that survival was much higher for patients undergoing ECPR in the prehospital setting than patients undergoing ECPR on arrival to hospital, suggesting that the prehospital approach, with its time to cannulation savings, should be considered in settings where rapid transport and hospital cannulation are logistically difficult.

Japan

Advanced endovascular procedures have been used for many years in Japan. A meta-analysis from Japan[43] demonstrated that between 1983 and 2008, 1282 patients received ECPR for OHCA with a survival rate of approximately 27%. A more recent prospective observational analysis concluded that patients with OHCA treated with ECPR had better neurologic outcomes at 1 and 6 months compared with those treated with CCPR.[27] Interestingly, in these reports a larger proportion of patients in the ECPR group receive therapeutic hypothermia (92% vs 54%, respectively) and an intra-aortic balloon pump (93% and 62%, respectively), compared with those in the CCPR group, which makes it impossible to determine if the large improvement in outcomes is related to ECMO or the other adjunctive therapies deployed in this patient population.

AREAS OF UNCERTAINTY AND CONTROVERSY
Timing of Cannulation

A primary postulated benefit of ECPR is that it can provide full cardiopulmonary support for days or weeks, providing time to address the underlying cause of the arrest. Although there are case series that demonstrate neurologically intact survival after greater than 60 minutes of conventional CPR in normothermic patients, the probability of neurologically intact survival after 20 minutes of CPR in adults is approximately less than 2%.[33] Accordingly, the arguments against the immediate use of ECPR relate to procedural risks, cost, and complexity of care. ECPR theoretically becomes increasingly beneficial during the course of CPR as the balance of risks and benefits shifts away from conventional CPR and toward ECPR. In the case of shockable rhythms, approximately 30% of patients will have neurologically favorable survival with conventional CPR if ROSC can be obtained within the first few minutes of arrest.[11] Thus, very early in the resuscitation, the benefits of ECPR are likely outweighed by risks. However, the likelihood of a favorable outcome decreases dramatically over time until, after approximately 30 minutes, it is around 5%. The cohort remaining in refractory cardiac arrest after this time becomes functionally enriched with unfavorable characteristics, such as metabolic acidosis, hypercarbia, hypoxemia, and traumatic injuries from CPR. At some point during resuscitation, the risks of ECPR are outweighed by the vanishing probability of survival with continued conventional CPR.

The determination of this inflection point is an area guided more by reasoning from observational data and practical limitations than rigorous data. Current data suggest that the duration of CPR (known as low-flow time) is inversely associated with survival.[34,35] Although some experts have suggested that 20 minutes is an appropriate time to mobilize the ECMO response, more data are needed on the potential benefit of ECPR when initiated at different time points before a definitive recommendation can be made. The time to initiation is lower bounded, in part, by the nature of OHCA, which requires a rapid emergency medical services (EMS) response, early recognition of potential candidates, and timely transport or rendezvous with hospital-based ECPR teams.

Although time is, perhaps, the most important predictor of neurologic recovery currently available, a more physiologic predictor of survival probability is needed. Physiologic proxy markers of ischemia (lactate, pH) and perfusion (Pao_2, $EtCO_2$) during low-flow time may be more reflective of CPR quality and downtime and therefore of the probability of neurologic survival.[35,36,44–46]

Selection Criteria

The indications' for ECPR are defined largely based on protocols from observational studies (**Table 1**), as no randomized trial data yet exist. Published opinions on indications for use have ranged from highly selective, including initial witnessed arrest, shockable rhythms with bystander CPR, and no comorbidities[47] to as broad as cannulator discretion.[41] The former are based on the philosophy that patient selection for this invasive and expensive therapy should be reserved for patients with optimal probability of neurologic survival using conventional CPR, whereas the latter are based on the rationale that even the lowest survival benefit from observational studies of ECPR may be an improvement over standard care.

During CPR, signs of neurologic viability such as gasping[48] and pupil reactivity[49] are associated with good neurologic outcomes if ROSC can be achieved. Such findings, along with spontaneous movements during CPR were reported as favorable signs in a cohort of patients with refractory cardiac arrest undergoing ECPR.[50] Such signs of life are included among eligibility criteria in some ECPR programs.[40]

Exclusions for ECPR are generally based on patient factors such as advanced age or poor prearrest quality of life, comorbidities such as liver failure or dementia, and arrest-specific variables associated with poor outcome such as an initial rhythm of asystole.[51,52]

Procedural Competency and Maintenance of Skills

ECPR is a time-dependent therapy that requires the ability to correctly and reliably access the common femoral artery and the femoral vein, confirm wire placement in the aorta and inferior vena cava (IVC), carefully dilate overlying tissue in order to

Table 1
Typical patient selection criteria for extracorporeal pulmonary resuscitation for treatment of refractory out-of-hospital cardiac arrest

Inclusion Criteria	Exclusion Criteria
Witnessed arrest	Advanced age
Initial rhythm other than asystole	Significant medical comorbidities
No return of spontaneous circulation within 15 minutes	(ie, cirrhosis, end-stage renal disease, metastatic cancer)
Cannulation can be Achieved within 60 minutes of collapse	Poor prearrest quality of life
Bystander CPR (or EMS arrival within 5 min)	Skin infections, including candidiasis, over the cannulation site

accommodate the large-bore venous and arterial cannulae, guide the venous catheter to the right atrium, rapidly prepare the ECMO machine and circuit for use, and correctly connect the cannulae to the circuit free of air bubbles. Potential errors in cannulation during ECPR include cannulation through the superficial or profundis femoral arteries, puncture of the posterior vessel wall leading to thigh or retroperitoneal hematoma, inadvertent A-A or V-V cannulation, kinking of introducer wires, vessel dissection or perforation, and failure to advance the venous catheter to the level of the right atrium. Further catastrophic errors can occur if air is entrapped within the circuit leading to massive air embolism; if the circuit is incorrectly assembled, leading to oxygenation and return of blood into the venous system; and if the cannula is displaced leading to exsanguination. There are no consensus recommendations regarding training and proficiency as there are with other emergency procedures, such as endotracheal intubation. ELSO has long recommended 24 to 36 hours of didactic training along with animal laboratory training for inexperienced centers.[53] ELSO offers a 1-day course in cannulation, but this training does not imply personal proficiency. The number of live cannulations required to acquire proficiency remains uncertain. An evidence-based process for maintenance of skills is also entirely unknown. Non-ELSO training courses in cannulation have proliferated in the last 10 years. However, in the authors' opinion, no simulation can currently model the difficulties of pulseless ECPR cannulation with sufficient fidelity to replace live tissue training. This generally requires high volumes or access to a swine laboratory and/or cadavers. The necessity of achieving rapid cannulation to reduce the low-flow state has led nonsurgeons to successfully learn and apply this procedure in clinical practice (eg, emergency physicians, intensivists, or cardiologists) in the prehospital and in-hospital setting.

Setting of Cannulation

In ELSO and other registry data, cannulation for IHCA has been reported in multiple settings including the emergency department, ICU, operating room, and cardiac catheterization laboratory (CCL). When used to treat OHCA, cannulation has been reported in the prehospital setting, the emergency department, the ICU, and the CCL. ECPR for IHCA and OHCA requires either rapidly mobilizing ECPR personnel and equipment to the location of the arrest or rapidly transporting the cardiac arrest patient to the location of ECPR equipment and expertise. This represents a fundamental logistical challenge that is most acute in OHCA.[54] In the United States and other countries where paramedics deliver prehospital care, the ability to rapidly and accurately identify potential ECPR candidates, transport the patient to an ECPR center with minimal interruption in CPR quality, and transfer care to the ECPR team before an unacceptable burden of ischemic brain injury has occurred requires a level of care coordination that rivals trauma systems of care.

In Europe, where physicians provide a substantial on-scene role in prehospital medicine, specialized, physician-led response teams have learned to perform cannulation in the less-controlled prehospital environment where OHCA occurs. The prehospital team from the SAMU de Paris has shown that implementing ECPR in the prehospital setting can be done successfully. Indeed, delivered by land or air (helicopter EMS or HEMS), this strategy has the potential to reduce low-flow time by curtailing patient packaging and transport times, which can be a significant advantage in traffic-congested urban areas and in rural areas far from in-hospital ECPR capabilities. As mentioned previously, in a large cohort of more than 13,000 patients with OHCA (525 of whom underwent ECPR), ECPR implementation was not associated with hospital survival when controlling for age, sex, location of arrest, bystander CPR, initial rhythm, collapse-to-CPR time, duration of resuscitation, and ROSC.[41] However,

ECPR cases started in the prehospital setting had an adjusted odds ratio for survival to hospital discharge of 2.9 (95% confidence interval [CI] 1.5–5.9) compared with hospital based ECPR.

FUTURE AREAS OF RESEARCH

In addition to the uncertainties and controversies discussed previously, substantial uncertainty remains with respect to care once the patient has been placed on a pump. Ischemia-reperfusion injury is likely the main pathophysiology driving complications and mortality associated with ECPR. ECPR allows providers to control critical parameters of the reperfusion phase. However, there is no evidence to guide ideal reperfusion parameters. What should be the target flow rate, sweep (CO_2 removal), Fio_2, and temperature of initial and subsequent blood returned by the ECMO circuit? Would pulsatile flow be better than laminar flow? What arterial blood pressure should be targeted by adjunctive vasopressors? How do clinicians perform neuroprognostication on patients treated with ECPR? There are currently no good answers to these questions.

A prolonged (6-hour) period of low-flow (30–35 mL/kg/min) ECPR was associated with reduced lactate clearance and lower carotid blood flow in a pig model when compared with high-flow (65–70 mL/kg/min) ECPR.[55] Neurologic survival was not measured in this study, however, and neither was a strategy of initial low flow followed by gradually increasing flows over time. Optimal blood pressure targets are equally unclear. In a pig model, targeting a supraphysiologic blood pressure (80–85 mm Hg) during ECPR was not superior to normal blood pressure target (65–70 mm Hg) on measures of organ perfusion.[56]

There are no randomized controlled trials evaluating the optimal temperature target in ECPR patients, either. Research in the pig model of ECPR supports the use of hypothermia. Animals resuscitated with a target core temperature of 33° C had less tissue injury and a better hemodynamic profile when compared to those with a core temperature of 36.8°C.[57] Although rapid cooling appears to be protective,[58] the ideal cooling speed remains unknown. ECPR offers the theoretical advantage of allowing for rapid cooling at the initiation of reperfusion and a lower target temperature while maintaining perfusion.

Hyperoxemia following the return of spontaneous circulation in patients undergoing conventional CPR has been associated with higher mortality.[59] Exposure to hyperoxemia ($Pao_2 \geq$ 300 mm Hg) was also associated with an increased risk of mortality in patients with out-of-hospital cardiac arrest treated with ECPR and admitted to the ICU.[60] In more recent studies, hyperoxemia (Pao_2 >201 mm Hg) at 24 hours had no association with 1-month survival in patients treated with ECPR.[61] Hyperoxia is considered beneficial in the setting of traumatic brain injury, where cellular energy failure leads to cell death. As of this writing, a clinical trial is recruiting patients to investigate hyperbaric oxygen for treatment of traumatic brain injury (ClinicalTrials.gov Identifier: NCT02407028).

Carbon dioxide arterial content is also likely to be a crucial reperfusion parameter as nonpulsatile blood flow increases vascular sensitivity to $Paco_2$.[62] Although this is a more well-studied concept with conventional CPR, optimal targets for $Paco_2$ are unclear in ECPR patients. Hypocarbia is likely to reduce cerebral perfusion through cerebral vasoconstriction and should be avoided, in the authors' opinion.

Postcardiac arrest neuroprognostication is currently guided by a multimodal approach based on low-quality studies.[63] Care teams are increasingly presented with ethical and legal challenges around withdrawal of life support for ECPR patients.[64] Following ECPR for refractory VF, the combination of computed tomography, neuron-specific enolase (but not S100B) levels, brainstem reflex evaluation, and electroencephalogram appeared to be promising tools for early neuroprognostication in the Minnesota Resuscitation Consortium experience.[65] Data from the laboratory of some of the authors support the use of MRI in combination with electroencephalogram to quantify brain injury in the first 2 hours following initiation of ECPR.[66] However, MRI is difficult to perform while the patient is on a pump, and further studies are needed to establish whether this combined anatomic and functional approach can predict long-term neurologic outcomes.

SUMMARY

The use of ECPR is growing around the world because of a perceived survival benefit, improvements in the technology, and the development of interdisciplinary ECRP teams. However, significant questions regarding patient selection, procedure implementation, and patient management remain. Both translational and clinical research are needed to answer these questions.

DISCLOSURE

The authors have nothing to disclose.

REFERENCES

1. Tay PJM, Pek PP, Fan Q, et al. Effectiveness of a community based out-of-hospital cardiac arrest (OHCA) interventional bundle: results of a pilot study. Resuscitation 2020;146:220–8. https://doi.org/10.1016/j.resuscitation.2019.10.015.

2. Alqahtani S, Nehme Z, Williams B, et al. Long-term trends in the epidemiology of out-of-hospital cardiac arrest precipitated by suspected drug overdose. Resuscitation 2019;144:17–24.

3. Lee SY, Song KJ, Shin SD. Effect of implementation of cardiopulmonary resuscitation-targeted multi-tier response system on outcomes after out-of-hospital cardiac arrest: a before-and-after population-based study. Prehosp Emerg Care 2020;24(2):220–31.

4. Zive DM, Schmicker R, Daya M, et al. Survival and variability over time from out of hospital cardiac arrest across large geographically diverse communities participating in the Resuscitation Outcomes Consortium. Resuscitation 2018;131: 74–82.

5. Adabag S, Hodgson L, Garcia S, et al. Outcomes of sudden cardiac arrest in a state-wide integrated resuscitation program: results from the Minnesota Resuscitation Consortium. Resuscitation 2017;110:95–100.

6. Chan PS, McNally B, Tang F, et al, CARES Surveillance Group. Recent trends in survival from out-of-hospital cardiac arrest in the United States. Circulation 2014; 130(21):1876–82.

7. CARES survival report. 2019. Available at: https://mycares.net/sitepages/uploads/2019/2018%20Non-Traumatic%20National%20Survival%20Report.pdf. Accessed January 15, 2020.

8. Duggal C, Weil MH, Gazmuri RJ, et al. Regional blood flow during closed-chest cardiac resuscitation in rats. J Appl Physiol (1985) 1993;74(1):147–52.

9. Lurie KG, Mulligan KA, McKnite S, et al. Optimizing standard cardiopulmonary resuscitation with an inspiratory impedance threshold valve. Chest 1998;113(4): 1084–90.

10. Eleff SM, Kim H, Shaffner DH, et al. Effect of cerebral blood flow generated during cardiopulmonary resuscitation in dogs on maintenance versus recovery of ATP and pH. Stroke 1993;24(12):2066–73.

11. Reynolds JC, Grunau BE, Rittenberger JC, et al. Association between duration of resuscitation and favorable outcome after out-of-hospital cardiac arrest: implications for prolonging or terminating resuscitation. Circulation 2016;134(25): 2084–94.

12. Grunau B, Reynolds JC, Scheuermeyer FX, et al. Comparing the prognosis of those with initial shockable and non-shockable rhythms with increasing durations of CPR: informing minimum durations of resuscitation. Resuscitation 2016; 101:50–6.

13. Tonna JE, Selzman CH, Mallin MP, et al. Development and implementation of a comprehensive, multidisciplinary emergency department extracorporeal membrane oxygenation program. Ann Emerg Med 2017;70(1):32–40.

14. Youngquist ST, Hartsell S, McLaren D, et al. The use of prehospital variables to predict acute coronary artery disease in failed resuscitation attempts for out-of-hospital cardiac arrest. Resuscitation 2015;92:82–7.

15. Yannopoulos D, Bartos JA, Raveendran G, et al. Coronary artery disease in patients with out-of-hospital refractory ventricular fibrillation cardiac arrest. J Am Coll Cardiol 2017;70(9):1109–17.

16. Lamhaut L, Tea V, Raphalen J-H, et al. Coronary lesions in refractory out of hospital cardiac arrest (OHCA) treated by extra corporeal pulmonary resuscitation (ECPR). Resuscitation 2018;126:154–9.

17. Salcido DD, Sundermann ML, Koller AC, et al. Incidence and outcomes of rear-rest following out-of-hospital cardiac arrest. Resuscitation 2015;86:19–24.

18. Trzeciak S, Jones AE, Kilgannon JH, et al. Significance of arterial hypotension after resuscitation from cardiac arrest. Crit Care Med 2009;37(11):2895–903.

19. Lee SW, Han KS, Park JS, et al. Prognostic indicators of survival and survival prediction model following extracorporeal cardiopulmonary resuscitation in patients with sudden refractory cardiac arrest. Ann Intensive Care 2017;7(1):87.

20. Yannopoulos D, Bartos JA, Martin C, et al. Minnesota resuscitation consortium's advanced perfusion and reperfusion cardiac life support strategy for out-of-hospital refractory ventricular fibrillation. J Am Heart Assoc 2016;5(6). https://doi.org/10.1161/JAHA.116.003732.

21. Chen Z, Liu C, Huang J, et al. Clinical efficacy of extracorporeal cardiopulmonary resuscitation for adults with cardiac arrest: meta-analysis with trial sequential analysis. Biomed Res Int 2019;2019:6414673.

22. Chen Y-S, Lin J-W, Yu H-Y, et al. Cardiopulmonary resuscitation with assisted extracorporeal life-support versus conventional cardiopulmonary resuscitation in adults with in-hospital cardiac arrest: an observational study and propensity analysis. Lancet 2008;372(9638):554–61.

23. Patricio D, Peluso L, Brasseur A, et al. Comparison of extracorporeal and conventional cardiopulmonary resuscitation: a retrospective propensity score matched study. Crit Care 2019;23(1):27.

24. Choi DS, Kim T, Ro YS, et al. Extracorporeal life support and survival after out-of-hospital cardiac arrest in a nationwide registry: a propensity score-matched analysis. Resuscitation 2016;99:26–32.

25. Shin TG, Choi J-H, Jo IJ, et al. Extracorporeal cardiopulmonary resuscitation in patients with inhospital cardiac arrest: a comparison with conventional cardiopulmonary resuscitation. Crit Care Med 2011;39(1):1–7.

26. Stub D, Bernard S, Pellegrino V, et al. Refractory cardiac arrest treated with mechanical CPR, hypothermia, ECMO and early reperfusion (the CHEER trial). Resuscitation 2015;86:88–94.

27. Sakamoto T, Morimura N, Nagao K, et al. Extracorporeal cardiopulmonary resuscitation versus conventional cardiopulmonary resuscitation in adults with out-of-hospital cardiac arrest: a prospective observational study. Resuscitation 2014; 85(6):762–8.

28. Maekawa K, Tanno K, Hase M, et al. Extracorporeal cardiopulmonary resuscitation for patients with out-of-hospital cardiac arrest of cardiac origin: a propensity-matched study and predictor analysis. Crit Care Med 2013;41(5): 1186–96.

29. Kim SJ, Kim HJ, Lee HY, et al. Comparing extracorporeal cardiopulmonary resuscitation with conventional cardiopulmonary resuscitation: a meta-analysis. Resuscitation 2016;103:106–16.

30. Ahn C, Kim W, Cho Y, et al. Efficacy of extracorporeal cardiopulmonary resuscitation compared to conventional cardiopulmonary resuscitation for adult cardiac arrest patients: a systematic review and meta-analysis. Sci Rep 2016;6:34208.

31. Lin J-W, Wang M-J, Yu H-Y, et al. Comparing the survival between extracorporeal rescue and conventional resuscitation in adult in-hospital cardiac arrests: propensity analysis of three-year data. Resuscitation 2010;81(7):796–803.

32. Goto Y, Funada A, Goto Y. Relationship between the duration of cardiopulmonary resuscitation and favorable neurological outcomes after out-of-hospital cardiac arrest: a prospective, nationwide, population-based cohort study. J Am Heart Assoc 2016;5(3):e002819.

33. Reynolds JC, Frisch A, Rittenberger JC, et al. Duration of resuscitation efforts and functional outcome after out-of-hospital cardiac arrest: when should we change to novel therapies? Circulation 2013;128(23):2488–94.

34. D'Arrigo S, Cacciola S, Dennis M, et al. Predictors of favourable outcome after in-hospital cardiac arrest treated with extracorporeal cardiopulmonary resuscitation: a systematic review and meta-analysis. Resuscitation 2017;121:62–70.

35. Debaty G, Babaz V, Durand M, et al. Prognostic factors for extracorporeal cardiopulmonary resuscitation recipients following out-of-hospital refractory cardiac arrest. A systematic review and meta-analysis. Resuscitation 2017;112:1–10.

36. Bartos JA, Grunau B, Carlson C, et al. Improved survival with extracorporeal cardiopulmonary resuscitation despite progressive metabolic derangement associated with prolonged resuscitation. Circulation 2020;141(11):877–86.

37. Bartlett RH, Gazzaniga AB, Fong SW, et al. Extracorporeal membrane oxygenator support for cardiopulmonary failure. Experience in 28 cases. J Thorac Cardiovasc Surg 1977;73(3):375–86.

38. Bellezzo JM, Shinar Z, Davis DP, et al. Emergency physician-initiated extracorporeal cardiopulmonary resuscitation. Resuscitation 2012;83(8):966–70.

39. Tonna JE, Johnson NJ, Greenwood J, et al. Practice characteristics of emergency department extracorporeal cardiopulmonary resuscitation (ECPR) programs in the United States: the current state of the art of emergency department extracorporeal membrane oxygenation (ED ECMO). Resuscitation 2016;107:38–46.

40. Lamhaut L, Hutin A, Puymirat E, et al. A Pre-hospital extracorporeal cardio pulmonary resuscitation (ECPR) strategy for treatment of refractory out hospital cardiac

arrest: an observational study and propensity analysis. Resuscitation 2017;117: 109–17.

41. Bougouin W, Dumas F, Lamhaut L, et al. Extracorporeal cardiopulmonary resuscitation in out-of-hospital cardiac arrest: a registry study. Eur Heart J 2020;41(21): 1961–71.

42. Andersen LW, Grossestreuer AV, Donnino MW. "Resuscitation time bias"-A unique challenge for observational cardiac arrest research. Resuscitation 2018;125: 79–82.

43. Morimura N, Sakamoto T, Nagao K, et al. Extracorporeal cardiopulmonary resuscitation for out-of-hospital cardiac arrest: a review of the Japanese literature. Resuscitation 2011;82(1):10–4. https://doi.org/10.1016/j.resuscitation.2010. 08.032.

44. Jung C, Bueter S, Wernly B, et al. Lactate clearance predicts good neurological outcomes in cardiac arrest patients treated with extracorporeal cardiopulmonary resuscitation. J Clin Med 2019;8(3). https://doi.org/10.3390/jcm8030374.

45. Mizutani T, Umemoto N, Taniguchi T, et al. The lactate clearance calculated using serum lactate level 6 h after is an important prognostic predictor after extracorporeal cardiopulmonary resuscitation: a single-center retrospective observational study. J Intensive Care 2018;6:33.

46. Bartos JA, Carlson K, Carlson C, et al. Surviving refractory out-of-hospital ventricular fibrillation cardiac arrest: critical care and extracorporeal membrane oxygenation management. Resuscitation 2018;132:47–55.

47. Bol ME, Suverein MM, Lorusso R, et al. Early initiation of extracorporeal life support in refractory out-of-hospital cardiac arrest: design and rationale of the INCEPTION trial. Am Heart J 2019;210:58–68.

48. Debaty G, Labarere J, Frascone RJ, et al. Long-term prognostic value of gasping during out-of-hospital cardiac arrest. J Am Coll Cardiol 2017;70(12):1467–76.

49. Steen-Hansen JE, Hansen NN, Vaagenes P, et al. Pupil size and light reactivity during cardiopulmonary resuscitation: a clinical study. Crit Care Med 1988; 16(1):69–70.

50. Debaty G, Nicol M, Aubert R, et al. Abstract 362: early signs of life as a prognostic factor for extracorporeal cardiopulmonary resuscitation in refractory out-of-hospital cardiac arrest. 2018;132(Suppl_2). Available at: https://www. ahajournals.org/doi/10.1161/circ.138.suppl_2.362. Accessed February 20, 2020.

51. Baldi E, Caputo ML, Savastano S, et al. An Utstein-based model score to predict survival to hospital admission: the UB-ROSC score. Int J Cardiol 2020;308:84–9.

52. Roth R, Stewart RD, Rogers K, et al. Out-of-hospital cardiac arrest: factors associated with survival. Ann Emerg Med 1984;13(4):237–43.

53. Extracorporeal Life Support Organization (ELSO) general guidelines for all ECLS cases. 2013. Available at: https://www.elso.org/Portals/0/IGD/Archive/FileManager/ 929122ae88cusersshyerdocumentselsoguidelinesgeneralalleclsversion1.3.pdf. Accessed January 21, 2020.

54. Chonde M, Escajeda J, Elmer J, et al. Challenges in the development and implementation of a healthcare system based extracorporeal cardiopulmonary resuscitation (ECPR) program for the treatment of out of hospital cardiac arrest. Resuscitation 2020;148:259–65.

55. Luo Y, Fritz C, Hammache N, et al. Low versus standard-blood-flow reperfusion strategy in a pig model of refractory cardiac arrest resuscitated with Extra Corporeal Membrane Oxygenation. Resuscitation 2018;133:12–7.

56. Fritz C, Kimmoun A, Vanhuyse F, et al. High versus low blood-pressure target in experimental ischemic prolonged cardiac arrest treated with extra corporeal life support. Shock 2017;47(6):759–64.

57. Ostadal P, Mlcek M, Kruger A, et al. Mild therapeutic hypothermia is superior to controlled normothermia for the maintenance of blood pressure and cerebral oxygenation, prevention of organ damage and suppression of oxidative stress after cardiac arrest in a porcine model. J Transl Med 2013;11:124.

58. Nagao K, Kikushima K, Watanabe K, et al. Early induction of hypothermia during cardiac arrest improves neurological outcomes in patients with out-of-hospital cardiac arrest who undergo emergency cardiopulmonary bypass and percutaneous coronary intervention. Circ J 2010;74(1):77–85.

59. Ni Y-N, Wang Y-M, Liang B-M, et al. The effect of hyperoxia on mortality in critically ill patients: a systematic review and meta analysis. BMC Pulm Med 2019; 19(1):53.

60. Halter M, Jouffroy R, Saade A, et al. Association between hyperoxemia and mortality in patients treated by ECPR after out-of-hospital cardiac arrest. Am J Emerg Med 2019. https://doi.org/10.1016/j.ajem.2019.07.008.

61. Kobayashi M, Kashiura M, Sugiyama K, et al. 1497: Association between hyperoxia and 1-month mortality in OHCA patients with ECPR. Crit Care Med 2020; 48(1):724.

62. Veraar CM, Rinosl H, Kuhn K, et al. Non-pulsatile blood flow is associated with enhanced cerebrovascular carbon dioxide reactivity and an attenuated relationship between cerebral blood flow and regional brain oxygenation. Crit Care 2019; 23(1):426.

63. Geocadin RG, Callaway CW, Fink EL, et al. Standards for studies of neurological prognostication in comatose survivors of cardiac arrest: a scientific statement from the American Heart Association. Circulation 2019;140(9):e517–42.

64. Grunau B, MacRedmond R, Gill J. A promising therapy in Jeopardy the need to define limits for extracorporeal cardiopulmonary resuscitation. Circulation 2019; 139(4).

65. Bartos JA, Nutting L, Carlson C, et al. Abstract 10: early neuroprognostication after refractory VF/VT cardiac arrest requiring ECPR. Circulation 2019; 140(Suppl_2):A10.

66. Peckham M, DeHavenon A, Alexander MD, et al. Abstract 11: early magnetic resonance imaging to quantify ischemic brain insult early following cardiac arrest in a swine model. Circulation 2019;140(Suppl_2):A11.

Precision Cardiac Arrest Resuscitation Based on Etiology

Cameron Dezfulian, MD[a,b,*], Eric J. Lavonas, MD, MS[c,d]

KEYWORDS

- Cardiac arrest • Etiology • Asphyxia • Sudden cardiac death • Hypoxia-ischemia
- Global ischemia • Ventricular fibrillation

KEY POINTS

- Most cardiac arrest etiologies fall into the broad groups of sudden or asphyxial. These etiologies require different resuscitation and postresuscitation strategies.
- Sudden cardiac arrest is generally of cardiac etiology, and the hallmark is rapid loss of perfusion at the same time or preceding cessation of breathing.
- Respiratory etiology asphyxia arrest results from progressive hypoxemia, which includes a period of hypoxic perfusion before loss of cardiac contractility.
- Outcomes and cause of in-hospital death differ between sudden and asphyxial etiology cardiac arrests.
- Present guidelines and therapies have not been based on etiology, but making these adjustments may optimize outcomes.

INTRODUCTION

Cardiac arrest (CA) has been classified by several descriptive means. Distinguishing out-of-hospital CA (OHCA) from in-hospital CA (IHCA) is typical within epidemiology,[1] as many important characteristics (eg, comorbidities, resuscitation time, and presence of monitoring) and ultimately outcomes track distinctly within these groups. After

Funding: Dr Dezfulian is supported by R01HL129722 and an investigator-initiated award from Mallinckrodt Pharmaceuticals, Inc.
[a] Critical Care Medicine, University of Pittsburgh School of Medicine, 4401 Penn Avenue, CHP Faculty Pavilion, Room 2119, Pittsburgh, PA 15224, USA; [b] Clinical and Translational Sciences, University of Pittsburgh School of Medicine, 4401 Penn Avenue, CHP Faculty Pavilion, Room 2119, Pittsburgh, PA 15224, USA; [c] Department of Emergency Medicine, Rocky Mountain Poison and Drug Safety, Denver Health, 777 Bannock Street, MC 0108, Denver, CO 80238, USA; [d] Department of Emergency Medicine, University of Colorado School of Medicine, Aurora, CO, USA
* Corresponding author. 4401 Penn Avenue, CHP Faculty Pavilion, Room 2119, Pittsburgh, PA 15224.
E-mail address: dezfulianc@upmc.edu
Twitter: @Dezfulian_CCM (C.D.)

Crit Care Clin 36 (2020) 737–752
https://doi.org/10.1016/j.ccc.2020.07.005
0749-0704/20/© 2020 Elsevier Inc. All rights reserved.

this characterization, CA is generally classified by presenting rhythm. This is pragmatically helpful, because it guides resuscitation and use (or lack of) of cardioversion, and loosely tracks with etiology. Yet etiology is rarely at the forefront. In the 2019 American Heart Association (AHA) Heart Disease and Stroke Statistics[1] section dedicated to CA, etiology appears 4 times, only in the references. The 2020 publication of these statistics[2] is the first time a figure was provided describing etiology of OHCA and IHCA. Using these same data, which were derived from the University of Pittsburgh Cardiac Arrest Registry, the authors characterize etiology of CA and broadly divide most cases into 2 groups (**Fig. 1**). Sudden CA (SCA) refers to abrupt

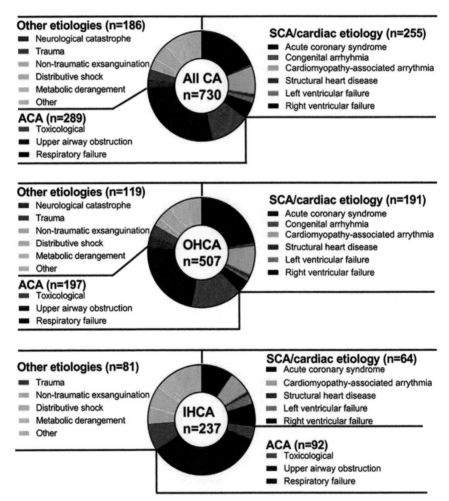

Fig. 1. Distribution of etiology after CA. Using data obtained from Chen and colleagues,[13] we have plotted the distribution of etiology in those patients with only a single identified cause of CA. The top panel reflects all CA, whereas the next 2 panels reflect OHCA and IHCA. Etiologies are broadly grouped into SCA, which reflects all cardiac causes and ACA, which reflects etiologies associated with loss of airway or cessation of breathing. (*Data from* Chen N, Callaway CW, Guyette FX, et al. Arrest etiology among patients resuscitated from cardiac arrest. Resuscitation. 2018;130:33-40.)

cessation of cardiac output and as defined here is synonymous with cardiac etiology CA. Asphyxial CA (ACA) refers to loss of airway or breathing that results in progressive hypoxemia and eventually loss of cardiac output.

CA etiology[3–5] is strongly linked to the extent of brain injury and consequently clinical outcome.[6,7] Characterizing CA based on etiology is difficult because of the challenges inherent to ascertaining the etiology, particularly early after CA, as well as the historical context. Three to 4 decades ago, most CA was because of a cardiac dysrhythmia causing sudden circulatory collapse and global ischemia (ie, SCA). Most patients with OHCA had ventricular fibrillation (VF) or pulseless ventricular tachycardia (VT).[8,9] In the past 30 years, the proportion of OHCA caused by ACA has steadily increased,[10] while the rate of SCA has decreased.[8,9,11,12] Although CA etiology has shifted, resuscitation and postresuscitation care guidelines remain largely etiology blind.[13–15] Furthermore, most existing knowledge on CA is not from ACA. In a systematic review, only 25% of published animal studies of CA involved ACA models.[16] Earlier reports are even more dominated by VF[17,18] or global ischemia (eg, 4 cerebral vessel occlusion with hypotension). Thus, knowledge of CA-mediated brain injury derives mostly from pure global ischemia (SCA), rather than hypoxia preceding ischemia (ACA).

This article will focus on the basic scientific and clinical distinctions between ACA and SCA, primarily within OHCA, with the goal of identifying clinically meaningful phenotypes of CA. These 2 broad phenotypes, ACA and SCA, deserve not only focused future investigation but perhaps modification of existing guidelines on resuscitation[19,20] and postresuscitation care.[14] In pediatric and neonatal CA, ACA has long predominated,[21–26] making these etiologic distinctions less relevant. Hence the focus will be on adults, in whom etiologic heterogeneity is the greatest.

PATHOPHYSIOLOGICAL DISTINCTIONS BETWEEN ASPHYXIAL CARDIAC ARREST AND SUDDEN CARDIAC ARREST
Anoxic Perfusion

Anoxia, as it will be referred to here, is a tissue oxygen concentration (Po_2) below which aerobic metabolism ceases. Within both heart and brain, anoxia occurs with drops of Po_2 below 22 mm Hg.[27,28] Yet heart and brain differ fundamentally in that tissue necrosis (infarction) within heart is absent when reperfusion occurs within 20 min of ischemia[29] whereas brain adenylate charge (ATP) is lost within 3 to 5 minutes of ischemia[30] with nearly 95% of the brain injured after 15 min of global ischemia.[31,32] The development of anoxic brain damage depends not only on Po_2 but also the cerebral blood flow (CBF) and glucose supply. Brain reflexively defends its oxygen delivery over all other organs; increases in CBF of 400% to 500% occur during hypoxia, which prevents neuronal death even with arterial Po_2 approaching 10 mm Hg.[30] Nonetheless, once Po_2 drops to the single digits, even large increases in CBF cannot provide adequate oxygen delivery to maintain brain function or neuronal viability despite the ability of the heart to keep pumping and high systemic blood pressures owing to cerebral vasoconstriction.[33]

Anoxic perfusion is the hallmark of ACA. By the time the heart has stopped, the brain has experienced several minutes of anoxic perfusion.[33] This differs significantly from SCA, where loss of cardiac output precedes any loss in Po_2 such that anoxic perfusion is absent.[34] Canine studies indicate that arterial oxygen saturation remains above 90% for at least 4 minutes after the onset of SCA,[35] permitting adequate oxygen delivery to the brain in the setting of chest compressions (CCs). On the other hand, CCs are unable to provide the brain any additional oxygen delivery in ACA because of the profound systemic depletion of oxygen. The implications of this on cardiopulmonary resuscitation will be discussed.

Impact of Anoxic Perfusion on Brain Injury

During anoxic perfusion, the delivery of energy substrates such as glucose continues despite the absence of oxygen needed to drive aerobic respiration. Anoxic perfusion exacerbates lactic acidosis, as ongoing glucose delivery drives anaerobic respiration, pushing brain tissue lactate concentrations to 32.8 plus or minus 3.8 mM/kg.[36] This is a far higher cerebral lactate concentration than produced by similar durations of hypoxia with preserved blood flow (10.7 ± 0.9 mM kg)[36] or global ischemia as seen in SCA (19.6 ± 1.9 mM/kg).[37] Greater glucose availability during anoxia and the increased acidosis seen after ACA worsen recovery of cerebral energy stores following reperfusion.[38–40] Greater cerebral acidosis in the setting of CA is likely to be pathophysiologically important as it is associated with greater neuronal cell death, whereas mild cerebral acidemia may be protective.[38–40] Consistent with this hypothesis, animal studies examined the impact of blood glucose in the setting of anoxia and found that higher glucose delivery is associated with greater brain injury after resuscitation from CA.[41,42]

Another mechanism responsible for the worsening of brain injury in ACA compared with SCA is free radical injury. It is unclear whether this is caused by the increase in cerebral acidosis, another mechanism, or a combination. Pure global ischemia, as seen in SCA up to even 15 minutes duration, produces minimal reperfusion reactive oxygen species (ROS).[43] By contrast, ACA results in iron delocalization, a driver of lipid peroxidation.[44] Numerous animal studies have confirmed that brain iron delocalization from plasma transferrin or cellular ferritin is associated with greater reperfusion ROS generation and lipid peroxidation.[45–51] The iron chelator deferoxamine has been shown to reduce cellular injury by reducing lipid peroxidation.[52–56]

There have now been several comparative animal studies that demonstrate that ACA results in more severe brain injury than SCA using differing models of matching the overall insult.[57–59] These findings may be the result of ROS injury as described previously. Alternatively, greater cerebral acidosis after ACA may result in activation of acid-sensitive ion channels (ASICs) expressed throughout the brain.[60–62] Activation of ASICs may induce glutamate-independent brain injury by potentiating Ca^{2+} overload in neurons.[49] Greater cerebral acidemia is also associated with increased endoplasmic reticulum protein misfolding and ionic imbalances resulting in ER stress,[63–65] which may worsen injury when comparing ACA with SCA. ACA has been demonstrated to result in greater CBF heterogeneity with hyperperfusion early after return of spontaneous circulation (ROSC) followed by subsequent hypoperfusion.[66]

CLINICAL DISTINCTIONS BETWEEN ASPHYXIAL CARDIAC ARREST AND SUDDEN CARDIAC ARREST
Epidemiology

The differing etiologies of OHCA and IHCA have been poorly reported in the past. This is the result of the absence of an accepted classification system and the challenges inherent to assigning etiology at the time of CA or shortly after resuscitation. The University of Pittsburgh Cardiac Arrest Registry recently created an etiologic classification scheme by a Delphi method and applied it to 982 patients seen after CA.[13] Using chart abstraction by a trained researcher and considering all data obtained prior to and throughout the hospitalization, etiology could be assigned to 899 of 982 (92%) cases.

An additional 169 of 982 cases (17%) had 2 or more likely etiologies assigned. **Fig. 1** presents the distribution of etiologies in all CA and for OHCA and IHCA separately in cases where only 1 etiology was assigned. Because most cardiac etiology CA presents as SCA, these have been grouped together, whereas toxicologic causes, most of which were opioid poisoning, have been grouped with other airway or breathing disturbances resulting in ACA. It is notable that ACA represents a slightly higher proportion of cases than SCA, which differs from numerous earlier studies and reflects the changing epidemiology of CA. Nonetheless, ischemic heart disease (acute coronary syndromes) remains a major etiologic factor, constituting nearly a quarter of OHCA cases. This finding underscores the role for urgent coronary angiography in OHCA, which is at present the only etiology-based recommendation in postresuscitation guidelines.[14]

It has been consistently noted that patients with SCA are considerably more likely to present with shockable rhythms such as VF/VT than those with ACA (**Fig. 2A**).[13,67–69] This finding is important for several reasons. First, presenting rhythm strongly correlates with outcome; higher survival and better neurologic outcome are noted when VF/VT is the initial rhythm both in OHCA[3,70] and IHCA.[71] Rhythm also correlates with other clinical factors linked to outcome; VF/VT, which is more commonly found in SCA, is more often noted in patients with CA who also more often receive bystander cardiopulmonary resuscitation (CPR).[67] Thus it is not surprising that degree of

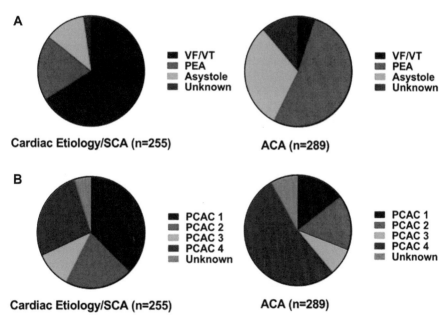

Fig. 2. Differences in presenting rhythm and early brain injury based on etiology. (*A*) The distribution of rhythms within SCA is contrasted with ACA. SCA constituted the bulk of ventricular fibrillation and pulseless ventricular tachycardia (VF/VT) which is the major presenting rhythm in this form of cardiac arrest whereas pulseless electrical activity (PEA) was the predominant rhythm in ACA. (*B*) SCA and ACA differ in terms of early post-resuscitation brain injury based on the Pittsburgh Cardiac Arrest Category (PCAC) assigned within 6 hours of return of spontaneous circulation. PCAC 1 patients have excellent (>80%) survival and are more frequently noted after SCA whereas PCAC 4 patients have very poor outcomes (<5% good neurologic survival) and constitute half of the ACA group.

neurologic injury, measured by the validated Pittsburgh Cardiac Arrest Category (PCAC),[72,73] is consistently worse in patients resuscitated from ACA compared with SCA (**Fig. 2**B). The PCAC is assigned within 6 hours of return of spontaneous circulation (ROSC), and strongly correlates with outcome,[72,73] which in turn is most strongly predicted by neurologic injury. The fact that ACA patients present with worse (higher) PCAC scores means they have more severe neurologic injury than resuscitated SCA patients shortly after ROSC.

Outcomes

Clinical reports of outcomes after SCA compared with ACA have been mixed. The University of Pittsburgh Post-Cardiac Arrest Service has previously reported worsened neurologic outcomes and survival associated with noncardiac etiology CA,[4] which was also noted in the Korean Hypothermia Network (KORHN) registry.[74] This finding would be expected based on the basic science and clinical factors reviewed previously, yet some contradictory reports exist. The Resuscitation Outcomes Consortium (ROC)[3] noted the opposite effect, with better outcomes noted in noncardiac etiology OHCA. The ROC study reported noncardiac etiology in less than 10% of all OHCA cases. Reports from primarily prehospital databases such as ROC suffer from the limitation that OHCA etiology cannot be fully determined at the time of resuscitation, and a substantially different proportion of causes of CA is reported when etiology is assigned at hospital discharge (see **Fig. 1**).[13] Reports on overdose-associated OHCA, which tends to be primarily opioid-mediated ACA, have likewise reported similar outcomes between SCA and overdose-related ACA,[75–77] in apparent contradiction to the notion that ACA results in greater brain injury. In these studies, the issue of etiology assignment remains a problem with an added nuance. In many cases of opioid poisoning, ROSC is achieved early in resuscitation after use of naloxone. However, it is likely that many of these patients were never pulseless, and others had only just experienced CA. These patients have excellent discharge outcomes. When averaging these outcomes with those from patients with longer durations of ACA, overall outcomes are far better than most ACA cases and thus approximate SCA. Animal studies offer the advantage of being able to match factors such as time to resuscitation, total insult duration, and resuscitation quality, and consistently show worse outcomes driven by brain injury after ACA compared with SCA.[57–59]

Although brain injury is the principal driver of in-hospital death after OHCA, shock effects on other organs affect many of these patients, and results in death in a smaller but significant minority.[6,7] In both animal models and human data, postresuscitation shock and myocardial dysfunction were more severe after SCA than ACA.[58] Prior data on the etiology of CA[13] demonstrate that postresuscitation intractable shock results in mortality after SCA in nearly the same proportion as brain injury (**Fig. 3**) and twice as often as in ACA. These deaths often occur early in the hospitalization (days 1 and 2), as opposed to neurologic deaths, which are often delayed because of the need to perform reliable prognostication. Strategies aimed at optimizing hemodynamics in patients after SCA may therefore yield improved outcomes that may not translate to ACA, in which neurologic injury may be more severe, and even those who can be managed through their shock may ultimately succumb to their brain injury.

IMPLICATIONS OF ETIOLOGY ON CLINICAL MANAGEMENT
Resuscitation

In an effort to increase rates of bystander CPR, the AHA has promoted compression-only CPR.[78] Of note, this recommendation was not intended for noncardiac etiology

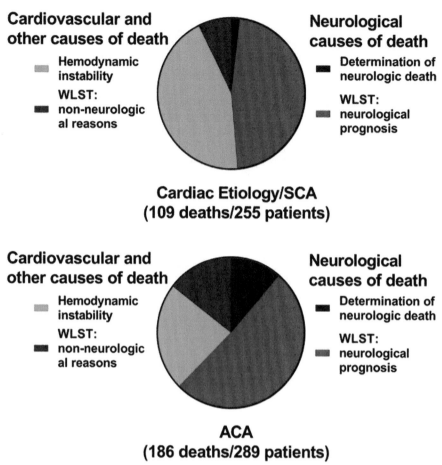

**Cardiac Etiology/SCA
(109 deaths/255 patients)**

**ACA
(186 deaths/289 patients)**

Fig. 3. Causes of in-hospital death after successful resuscitation from cardiac arrest. Patients successfully resuscitated from sudden cardiac arrest (SCA) have an equal chance of dying from neurologic injury as compared to other causes. Those with ACA are more likely to die because of withdrawal of life-sustaining therapies based on a poor neurologic prognosis or brain death.

OHCA or OHCA in children, where ACA predominates.[24–26] Observational studies that have examined compression-only CPR in SCA only (excluding ACA) have reported improved survival compared with conventional CPR.[79,80] This may be the result of hands-only CPR providing a greater chest compression fraction than compression-ventilation CPR and the ease with which layperson resuscitators can provide it effectively. Because SCA patients have a blood reservoir of oxygen at the time of collapse,[35] restoration of blood flow is the most critical intervention. However, broader analyses that include all OHCA cases confirm that conventional CPR is associated with better outcomes in ACA, likely because critical oxygen reserves are replenished when ventilation is provided.[81,82] Likewise, in randomized trials of telecommunicator-instructed CPR for OHCA, the use of compression-only CPR resulted in similar or better outcomes than conventional CPR.[83–86] A closer look at these studies demonstrates that some excluded ACA from causes such as alcohol intoxication or opioid poisoning.[84,86] In the studies where subgroup analyses were performed, dispatcher instructions for compression-only CPR were superior when restricting to SCA, whereas conventional CPR performed better in ACA.[83,85]

These clinical findings are consistent with the findings of the animal studies noted previously that demonstrate anoxic perfusion in ACA and the presence of a significant blood oxygen reservoir in SCA.[35] There is, however, an important question that remains. If the deleterious impact of anoxic perfusion noted in animal studies is to be believed, the implication is that compression-only CPR is potentially harmful in patients suffering from ACA. In ACA, it is clear that for resuscitation to be successful, oxygenation is essential. What is less clear is whether just providing circulation via compressions in the absence of ventilation is neutral, as commonly believed, or in fact worsens cerebral acidosis and ROS generation on reperfusion. At present, many 911 dispatchers and layperson educational campaigns are promoting compression-only CPR due to the ease of just-in-time teaching and the common reluctance or inability of bystanders to provide mouth-to-mouth ventilation. The indiscriminate application of compression-only CPR to those suffering ACA may not in fact be a benign event. The animal studies certainly provide reason for pause and demand further investigations, which, if this initial suspicion is confirmed, could change recommendations and policy. However, in the absence of high-quality evidence to the contrary, CPR, to the extent the rescuer can provide it, is currently recommended for all victims of CA.

Postresuscitation Care

In the postresuscitation setting, out-of-hospital SCA is often the result of coronary ischemia (see **Fig. 1**), and the administration of urgent coronary angiography followed by percutaneous intervention (PCI) has been consistently associated with improved outcomes in patients with coronary occlusion.[87–90] A recent randomized trial of urgent versus delayed coronary angiography failed to show a benefit for urgent timing of this intervention.[91] This trial underscores the need for further phenotyping. The investigators enrolled OHCA patients presenting with VF/VT as a surrogate for coronary occlusion but as previously noted (see **Fig. 1**),[13] several other causes of SCA including arrhythmia due to cardiomyopathy can present similarly. Better pragmatic diagnostic tools are needed to determine the subgroup of patients with SCA likely to have acute coronary occlusion and thus to benefit from urgent PCI.

Mild therapeutic hypothermia to 33°C was shown to be beneficial over normothermia which was really on average 37.5° to 37.9°C in 2 landmark randomized trials in 2002.[92,93] These studies enrolled exclusively out-of-hospital SCA patients presenting in VF/VT. A subsequent randomized study of therapeutic temperature management (TTM) of 33°C compared with 36°C, which again enrolled only out-of-hospital SCA patients (80% VF/VT), demonstrated equivalence between these 2 arms,[94] with perhaps some improvements in hemodynamics at 36°C.[95] The application of TTM to patients after ACA and IHCA was adopted at some centers based on these data from out-of-hospital SCA, but until recently, no data existed within these populations. A recent randomized study (HYPERION) enrolling OHCA and IHCA patients (approximately 70% OHCA) presenting with nonshockable rhythms was enriched for ACA (60%–70% of the cohort).[96] This study randomized patients to 33°C compared with 37°C and demonstrated improved neurologic outcome at 90 days in those cooled to 33°C. At this point, no comparison has been made between TTM at 33°C and 36°C in ACA, but these studies are ongoing. HYPERION, unlike the 2002 hypothermia trials, enforced true normothermia in the comparison arm and showed the lower temperature was superior. These findings leave open many questions including whether the goal temperature for TTM after ACA and SCA should be the same.

Additional questions remain for TTM such as the optimal duration based on etiology. A comparison of 24 hours to 48 hours of TTM at 33°C in out-of-hospital SCA patients showed a nonsignificant trend toward benefit in the 48-hour group.[97] Whether this trend would be more significant in ACA patients who may have a better response to the lower temperature target[96] demands consideration, as it could yield important changes in management.

Neuroprotection and Cardioprotection Based on Etiology

Attempts to provide pharmacologic neuroprotection after CA have been fraught with failure in clinical trials[98–101] despite promising animal results. One hypothesis to explain these failures is the significant degree of heterogeneity noted in human CA compared with well controlled animal models. Based on the animal studies, it is clear that ACA compared with SCA results in significant differences in cerebral lactic acidosis, reperfusion ROS and CBF.[36,39,40,49,58,64,66] These early differences in the brain may then result in fundamental differences in later CBF and cell survival signaling that impact delayed neuronal death. For example, specific forms of programmed cell death such as apoptosis and ferroptosis are known to be driven by lipid peroxidation (specifically cardiolipin[102] and phosphatidylethanolamine,[103,104] respectively). Targeting these cell death pathways may yield improved outcomes after ACA compared with SCA.

SCA, which often presents in VF/VT (see **Fig. 2**A) and is often caused by focal myocardial ischemia or prior cardiomyopathy (see **Fig. 1**), likely results in more significant myocardial stunning than CA from other causes.[58,105,106] This stunning, combined with distributive shock driven by cytokine release after CA,[107–109] may cause refractory shock resulting in death after SCA. Indeed, nearly half of the in-hospital deaths noted after SCA are the result of shock (see **Fig. 3**). This number is likely an underestimate given that the most severe forms of myocardial dysfunction will result in an inability to achieve ROSC. As such, the application of cardioprotective therapies as early as possible in SCA may provide significant improvements in outcome.

SUMMARY

CA results from a broad range of etiologies that can be broadly grouped into SCA and ACA. These distinctions are important, as there is evidence for fundamental differences in injury pathways in the heart and brain that drive clinical outcomes. Present guidelines largely ignore etiology in their management recommendations, and many clinical trials consider this minimally during enrollment with a strong bias to inclusion of the SCA population who have better outcomes. This heterogeneity demands exploration in determining how best to apply presently employed resuscitation and postresuscitation strategies such as CPR and TTM to optimize outcomes. Furthermore, the development of neuroprotective and cardioprotective therapies should take etiology into consideration when attempting to translate from bench to bedside in hopes of achieving success.

CRITICAL CARE POINTS

SCA generally results from cardiac etiology and often presents in VF/VT; death results as often from shock as brain injury. ACA results in fundamental differences in neurochemistry, which result in greater brain injury than SCA of similar duration and may portend poor prognosis even after brief CPR times.

Compression-only CPR is most effective in SCA, and animal studies lead to concern of potential harm in ACA. Conventional CPR is superior for resuscitation of ACA.

OHCA patients achieving ROSC after SCA appear to benefit equally from TTM at 33 to 36°C, whereas ACA patients have only had demonstrated benefits with TTM at 33°C compared with 37°C.

DISCLOSURE

The author has nothing to disclose.

REFERENCES

1. Benjamin EJ, Muntner P, Alonso A, et al. Heart disease and stroke statistics-2019 update: a report from the American Heart Association. Circulation 2019; 139(10):e56–528.
2. Virani SS, Alonso A, Benjamin EJ, et al. Heart disease and stroke statistics—2020 update: a report from the American Heart Association. Circulation 2020; 141(9):e139–596.
3. Daya MR, Schmicker RH, Zive DM, et al. Out-of-hospital cardiac arrest survival improving over time: results from the Resuscitation Outcomes Consortium (ROC). Resuscitation 2015;91:108–15.
4. Uray T, Mayr FB, Fitzgibbon J, et al. Socioeconomic factors associated with outcome after cardiac arrest in patients under the age of 65. Resuscitation 2015;93(0):14–9.
5. Rea TD, Cook AJ, Stiell IG, et al. Predicting survival after out-of-hospital cardiac arrest: role of the Utstein data elements. Ann Emerg Med 2010;55(3):249–57.
6. Laver S, Farrow C, Turner D, et al. Mode of death after admission to an intensive care unit following cardiac arrest. Intensive Care Med 2004;30(11):2126–8.
7. Lemiale V, Dumas F, Mongardon N, et al. Intensive care unit mortality after cardiac arrest: the relative contribution of shock and brain injury in a large cohort. Intensive Care Med 2013;39(11):1972–80.
8. Bunch TJ, White RD. Trends in treated ventricular fibrillation in out-of-hospital cardiac arrest: ischemic compared to non-ischemic heart disease. Resuscitation 2005;67(1):51–4.
9. Cobb LA, Fahrenbruch CE, Olsufka M, et al. Changing incidence of out-of-hospital ventricular fibrillation, 1980-2000. JAMA 2002;288(23):3008–13.
10. Hess EP, Campbell RL, White RD. Epidemiology, trends, and outcome of out-of-hospital cardiac arrest of non-cardiac origin. Resuscitation 2007;72(2):200–6.
11. Herlitz J, Engdahl J, Svensson L, et al. Decrease in the occurrence of ventricular fibrillation as the initially observed arrhythmia after out-of-hospital cardiac arrest during 11 years in Sweden. Resuscitation 2004;60(3):283–90.
12. Polentini MS, Pirrallo RG, McGill W. The changing incidence of ventricular fibrillation in Milwaukee, Wisconsin (1992-2002). Prehosp Emerg Care 2006;10(1): 52–60.
13. Chen N, Callaway CW, Guyette FX, et al. Arrest etiology among patients resuscitated from cardiac arrest. Resuscitation 2018;130:33–40.
14. Callaway CW, Donnino MW, Fink EL, et al. Part 8: post-cardiac arrest care 2015 American Heart Association guidelines update for cardiopulmonary resuscitation and emergency cardiovascular care. Circulation 2015;132(18):S465–82.
15. Lavonas EJ, Drennan IR, Gabrielli A, et al. Part 10: special circumstances of resuscitation: 2015 American Heart Association guidelines update for cardiopulmonary resuscitation and emergency cardiovascular care. Circulation 2015; 132(18 suppl 2):S501–18.

16. Vognsen M, Fabian-Jessing BK, Secher N, et al. Contemporary animal models of cardiac arrest: a systematic review. Resuscitation 2017;113:115–23.
17. Idris AH, Becker LB, Wenzel V, et al. Lack of uniform definitions and reporting in laboratory models of cardiac arrest: a review of the literature and a proposal for guidelines. Ann Emerg Med 1994;23(1):9–16.
18. Reynolds JC, Rittenberger JC, Menegazzi JJ. Drug administration in animal studies of cardiac arrest does not reflect human clinical experience. Resuscitation 2007;74(1):13–26.
19. Kleinman ME, Brennan EE, Goldberger ZD, et al. Part 5: adult basic life support and cardiopulmonary resuscitation quality: 2015 American Heart Association guidelines update for cardiopulmonary resuscitation and emergency cardiovascular care. Circulation 2015;132(18 suppl 2):S414–35.
20. Link MS, Berkow LC, Kudenchuk PJ, et al. Part 7: adult advanced cardiovascular life support: 2015 american heart association guidelines update for cardiopulmonary resuscitation and emergency cardiovascular care. Circulation 2015;132(18 Suppl 2):S444–64.
21. Atkins DL, Berger S, Duff JP, et al. Part 11: pediatric basic life support and cardiopulmonary resuscitation quality: 2015 American Heart Association guidelines update for cardiopulmonary resuscitation and emergency cardiovascular care. Circulation 2015;132(18 Suppl 2):S519–25.
22. de Caen AR, Berg MD, Chameides L, et al. Part 12: pediatric advanced life support: 2015 American Heart Association guidelines update for cardiopulmonary resuscitation and emergency cardiovascular care. Circulation 2015;132(18 suppl 2):S526–42.
23. Wyckoff MH, Aziz K, Escobedo MB, et al. Part 13: neonatal resuscitation: 2015 American Heart Association guidelines update for cardiopulmonary resuscitation and emergency cardiovascular care. Circulation 2015;132(18 Suppl 2): S543–60.
24. Moler FW, Donaldson AE, Meert K, et al. Multicenter cohort study of out-of-hospital pediatric cardiac arrest. Crit Care Med 2011;39(1):141–9.
25. Moler FW, Meert K, Donaldson AE, et al. In-hospital versus out-of-hospital pediatric cardiac arrest: a multicenter cohort study. Crit Care Med 2009;37(7): 2259–67.
26. Moler FW, Silverstein FS, Holubkov R, et al. Therapeutic hypothermia after out-of-hospital cardiac arrest in children. N Engl J Med 2015;372(20):1898–908.
27. Carrier M, Trudelle S, Thai P, et al. Ischemic threshold during cold blood cardioplegic arrest: monitoring with tissue pH and pO2. J Cardiovasc Surg 1998; 39(5):593–7.
28. Doppenberg EM, Zauner A, Watson JC, et al. Determination of the ischemic threshold for brain oxygen tension. Acta Neurochir Suppl 1998;71:166–9.
29. Jennings RB, Reimer KA. Factors involved in salvaging ischemic myocardium: effect of reperfusion of arterial blood. Circulation 1983;68(2 Pt 2):I25–36.
30. Siesjö BK, Ljunggren B. Cerebral energy reserves after prolonged hypoxia and ischemia. Arch Neurol 1973;29(6):400–7.
31. Busl KM, Greer DM. Hypoxic-ischemic brain injury: pathophysiology, neuropathology and mechanisms. NeuroRehabilitation 2010;26:5–13.
32. Ames A 3rd, Wright RL, Kowada M, et al. Cerebral ischemia. II. The no-reflow phenomenon. Am J Pathol 1968;52(2):437–53.
33. Elmer J, Flickinger KL, Anderson MW, et al. Effect of neuromonitor-guided titrated care on brain tissue hypoxia after opioid overdose cardiac arrest. Resuscitation 2018;129:121–6.

34. Cavus E, Bein B, Dörges V, et al. Brain tissue oxygen pressure and cerebral metabolism in an animal model of cardiac arrest and cardiopulmonary resuscitation. Resuscitation 2006;71(1):97–106.

35. Chandra NC, Gruben KG, Tsitlik JE, et al. Observations of ventilation during resuscitation in a canine model. Circulation 1994;90(6):3070–5.

36. Salford LG, Siesjo BK. The influence of arterial hypoxia and unilateral carotid artery occlusion upon regional blood flow and metabolism in the rat brain. Acta Physiol Scand 1974;92(1):130–41.

37. Eklof B, Siesjo BK. The effect of bilateral carotid artery ligation upon acid-base parameters and substrate levels in the rat brain. Acta Physiol Scand 1972;86(4):528–38.

38. Gardiner M, Smith ML, Kagstrom E, et al. Influence of blood glucose concentration on brain lactate accumulation during severe hypoxia and subsequent recovery of brain energy metabolism. J Cereb Blood Flow Metab 1982;2(4):429–38.

39. Siesjo BK. Lactic acidosis in the brain: occurrence, triggering mechanisms and pathophysiological importance. Ciba Found Symp 1982;87:77–100.

40. Salford LG, Plum F, Siesjö BK. Graded hypoxia-oligemia in rat brain: I. biochemical alterations and their implications. Arch Neurol 1973;29(4):227–33.

41. Kawai N, Keep RF, Betz AL. Hyperglycemia and the vascular effects of cerebral ischemia. Stroke 1997;28(1):149–54.

42. Chopp M, Welch KM, Tidwell CD, et al. Global cerebral ischemia and intracellular pH during hyperglycemia and hypoglycemia in cats. Stroke 1988;19(11):1383–7.

43. Lundgren J, Zhang H, Agardh CD, et al. Acidosis-induced ischemic brain damage: are free radicals involved? J Cereb Blood Flow Metab 1991;11(4):587–96.

44. Bralet J, Schreiber L, Bouvier C. Effect of acidosis and anoxia on iron delocalization from brain homogenates. Biochem Pharmacol 1992;43(5):979–83.

45. Krause GS, Joyce KM, Nayini NR, et al. Cardiac arrest and resuscitation: brain iron delocalization during reperfusion. Ann Emerg Med 1985;14(11):1037–43.

46. Krause GS, Nayini NR, White BC, et al. Natural course of iron delocalization and lipid peroxidation during the first eight hours following a 15-minute cardiac arrest in dogs. Ann Emerg Med 1987;16(11):1200–5.

47. White BC, Krause GS, Aust SD, et al. Postischemic tissue injury by iron-mediated free radical lipid peroxidation. Ann Emerg Med 1985;14(8):804–9.

48. Nayini NR, White BC, Aust SD, et al. Post resuscitation iron delocalization and malondialdehyde production in the brain following prolonged cardiac arrest. J Free Radic Biol Med 1985;1(2):111–6.

49. Siesjo BK, Agardh CD, Bengtsson F. Free radicals and brain damage. Cerebrovasc Brain Metab Rev 1989;1(3):165–211.

50. Komara JS, Nayini NR, Bialick HA, et al. Brain iron delocalization and lipid peroxidation following cardiac arrest. Ann Emerg Med 1986;15(4):384–9.

51. Babbs CF. Role of iron ions in the genesis of reperfusion injury following successful cardiopulmonary resuscitation: preliminary data and a biochemical hypothesis. Ann Emerg Med 1985;14(8):777–83.

52. White BC, Nayini NR, Krause GS, et al. Effect on biochemical markers of brain injury of therapy with deferoxamine or superoxide dismutase following cardiac arrest. Am J Emerg Med 1988;6(6):569–76.

53. Kompala SD, Babbs CF, Blaho KE. Effect of deferoxamine on late deaths following CPR in rats. Ann Emerg Med 1986;15(4):405–7.

54. Rosenthal RE, Chanderbhan R, Marshall G, et al. Prevention of post-ischemic brain lipid conjugated diene production and neurological injury by hydroxyethyl starch-conjugated deferoxamine. Free Radic Biol Med 1992;12(1):29–33.

55. Cerchiari EL, Hoel TM, Safar P, et al. Protective effects of combined superoxide dismutase and deferoxamine on recovery of cerebral blood flow and function after cardiac arrest in dogs. Stroke 1987;18(5):869–78.

56. Kumar K, White BC, Krause GS, et al. A quantitative morphological assessment of the effect of lidoflazine and deferoxamine therapy on global brain ischaemia. Neurol Res 1988;10(3):136–40.

57. Vaagenes P, Safar P, Moossy J, et al. Asphyxiation versus ventricular fibrillation cardiac arrest in dogs.: differences in cerebral resuscitation effects—a preliminary study. Resuscitation 1997;35(1):41–52.

58. Uray T, Lamade A, Elmer J, et al. Phenotyping cardiac arrest: bench and bedside characterization of brain and heart injury based on etiology. Crit Care Med 2018;46(6):e508–15.

59. Kamohara T, Weil MH, Tang W, et al. A comparison of myocardial function after primary cardiac and primary asphyxial cardiac arrest. Am J Respir Crit Care Med 2001;164(7):1221–4.

60. Isaev NK, Stelmashook EV, Plotnikov EY, et al. Role of acidosis, NMDA receptors, and acid-sensitive ion channel 1a (ASIC1a) in neuronal death induced by ischemia. Biochemistry (Mosc) 2008;73(11):1171–5.

61. Wemmie JA, Taugher RJ, Kreple CJ. Acid-sensing ion channels in pain and disease. Nat Rev Neurosci 2013;14(7):461–71.

62. Xiong ZG, Zhu XM, Chu XP, et al. Neuroprotection in ischemia: blocking calcium-permeable acid-sensing ion channels. Cell 2004;118(6):687–98.

63. Narasimhan P, Swanson RA, Sagar SM, et al. Astrocyte survival and HSP70 heat shock protein induction following heat shock and acidosis. Glia 1996;17(2):147–59.

64. Siesjo BK, Katsura KI, Kristian T, et al. Molecular mechanisms of acidosis-mediated damage. Acta Neurochir Suppl 1996;66:8–14.

65. Wolosker H, Rocha JB, Engelender S, et al. Sarco/endoplasmic reticulum Ca2+-ATPase isoforms: diverse responses to acidosis. Biochem J 1997;321(Pt 2):545–50.

66. Drabek T, Foley LM, Janata A, et al. Global and regional differences in cerebral blood flow after asphyxial versus ventricular fibrillation cardiac arrest in rats using ASL-MRI. Resuscitation 2014;85(7):964–71.

67. Granfeldt A, Wissenberg M, Hansen SM, et al. Clinical predictors of shockable versus non-shockable rhythms in patients with out-of-hospital cardiac arrest. Resuscitation 2016;108:40–7.

68. Kitamura T, Kiyohara K, Sakai T, et al. Epidemiology and outcome of adult out-of-hospital cardiac arrest of non-cardiac origin in Osaka: a population-based study. BMJ Open 2014;4(12):e006462.

69. Patil KD, Halperin HR, Becker LB. Cardiac arrest: resuscitation and reperfusion. Circ Res 2015;116(12):2041–9.

70. Chan PS, McNally B, Tang F, et al. Recent trends in survival from out-of-hospital cardiac arrest in the United States. Circulation 2014;130(21):1876–82.

71. Nadkarni VM, Larkin GL, Peberdy MA, et al. First documented rhythm and clinical outcome from in-hospital cardiac arrest among children and adults. JAMA 2006;295(1):50–7.

72. Rittenberger JC, Tisherman SA, Holm MB, et al. An early, novel illness severity score to predict outcome after cardiac arrest. Resuscitation 2011;82(11):1399–404.
73. Coppler PJ, Elmer J, Calderon L, et al. Validation of the Pittsburgh cardiac arrest category illness severity score. Resuscitation 2015;89:86–92.
74. Lee SJ, Jeung KW, Lee BK, et al. Impact of case volume on outcome and performance of targeted temperature management in out-of-hospital cardiac arrest survivors. Am J Emerg Med 2015;33(1):31–6.
75. Smith G, Beger S, Vadeboncoeur T, et al. Trends in overdose-related out-of-hospital cardiac arrest in Arizona. Resuscitation 2019;134:122–6.
76. Salcido DD, Torres C, Koller AC, et al. Regional incidence and outcome of out-of-hospital cardiac arrest associated with overdose. Resuscitation 2016;99:13–9.
77. Orkin AM, Zhan C, Buick JE, et al. Out-of-hospital cardiac arrest survival in drug-related versus cardiac causes in Ontario: a retrospective cohort study. PLoS One 2017;12(4):e0176441.
78. Sayre MR, Berg RA, Cave DM, et al. Hands-only (compression-only) cardiopulmonary resuscitation: a call to action for bystander response to adults who experience out-of-hospital sudden cardiac arrest: a science advisory for the public from the American Heart Association Emergency Cardiovascular Care Committee. Circulation 2008;117(16):2162–7.
79. Bobrow BJ, Spaite DW, Berg RA, et al. Chest compression-only CPR by lay rescuers and survival from out-of-hospital cardiac arrest. JAMA 2010;304(13):1447–54.
80. Iwami T, Kitamura T, Kawamura T, et al. Chest compression–only cardiopulmonary resuscitation for out-of-hospital cardiac arrest with public-access defibrillation: a nationwide cohort study. Circulation 2012;126(24):2844–51.
81. SOS-KANTO study group. Cardiopulmonary resuscitation by bystanders with chest compression only (SOS-KANTO): an observational study. Lancet 2007;369(9565):920–6.
82. Ogawa T, Akahane M, Koike S, et al. Outcomes of chest compression only CPR versus conventional CPR conducted by lay people in patients with out of hospital cardiopulmonary arrest witnessed by bystanders: nationwide population based observational study. BMJ 2011;342:c7106.
83. Dumas F, Rea TD, Fahrenbruch C, et al. Chest compression alone cardiopulmonary resuscitation is associated with better long-term survival compared with standard cardiopulmonary resuscitation. Circulation 2013;127(4):435–41.
84. Hallstrom A, Cobb L, Johnson E, et al. Cardiopulmonary resuscitation by chest compression alone or with mouth-to-mouth ventilation. N Engl J Med 2000;342(21):1546–53.
85. Rea TD, Fahrenbruch C, Culley L, et al. CPR with chest compression alone or with rescue breathing. N Engl J Med 2010;363(5):423–33.
86. Svensson L, Bohm K, Castrèn M, et al. Compression-only CPR or standard CPR in out-of-hospital cardiac arrest. N Engl J Med 2010;363(5):434–42.
87. Dumas F, Cariou A, Manzo-Silberman S, et al. Immediate percutaneous coronary intervention is associated with better survival after out-of-hospital cardiac arrest: insights from the PROCAT (Parisian Region Out of hospital Cardiac ArresT) registry. Circ Cardiovasc Interv 2010;3(3):200–7.
88. Geri G, Dumas F, Bougouin W, et al. Immediate percutaneous coronary intervention is associated with improved short- and long-term survival after out-of-hospital cardiac arrest. Circ Cardiovasc Interv 2015;8(10):e002303.

89. Vyas A, Chan PS, Cram P, et al. Early coronary angiography and survival after out-of-hospital cardiac arrest. Circ Cardiovasc Interv 2015;8(10):e002321.

90. Jentzer JC, Scutella M, Pike F, et al. Early coronary angiography and percutaneous coronary intervention are associated with improved outcomes after out of hospital cardiac arrest. Resuscitation 2018;123:15–21.

91. Lemkes JS, Janssens GN, van der Hoeven NW, et al. Coronary angiography after cardiac arrest without ST-segment elevation. N Engl J Med 2019;380(15): 1397–407.

92. Bernard SA, Gray TW, Buist MD, et al. Treatment of comatose survivors of out-of-hospital cardiac arrest with induced hypothermia. N Engl J Med 2002;346:: 557–63.

93. Hypothermia after Cardiac Arrest Study Group. Mild therapeutic hypothermia to improve the neurologic outcome after cardiac arrest. N Engl J Med 2002;346(8): 549–56.

94. Nielsen N, Wetterslev J, Cronberg T, et al. Targeted temperature management at 33 degrees C versus 36 degrees C after cardiac arrest. N Engl J Med 2013; 369(23):2197–206.

95. Bro-Jeppesen J, Annborn M, Hassager C, et al. Hemodynamics and vasopressor support during targeted temperature management at 33°C versus 36°C after out-of-hospital cardiac arrest: a post hoc study of the target temperature management trial. Crit Care Med 2015;43(2):318–27.

96. Lascarrou J-B, Merdji H, Le Gouge A, et al. Targeted temperature management for cardiac arrest with nonshockable rhythm. N Engl J Med 2019;381(24): 2327–37.

97. Kirkegaard H, Søreide E, de Haas I, et al. Targeted temperature management for 48 vs 24 hours and neurologic outcome after out-of-hospital cardiac arrest: a randomized clinical trial. JAMA 2017;318(4):341–50.

98. Brain Resuscitation Clinical Trial I Study Group. Randomized clinical study of thiopental loading in comatose survivors of cardiac arrest. N Engl J Med 1986;314(7):397–403.

99. Brain Resuscitation Clinical Trial II Study Group. A randomized clinical study of a calcium-entry blocker (lidoflazine) in the treatment of comatose survivors of cardiac arrest. N Engl J Med 1991;324(18):1225–31.

100. Cariou A, Deye N, Vivien B, et al. Early high-dose erythropoietin therapy after out-of-hospital cardiac arrest: a multicenter, randomized controlled trial. J Am Coll Cardiol 2016;68(1):40–9.

101. Wiberg S, Hassager C, Schmidt H, et al. Neuroprotective effects of the glucagon-like peptide-1 analog exenatide after out-of-hospital cardiac arrest: a randomized controlled trial. Circulation 2016;134(25):2115–24.

102. Ji J, Kline AE, Amoscato A, et al. Lipidomics identifies cardiolipin oxidation as a mitochondrial target for redox therapy of brain injury. Nat Neurosci 2012;15(10): 1407–13.

103. Anthonymuthu TS, Kenny EM, Lamade AM, et al. Oxidized phospholipid signaling in traumatic brain injury. Free Radic Biol Med 2018;124:493–503.

104. Kenny EM, Fidan E, Yang Q, et al. Ferroptosis contributes to neuronal death and functional outcome after traumatic brain injury. Crit Care Med 2018;47(3):410–8.

105. Kern KB, Hilwig RW, Rhee KH, et al. Myocardial dysfunction after resuscitation from cardiac arrest: an example of global myocardial stunning. J Am Coll Cardiol 1996;28(1):232–40.

106. Yang L, Li C, Gao C, et al. Investigation of myocardial stunning after cardiopulmonary resuscitation in pigs. Biomed Environ Sci 2011;24(2):155–62.

107. Adrie C, Adib-Conquy M, Laurent I, et al. Successful cardiopulmonary resuscitation after cardiac arrest as a "sepsis-like" syndrome. Circulation 2002;106(5): 562–8.
108. Bro-Jeppesen J, Johansson PI, Kjaergaard J, et al. Level of systemic inflammation and endothelial injury is associated with cardiovascular dysfunction and vasopressor support in post-cardiac arrest patients. Resuscitation 2017;121: 179–86.
109. Bro-Jeppesen J, Kjaergaard J, Wanscher M, et al. Systemic inflammatory response and potential prognostic implications after out-of-hospital cardiac arrest: a substudy of the target temperature management trial. Crit Care Med 2015;43(6):1223–32.

Impact of the Opioid Epidemic

Eric J. Lavonas, MD, MS[a,b,*], Cameron Dezfulian, MD[c,d]

KEYWORDS

- Opioid analgesics • Overdose • Opioid use disorder • Respiratory arrest
- Cardiac arrest • Naloxone • Resuscitation • Critical care

KEY POINTS

- Naloxone rapidly reverses central nervous system and respiratory depression / respiratory arrest caused by opioid overdose.
- Patients with opioid overdose who are sleepy but have adequate respiratory drive and protective airway reflexes can be observed with pulse oximetry and waveform capnography until spontaneous recovery occurs.
- When naloxone administration is required, the lowest dose necessary to restore adequate minute ventilation and airway protection should be used.
- Patients who use fentanyl and fentanyl analogues may require higher doses of naloxone than those who use heroin or other opioids.
- Secondary prevention programs, such as referral to therapy, medication assisted therapy, and naloxone distribution programs may prevent subsequent mortality.

INTRODUCTION

Opioid misuse is endemic in the United States. In a 2017 survey, an estimated 11.4 million Americans (4.2% of US persons aged 12 years or older) reported opioid misuse in the past year.[1] This resulted in 47,600 drug overdose deaths, 91,840 hospital admissions, and 197,970 emergency department encounters involving opioid overdose in 2016.[1]

The epidemic of deaths from opioid overdose is now in entering its third decade, with approximately 600,000 lives lost in the United States since 1999. Although the

[a] Department of Emergency Medicine, Rocky Mountain Poison and Drug Safety, Denver Health, 777 Bannock Street, MC 0108, Denver, CO 80238, USA; [b] Department of Emergency Medicine, University of Colorado School of Medicine, Aurora, CO, USA; [c] Critical Care Medicine, University of Pittsburgh School of Medicine, 4401 Penn Avenue, CHP Faculty Pavilion, Room 2119, Pittsburgh, PA 15224, USA; [d] Clinical and Translational Sciences, University of Pittsburgh School of Medicine, 4401 Penn Avenue, CHP Faculty Pavilion, Room 2119, Pittsburgh, PA 15224, USA
* Corresponding author. 777 Bannock Street, MC 0108, Denver, CO 80204.
E-mail address: eric.lavonas@dhha.org

Crit Care Clin 36 (2020) 753–769
https://doi.org/10.1016/j.ccc.2020.07.006
0749-0704/20/© 2020 Elsevier Inc. All rights reserved.
criticalcare.theclinics.com

modal patient who dies from opioid overdose in the United States is a non-Hispanic White man in the fourth decade of life, the opioid epidemic includes people of all ages, sex, race, ethnicity, and environment.

The first wave of this epidemic, which began in approximately 1999, involved an increase in prescribing of, misuse of, and poisoning from prescription opioids, including oxycodone, hydrocodone, hydromorphone, and fentanyl.[1] Death rates from heroin overdose began to rise in 2010, as users switched because of decreasing availability of prescription opioids and the attractive, lower price of high-purity heroin. Since 2013, an enormous increase in deaths has been caused by the presence of illicitly manufactured fentanyl and fentanyl analogues in the illicit opioid supply, often sold in the form of counterfeit prescription opioid tablets or heroin. Although death rates because of prescription opioids, heroin, and opioids overall decreased from 2017 to 2018, deaths caused by synthetic opioids increased by 10% (**Fig. 1**).[1] Coingestion of other sedating substances is common; in 2017, ethanol was detected in 15% of opioid fatalities, and benzodiazepines in 21%.[2] The incidence of polypharmacy in fentanyl and other synthetic opioid poisonings may be 80%.[3] Although it is possible that the opioid overdose epidemic is decreasing, the age-adjusted death rate because of unintentional opioid overdose remains more than five times the rate in 1999.[1]

CLINICAL FEATURES

Opioid overdose causes central nervous system (CNS) and respiratory depression through agonism at μ-opioid receptors in the brain and spinal cord. Additional mechanisms involve modulation of κ, δ, and ORL-1 opioid receptors and GABA-A chloride channels, and opioids and benzodiazepines have synergistic effects on respiratory depression.[4] If untreated, this can progress to loss of protective airway reflexes,

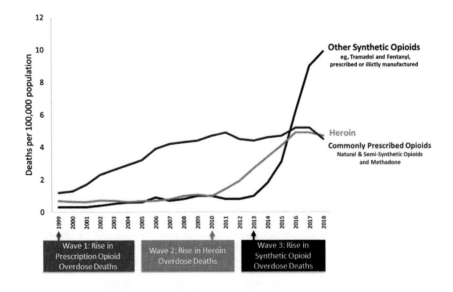

Fig. 1. Three waves of opioid overdose deaths. (*From* Centers for Disease Control. Opioid Overdose: Understanding the Epidemic. 2020. Available at: https://www.cdc.gov/drugoverdose/epidemic/index.html. Accessed June 19, 2020.)

impaired sensitivity to hypoxemia and hypercapnia, and loss of respiratory drive. The end result of this process is respiratory arrest, followed by cardiac arrest. In a minority of cases, mostly involving methadone, the cause of cardiac arrest may be arrhythmia precipitated by QT prolongation.[5–7]

The opioid overdose toxidrome is generally considered to be miotic pupils, CNS depression, and hypoventilation.[8] Although the presence of miosis strongly suggests the diagnosis of opioid overdose in patients with drug-related altered mental status (sensitivity, 91%; odds ratio, 20.0; 95% confidence interval, 1.9–216),[9] miosis is sometimes absent if opioids with serotonin agonism (eg, tramadol, tapentadol) are ingested. Many commonly ingested nonopioid drugs (eg, quetiapine, clonidine) cause CNS depression and miosis. There is no accepted gold standard to define a history suggestive of unintentional opioid overdose, and the diagnostic value of historical elements, such as bystander history and the presence of drug paraphernalia, is unknown. To date, no clinical decision rule has proven to be highly sensitive and specific for the diagnosis of opioid intoxication.[9]

The spectrum of opioid overdose severity ranges from mild CNS depression to respiratory depression, respiratory arrest, and cardiac arrest.

PREHOSPITAL AND EMERGENCY MANAGEMENT OF OPIOID OVERDOSE

In addition to an initial assessment to exclude other causes of altered mental status (eg, hypoglycemia, sepsis, trauma), patients with suspected opioid overdose should be assessed for the presence of protective airway reflexes and adequate respiratory drive. Because assessment of the gag reflex has poor specificity, poor reproducibility, and can lead to vomiting with aspiration, gag reflex testing is no longer recommended.[10–15] Evaluation of the patient's ability to coordinate spontaneous swallowing with respiration may be a more accurate assessment of the presence of airway protective reflexes.[16] In addition, coordination of swallow and respiration is impaired when the P_aCO_2 is high, as occurs with opioid-induced hypoventilation.[17]

In addition to counting respiratory rate, assessing for the adequacy of tidal volume by physical examination, and measuring arterial oxygen saturation with pulse oximetry, waveform capnography is useful to assess and monitor patients for opioid-induced hypoventilation.[18]

Patients who are somnolent with adequate respiratory rate and volume and intact airway reflexes may be observed with continuous pulse oximetry and capnography monitoring until they are awake (**Fig. 2**). Patients who are not breathing adequately or who are unable to maintain a patent airway should receive naloxone therapy.

Naloxone

Naloxone, first approved by the US Food and Drug administration in 1971 as Narcan, is a potent, competitive μ-opioid receptor antagonist.[18] When given in adequate doses, naloxone rapidly reverses all effects of opioid intoxication. Responsiveness to naloxone is generally considered the sine qua non of opioid overdose. Although coingestion and/or multiple medical conditions may lead to incomplete response to naloxone, naloxone administration is the mainstay of therapy for life-threatening CNS and respiratory depression potentially because of opioid overdose.[19]

When given in adequate doses, naloxone reverses all the clinical effects of opioid intoxication, restoring consciousness, protective airway reflexes, and normal minute ventilation. Patients who have life-threatening respiratory depression should receive naloxone, with bag-mask ventilation provided until naloxone is administered and takes

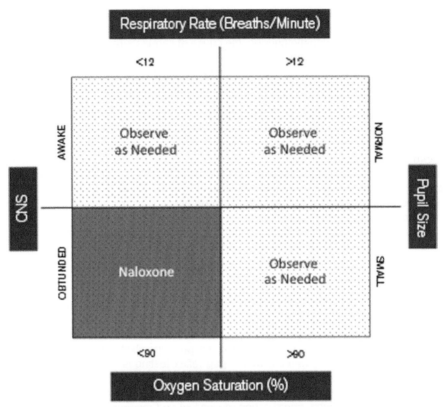

Fig. 2. Indications for naloxone in opioid overdose. (*From* Hack J. A Unified Naloxone Guideline Graph. ACEPNow. 2019: 38(7), July 26, 2019. Available at: https://www.acepnow. com/article/a-unified-naloxone-guideline-graph/. With permission.)

effect. However, naloxone administration is not risk-free. Naloxone administration often produces acute opioid withdrawal. This is intensely uncomfortable for patients, reducing faith in the health care system,[20] and sometimes leading to agitation and violence. In addition, naloxone administration can precipitate noncardiogenic pulmonary edema.[21–25] Furthermore, once a patient has undergone full opioid reversal with naloxone, the minimum safe observation period is unclear (see later). For patients who are sleepy but have adequate respiration and exhibit airway protection, observation with continuous pulse oximetry and capnography monitoring is simpler and likely safer.

Naloxone is administered by a variety of routes, including intravenous (IV), intramuscular, subcutaneous, intranasal, or aerosolized into the respiratory tree.[26] A prehospital clinical trial showed that the time to awakening of IV and subcutaneous naloxone were similar, because the more rapid time of drug administration in the subcutaneous group was offset by a slight delay in clinical effect.[27]

Naloxone is titrated to the clinical end point of restoring adequate spontaneous ventilation and airway reflexes. Although a randomized clinical trial found that larger doses of naloxone are likely required when using the intranasal route compared with intramuscular administration, the ideal starting dose of naloxone is unknown, and may vary by the situation.[28] Naloxone products intended for use in the community, administered by lay-persons who are not capable of providing assisted ventilation or titrating the administered dose, carry a larger naloxone dose (2 mg for intramuscular/subcutaneous formulations) than the commonly recommended starting dose for IV administration in a health care setting.[29] The 2015 American Heart Association recommendations suggest an initial naloxone dose of 0.04 to 0.4 mg IV or intramuscular, or 2 mg if the intranasal route is chosen, with repeat dosing or dose escalation as needed.[30]

Because fentanyl and fentanyl analogues (fentalogues) have a much greater affinity for the μ-opioid receptor than morphine, heroin, and other opioids, larger doses of naloxone may be required to reverse opioid intoxication when fentanyl or fentalogues are involved.[31] In the United States, forensic laboratory reports of fentanyl and fentalogues increased 60-fold from 2013 to 2017, and in some regions, particularly the Great Lakes and Northeast, most samples of white powder "heroin" are actually fentanyl or fentanyl-heroin combinations.[32] Fentanyl-containing counterfeit prescription opioid tablets are also common. Estimates of the proportion of opioid overdose patients who require more than one dose of naloxone in locations with a high prevalence of fentalogue overdose vary widely. A proposed dose-escalation algorithm for IV naloxone administration is shown in **Fig. 3**.

Most patients with opioid overdose are treated in and released from the emergency department, without involvement of the critical care team. In fact, several studies, conducted predominately in populations of patients who used heroin, demonstrated apparent safety (ie, low detected short-term mortality) when patients who received naloxone from paramedics were allowed to refuse care directly from the ambulance.[33–35] Applying the results of these studies to patients who ingested long-acting opioids (eg, buprenorphine; methadone; or sustained-release formulations of oxycodone, hydromorphone, or morphine) is probably unwise. Naltrexone, a long-acting μ-opioid antagonist, has been proposed and studied as an agent to counteract the effect of methadone, an opioid with a long effective half-life.[36] The safety of this approach is not well-established.

Naloxone has an apparent duration of action of 20 to 90 minutes, which is less than many opioids.[37] As a result, when patients experience complete reversal of opioid clinical effects following naloxone administration, a period of observation is required to watch for recurrent opioid toxicity when the naloxone is metabolized. Unfortunately, the minimum safe duration of this observation period is not known. The simplest solution is to give small doses of naloxone titrated to the clinical end point of a somnolent but breathing patient with intact airway reflexes. The patient can then wake up gradually as the opioid is metabolized and be safely discharged. When patients present fully awake after naloxone reversal, an empiric period of observation of at least 2 to 4 hours is recommended, and a longer period in patients whose toxicity is caused by a long-acting opioid.[38] However, several studies demonstrate a low risk of mortality in patients who respond to naloxone discharged after meeting clinical criteria for discharge after 1 hour of observation.[33,39,40] Following this observation period, clinical criteria for discharge from the emergency department are shown in **Box 1**.

In the original derivation and subsequent validation cohorts of this rule, only 2 of 1111 patients required additional naloxone after fulfilling the rule.[39,40]

Unfortunately, a similar data-driven approach to the observation and safe discharge of patients with an overdose of long-acting opioids (eg, buprenorphine; methadone; or sustained-release formulations of oxycodone, hydromorphone, or morphine) is not available. Similarly, data are lacking to recommend an observation period for opioid-intoxicated infants and children, nor for patients intoxicated with fentanyl and the ultrahigh-potency fentalogues.

CRITICAL CARE MANAGEMENT OF OPIOID OVERDOSE

In most studies, fewer than 15% of patients presenting to the emergency department for treatment of opioid overdose require intensive care unit (ICU) admission, and most of these admissions are because of multiple substance ingestion or other medical conditions (eg, infection, trauma). The most common opioid-specific reasons for ICU admissions are discussed next.

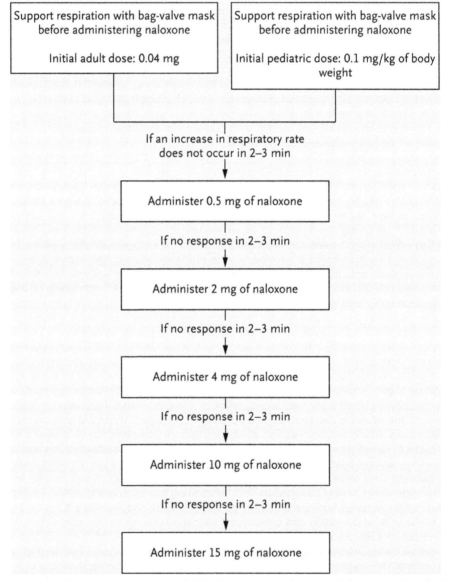

Fig. 3. Sample escalating dose protocol for intravenous naloxone administration in opioid overdose. (*From* Boyer EW. Management of Opioid Analgesic Overdose. *New Engl J Med* 2012; 367(2):146-55. Copyright © 2012 Massachusetts Medical Society. Reprinted with permission from Massachusetts Medical Society.)

Box 1
St. Paul's early discharge rule for adult emergency department patients who respond to naloxone administration

- Able to ambulate as usual

- Normal oxygen saturation

- Normal respiratory rate (>10 and <20 breaths/min)

- Normal temperature (>35.0°C and <37.5°C)

- Normal heart rate (>50 and <100 beats/min)

- Glasgow Coma Score of 15

- At least 1 hour after last dose of naloxone

From Christenson J, Etherington J, Grafstein E, et al. Early discharge of patients with presumed opioid overdose: development of a clinical prediction rule. Academic emergency medicine: official journal of the Society for Academic Emergency Medicine. 2000;7(10):1110-1118; with permission.

Recurrent Sedation

Some patients who respond to naloxone develop resedation requiring multiple doses of naloxone. Treatment options include repeat IV naloxone dosing or continuous naloxone infusion. The starting infusion rate for a naloxone infusion is two-thirds of the "waking" dose per hour.[41] Patients who develop resedation while on a naloxone infusion should receive additional naloxone bolus therapy, up-titration of the infusion, and examination for other causes of CNS and/or respiratory depression.

After an appropriate period of time (arbitrarily, 2–3 half-lives of the ingested opioid, if the substance is known), patients can have a trial of discontinuation of the naloxone drip. Down-titration is not necessary. Pulse oximetry and end-tidal carbon dioxide monitoring should continue during this trial. Although there does not seem to be any literature to define the minimum safe observation period following discontinuation of a naloxone infusion, a patient who remains awake and alert, normoxemic, with adequate respiratory drive for 6 to 12 hours after discontinuation is unlikely to experience resedation.

Opioid-Associated Pulmonary Edema

Some patients rapidly develop noncardiogenic pulmonary edema following opioid overdose, with or without reversal with naloxone. The pathophysiology of opioid-associated pulmonary edema is uncertain; some authors describe the phenomenon as a form of neurogenic pulmonary edema,[24] whereas other authors attribute it to increased capillary permeability,[42] a rapid increase in sympathetic response,[43] histamine release,[44] or to acutely generated negative pressure as patients attempt to inspire against a closed glottis.[21,45] The cause may be multifactorial, and the cause may differ between patients who develop pulmonary edema after using opioids alone and those in whom it develops following naloxone administration. There is some evidence that the development of pulmonary edema is dose dependent with higher associations when initial IV dose exceeds 0.4 mg and total dose exceeds 4.4 mg.[25] The largest modern case series reported an incidence of 2.1% of patients treated for heroin overdose,[23] although rates of 10% have been reported.[46] Signs of noncardiogenic pulmonary edema usually appear within minutes of naloxone administration, and include hypoxemia, respiratory distress, and rales. Chest radiography commonly shows bilateral fluffy pulmonary infiltrates. Not all patients require treatment; successful use is reported of bilevel positive airway pressure (BiPAP),[47] or with some combination of nitrates, diuretics, and/or low-dose opioids.[21] Most patients respond rapidly and do not require intubation.

Cardiovascular Instability

Naloxone administration can precipitate a severe acute withdrawal syndrome in opioid-dependent patients. Although self-limited tachycardia and transient hypertension are common, a small proportion of patients develop atrial[48] or ventricular[49] arrhythmias. These may be caused by catecholamine release; hypoxemia; or the effects of other intoxicants, such as cocaine or methamphetamine. In the absence of evidence-supported alternative approaches, treatment is supportive, with the possible careful addition of low doses of opioids, benzodiazepines, or clonidine to reduce withdrawal severity.

Hypoxemic-Ischemic Encephalopathy

Opioid overdose causes respiratory depression leading to respiratory arrest and ultimately cardiac arrest. The cellular injury from progressive hypoxia and hypercapnia with preserved blood flow and glucose delivery differs fundamentally from that caused by sudden global ischemia with simultaneous loss of blood flow, as is seen in sudden cardiac arrest.[50] Reperfusion injury after hypoxemia-ischemia is more severe than following sudden cardiac arrest. Although the pragmatic implications of this observation are unknown, a large proportion of opioid-associated cardiac arrest survivors develop ischemic injury to the brain and heart.[51,52] The hippocampus, basal ganglia, and globus pallidus seem particularly susceptible to injury.[53–55] The field of neuroprotection after hypoxemic-ischemic or ischemic insult is evolving rapidly, but no specific neuroprotective agents are yet approved.

Cardiac Arrest

Some patients with opioid overdose suffer cardiac arrest from which they are successfully resuscitated. In patients who are intubated and ventilated, naloxone administration has no known or theoretic benefit in this situation, and there are several theoretic reasons to suspect that opioid reversal may be harmful to cells that have just suffered severe hypoxemia-ischemia.[50] Standard post–cardiac arrest care, including targeted temperature management, and prevention of hypoxemia, hyperoxia, or hypertension, is appropriate in this situation. A diagnostic trial of naloxone to assess for opioid intoxication as a reversible cause of coma may be reasonable, but there is no evidence around this practice in the postarrest period.

Other Direct Complications of Opioid Use and Overdose

As with any overdose that causes CNS depression, patients with opioid overdose may develop aspiration pneumonitis.

Some opioids, particularly methadone, cause QT interval prolongation and torsades de pointes from blockade of the inward potassium rectifier (iKr; hERG) channel.[56,57] In addition, loperamide, which when taken in massive doses has mild euphoric effects and is sometimes used for self-medication of opioid withdrawal symptoms, can cause QT prolongation and torsades.[58–60] Management of QT prolongation includes cardiac monitoring, correction of hypokalemia and hypomagnesemia, avoidance of other QT prolonging medications, and avoidance of iatrogenic bradycardia. An up-to-date list of medications associated with QT prolongation or torsades is maintained by the Arizona Center for Education and Research on Therapeutics at www.qtdrugs.org. The risk that a given patient with QT prolongation will develop torsades can be estimated based on the heart rate and the absolute QT interval.[61] In severe cases, prophylactic overdrive pacing may be instituted to prevent torsades. If torsades de pointes develops, treatment includes IV magnesium sulfate boluses, overdrive pacing, or cardioversion.

Infective Endocarditis

People who inject drugs may develop bacterial endocarditis. Staphylococcal endocarditis in people who inject drugs is now the dominant form of the disease in many communities.[62] People who inject drugs are at increased risk of developing tricuspid valve (right-sided) endocarditis. In recent years, several clusters of patients with right-sided endocarditis were identified in persons who inject hydromorphone, and persons who inject extended-release hydromorphone may be at especially high risk.[63] Some evidence suggests that specific controlled-release opioids may facilitate the survival of *Staphylococcus aureus* in injection drug "cookers" and filters.[64] Drug use–associated infective endocarditis hospitalizations have increased markedly with the opioid epidemic, and the demographics have changed from an urban-predominate to a rural-predominate disease.[65–68] People who inject drugs seem to be at increased risk for methicillin-resistant *S aureus* infections, including endocarditis,[69] so initial therapy with vancomycin seems prudent until culture and sensitivity results are complete.

Other Infectious Diseases

People who inject drugs are at increased risk of developing blood-borne infections, including human immunodeficiency virus (HIV) and hepatitis C. Large local outbreaks of HIV have been associated with injection drug use clusters.[53,70] Testing for hepatitis B, hepatitis C, and HIV should routinely be offered to persons who inject drugs who present for care for opioid overdose or other reasons, and hepatitis B vaccination should be offered to persons who inject drugs who are not already infected or immune.

MODIFICATIONS TO RESUSCITATION

Resuscitation of the patient with opioid-associated cardiac arrest includes standard resuscitation with the addition of naloxone in specific circumstances.[30] Two simple guiding principles overlap to influence resuscitation decisions.

The first consideration is that naloxone effectively reverses respiratory arrest from opioid overdose, but has no known or theoretic benefit for the patient with cardiac arrest. The second is that lay rescuers have difficulty accurately assessing for the presence of a pulse, and resuscitation guidelines no longer recommend that lay rescuers perform health checks.[71]

As a result of these factors, the American Heart Association recommends that non–health care providers assume that any unresponsive patient is in cardiac arrest, and initiate cardiopulmonary resuscitation (CPR) without attempting to determine whether a pulse is present.[71] When opioid overdose is suspected, naloxone administration is recommended (**Fig. 4**).[30] In this situation, the potential benefit from naloxone administration supersedes the theoretic harm of administering naloxone to a pulseless patient. Because opioids cause cardiac arrest as a result of respiratory arrest, CPR with compressions and ventilations is preferred over compression-only CPR whenever the rescuer is capable of providing ventilations.[30]

When a health care provider is able to reliably assess for the presence of a pulse, such as in an EMS or hospital setting, naloxone administration is recommended for patients who have a pulse (ie, for those in respiratory arrest), but not for pulseless patients (ie, cardiac arrest).[30]

Opioid-Associated Life-Threatening Emergency (Adult) Algorithm—New 2015

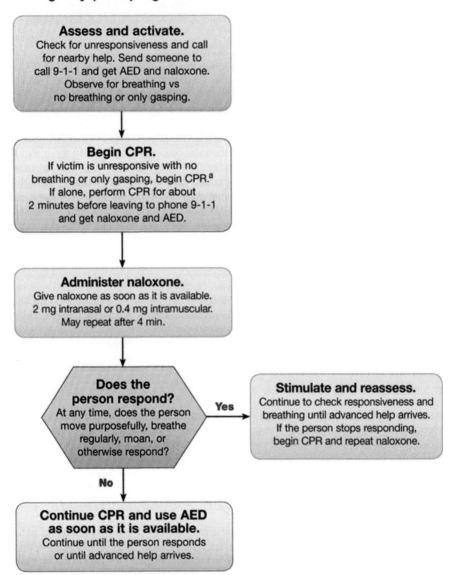

Fig. 4. American Heart Association opioid-associated emergency (adult) for lay responders algorithm (2015). [a] CPR technique based on rescuer's level of training. AED, automated external defibrillator. (*From* Lavonas EJ, Drennan IR, Gabrielli A, Heffner AC, et al. Part 10: special circumstances of resuscitation: 2015 American Heart Association guidelines update for cardiopulmonary resuscitation and emergency cardiovascular care. Reprinted with permission Circulation.2015;132:s501-s518 ©2015 American Heart Association, Inc.)

PRIMARY PREVENTION

The US opioid overdose epidemic grew in parallel with increases in opioid prescribing. The overall opioid prescribing rate in the United States peaked in 2010 to 2012 and had been decreasing since 2012, but the amount of opioids in milligrams of morphine-equivalent per capita is still approximately three times the 1999 prescribing levels.[72] Recent attention and program development have focused on alternatives to opioids (ALTO) approaches to pain control.[73] Intervention tactics include increasing the use of topical therapy, trigger point injections, regional anesthesia, low-dose intranasal or IV ketamine, nitrous oxide, and IV lidocaine,[74] combined with scripting and nonpharmaceutical interventions.[75] In Colorado, the introduction of ALTO training and protocols into 10 emergency departments was associated with a 36% decrease in opioid usage in those departments.[73]

Because high-dose opioids are ineffective for the treatment of chronic pain, thoughtful tapering of opioids for chronic pain may decrease the risk of overdose.[76–78]

SECONDARY PREVENTION AND TAKE-HOME MORPHINE-EQUIVALENT NALOXONE

Patients who survive an opioid overdose are at high risk for another overdose event and death. The 1-year mortality rate in opioid overdose survivors is 5.5%, with 1.1% of patients dying within a month of the index treated overdose, and 0.25% within 2 days.[79] Prevention of subsequent overdose and/or reducing the risk that a subsequent overdose will lead to death is therefore a critical portion of opioid overdose care.

Structured approaches to counseling, such as Screening, Brief Intervention, and Referral to Treatment (SBIRT), the Brief Negotiation Interview (BNI), and other motivational interviewing techniques are associated with a mild reduction in ongoing opioid use among persons with opioid use disorder.[80] Coupling these interventions with medication for opioid use disorder and referral to ongoing therapy significantly improves treatment success.[81] More importantly, medication use for opioid use disorder, whether methadone or buprenorphine, has resulted in more than 50% reduction in mortality in those with opioid use disorder.[82] A growing number of emergency departments offer buprenorphine treatment initiation on demand.[83–86]

The US Centers for Disease Control recommends coprescribing naloxone for patients on prescription opioids who are at increased risk of overdose, including those with a history of overdose or substance use disorder, higher opioid dosages (≥50 mg of morphine-equivalent/d), or concurrent benzodiazepine use.[87] Some US states now require naloxone to be coprescribed with high-dose opioids.[88] Opioid overdose survivors and persons with active opioid use disorder may also benefit from naloxone prescribing. Naloxone distribution from the emergency department is practical and well-accepted.[89] In an emergency department population, take-home naloxone seems to be more effective than naloxone prescribing; in one study, less than 2% of prescriptions for low-cost intranasal naloxone kits sent to a pharmacy 200 meters from the emergency department were filled.[90] Overdose education and naloxone distributions are also pragmatic following inpatient admissions and in the outpatient clinic setting.[91,92]

SUMMARY

In recent years the prescription opioid overdose epidemic has decreased, but has been more than offset by increases in overdose because of fentanyl and fentanyl analogues. Opioid overdose patients should receive naloxone if they have significant respiratory depression and/or loss of protective airway reflexes. Patients who receive naloxone should be observed for recurrent opioid effects. Patients with opioid overdose may be admitted to the ICU for naloxone infusions, treatment of noncardiogenic pulmonary edema, autonomic instability, or the sequelae of hypoxia-ischemia or cardiac arrest. Primary and secondary prevention are important to reduce the number of people with life-threatening opioid overdose.

DISCLOSURE

Dr. Lavonas has served as a paid consultant for the American Heart Association.

REFERENCES

1. Centers for Disease Control and Prevention. Annual surveillance report of drug-related risks and outcomes — United States surveillance special report. Atlanta (GA): Centers for Disease Control and Prevention, U.S. Department of Health and Human Services; 2019. Available at: https://www.cdc.gov/drugoverdose/pdf/pubs/2019-cdc-drug-surveillancereport.pdf. Accessed June 19, 2020.
2. Tori ME, Larochelle MR, Naimi TS. Alcohol or benzodiazepine co-involvement with opioid overdose deaths in the United States, 1999-2017. JAMA Netw Open 2020; 3(4):e202361.
3. Jones CM, Einstein EB, Compton WM. Changes in synthetic opioid involvement in drug overdose deaths in the United States, 2010-2016. JAMA 2018;319(17): 1819–21.
4. Valentino RJ, Volkow ND. Untangling the complexity of opioid receptor function. Neuropsychopharmacology 2018;43(13):2514–20.
5. Butler B, Rubin G, Lawrance A, et al. Estimating the risk of fatal arrhythmia in patients in methadone maintenance treatment for heroin addiction. Drug Alcohol Rev 2011;30(2):173–80.
6. Kim HK, Manini A. Methadone-associated sudden cardiac death? Am J Med 2008;121(9):e11.
7. Leece P, Cavacuiti C, Macdonald EM, et al. Predictors of opioid-related death during methadone therapy. J Subst Abuse Treat 2015;57:30–5.
8. Hoffman JR, Schriger DL, Luo JS. The empiric use of naloxone in patients with altered mental status: a reappraisal. Ann Emerg Med 1991;20(3):246–52.
9. Friedman MS, Manini AF. Validation of criteria to guide prehospital naloxone administration for drug-related altered mental status. J Med Toxicol 2016;12(3): 270–5.
10. Lim KS, Hew YC, Lau HK, et al. Bulbar signs in normal population. Can J Neurol Sci 2009;36(1):60–4.
11. Davies AE, Kidd D, Stone SP, et al. Pharyngeal sensation and gag reflex in healthy subjects. Lancet 1995;345(8948):487–8.
12. Leder SB. Videofluoroscopic evaluation of aspiration with visual examination of the gag reflex and velar movement. Dysphagia 1997;12(1):21–3.
13. Mackway-Jones K, Moulton C. Towards evidence based emergency medicine: best BETs from the Manchester Royal Infirmary. Gag reflex and intubation. J Accid Emerg Med 1999;16(6):444–5.
14. Kulig K, Rumack BH, Rosen P. Gag reflex in assessing level of consciousness. Lancet 1982;1(8271):565.
15. Burket GA, Horowitz BZ, Hendrickson RG, et al. Endotracheal intubation in the pharmaceutical-poisoned patient: a narrative review of the literature. J Med Toxicol 2020. https://doi.org/10.1007/s13181-020-00779-3.

16. Hårdemark Cedborg AI, Sundman E, Bodén K, et al. Effects of morphine and midazolam on pharyngeal function, airway protection, and coordination of breathing and swallowing in healthy adults. Anesthesiology 2015;122(6):1253–67.

17. Hårdemark Cedborg AI, Sundman E, Bodén K, et al. Co-ordination of spontaneous swallowing with respiratory airflow and diaphragmatic and abdominal muscle activity in healthy adult humans. Exp Physiol 2009;94(4):459–68.

18. Dahan A, Aarts L, Smith TW. Incidence, reversal, and prevention of opioid-induced respiratory depression. Anesthesiology 2010;112(1):226–38.

19. Boyer EW. Management of opioid analgesic overdose. N Engl J Med 2012; 367(2):146–55.

20. Neale J, Strang J. Naloxone—does over-antagonism matter? Evidence of iatrogenic harm after emergency treatment of heroin/opioid overdose. Addiction 2015;110(10):1644–52.

21. Schwartz JA, Koenigsberg MD. Naloxone-induced pulmonary edema. Ann Emerg Med 1987;16(11):1294–6.

22. Jiwa N, Sheth H, Silverman R. Naloxone-induced non-cardiogenic pulmonary edema: a case report. Drug Saf Case Rep 2018;5(1):20.

23. Sporer KA, Dorn E. Heroin-related noncardiogenic pulmonary edema: a case series. Chest 2001;120(5):1628–32.

24. Rzasa Lynn R, Galinkin JL. Naloxone dosage for opioid reversal: current evidence and clinical implications. Ther Adv Drug Saf 2018;9(1):63–88.

25. Farkas A, Lynch MJ, Westover R, et al. Pulmonary complications of opioid overdose treated with naloxone. Ann Emerg Med 2020;75(1):39–48.

26. Clarke SFJ, Dargan PI, Jones AL. Naloxone in opioid poisoning: walking the tightrope. Emerg Med J 2005;22(9):612.

27. Wanger K, Brough L, Macmillan I, et al. Intravenous vs subcutaneous naloxone for out-of-hospital management of presumed opioid overdose. Acad Emerg Med 1998;5(4):293–9.

28. Dietze P, Jauncey M, Salmon A, et al. Effect of intranasal vs intramuscular naloxone on opioid overdose: a randomized clinical trial. JAMA Netw Open 2019;2(11):e1914977.

29. Jiang T. Clinical and regulatory overview of naloxone products intended for use in the community. Washington, DC: Division of Anesthesia, Analgesia, and Addiction Products, Center for Drug Evaluation and Research, US Food and Drug Administration; 2018. Available at: https://www.fda.gov/media/121189/download. Accessed June 19, 2020.

30. Lavonas EJ, Drennan IR, Gabrielli A, et al. Part 10: special circumstances of resuscitation. Circulation 2015;132(18_suppl_2):S501–18.

31. Moss RB, Carlo DJ. Higher doses of naloxone are needed in the synthetic opioid era. Subst Abuse Treat Prev Policy 2019;14(1):6.

32. US Drug Enforcement Administration. 2019 Drug Enforcement Administration National Drug Threat Assessment. 2019. Available at: https://www.dea.gov/sites/default/files/2020-01/2019-NDTA-final-01-14-2020_Low_Web-DIR-007-20_2019.pdf. Accessed June 19, 2019.

33. Willman MW, Liss DB, Schwarz ES, et al. Do heroin overdose patients require observation after receiving naloxone? Clin Toxicol 2017;55(2):81–7.

34. Greene JA, Deveau BJ, Dol JS, et al. Incidence of mortality due to rebound toxicity after 'treat and release' practices in prehospital opioid overdose care: a systematic review. Emerg Med J 2019;36(4):219–24.

35. Kolinsky D, Keim SM, Cohn BG, et al. Is a prehospital treat and release protocol for opioid overdose safe? J Emerg Med 2017;52(1):52–8.

36. Aghabiklooei A, Hassanian-Moghaddam H, Zamani N, et al. Effectiveness of naltrexone in the prevention of delayed respiratory arrest in opioid-naive methadone-intoxicated patients. Biomed Res Int 2013;2013:903172.

37. Berkowitz BA. The relationship of pharmacokinetics to pharmacological activity: morphine, methadone and naloxone. Clin Pharmacokinet 1976;1(3):219–30.

38. Abuse NIoD. Opioid overdose reversal with naloxone (Narcan, Evzio). 2020. Available at: https://www.drugabuse.gov/drug-topics/opioids/opioid-overdose-reversal-naloxone-narcan-evzio. Accessed June 19, 2020.

39. Christenson J, Etherington J, Grafstein E, et al. Early discharge of patients with presumed opioid overdose: development of a clinical prediction rule. Acad Emerg Med 2000;7(10):1110–8.

40. Clemency BM, Eggleston W, Shaw EW, et al. Hospital observation upon reversal (HOUR) with naloxone: a prospective clinical prediction rule validation study. Acad Emerg Med 2019;26(1):7–15.

41. Goldfrank L, Weisman RS, Errick JK, et al. A dosing nomogram for continuous infusion intravenous naloxone. Ann Emerg Med 1986;15(5):566–70.

42. Katz S, Aberman A, Frand UI, et al. Heroin pulmonary edema. Am Rev Respir Dis 1972;106(3):472–4.

43. Kienbaum P, Thürauf N, Michel MC, et al. Profound increase in epinephrine concentration in plasma and cardiovascular stimulation after mu-opioid receptor blockade in opioid-addicted patients during barbiturate-induced anesthesia for acute detoxification. Anesthesiology 1998;88(5):1154–61.

44. Hakim TS, Grunstein MM, Michel RP. Opiate action in the pulmonary circulation. Pulm Pharmacol 1992;5(3):159–65.

45. Olsen KS. Naloxone administration and laryngospasm followed by pulmonary edema. Intensive Care Med 1990;16(5):340–1.

46. Sterrett C, Brownfield J, Korn CS, et al. Patterns of presentation in heroin overdose resulting in pulmonary edema. Am J Emerg Med 2003;21(1):32–4.

47. Ridgway ZA, Pountney AJ. Acute respiratory distress syndrome induced by oral methadone managed with non-invasive ventilation. Emerg Med J 2007;24(9):681.

48. Dela Cruz M, Slutsky J, Gillespie M, et al. Atrial fibrillation after naloxone administration: a rare complication of opioid feversal. J Emerg Med Trauma Surg Care 2017;1. Available at: https://www.henrypublishinggroups.com/wp-content/uploads/2017/09/atrial-fibrillation-after-naloxone-administration-a-rare-complication-of-opioid-reversal.pdf.

49. Lameijer H, Azizi N, Ligtenberg JJM, et al. Ventricular tachycardia after naloxone administration: a drug related complication? case report and literature review. Drug Saf Case Rep 2014;1(1):2.

50. Dezfulian C, Orkin A, Maron B, et al. Opioid-associated out-of-hospital cardiac arrest: distinctive clinical features and implications for healthcare and public responses: a scientific statement from the American Heart Association. Circulation, in press.

51. Jamshidi F, Sadighi B, Aghakhani K, et al. Brain computed tomographic scan findings in acute opium overdose patients. Am J Emerg Med 2013;31(1):50–3.

52. Doshi R, Majmundar M, Kansara T, et al. Frequency of cardiovascular events and in-hospital mortality with opioid overdose hospitalizations. Am J Cardiol 2019; 124(10):1528–33.

53. Zibbell JE, Iqbal K, Patel RC, et al. Increases in hepatitis C virus infection related to injection drug use among persons aged ≤30 years - Kentucky, Tennessee, Virginia, and West Virginia, 2006-2012. MMWR Morb Mortal Wkly Rep 2015;64(17): 453–8.

54. Hassan A, Al Jawad M, AA, et al. Bilateral basal ganglia lesions in patients with heroin overdose: a report of two cases. Case Rep Acute Med 2019;2019(2):62–8.
55. Andersen SN, Skullerud K. Hypoxic/ischaemic brain damage, especially pallidal lesions, in heroin addicts. Forensic Sci Int 1999;102(1):51–9.
56. Krantz MJ, Mehler PS. QTc prolongation: methadone's efficacy-safety paradox. Lancet 2006;368(9535):556–7.
57. Isbister GK, Brown AL, Gill A, et al. QT interval prolongation in opioid agonist treatment: analysis of continuous 12-lead electrocardiogram recordings. Br J Clin Pharmacol 2017;83(10):2274–82.
58. Wightman RS, Hoffman RS, Howland MA, et al. Not your regular high: cardiac dysrhythmias caused by loperamide. Clin Toxicol (Phila) 2016;54(5):454–8.
59. Katz KD, Cannon RD, Cook MD, et al. Loperamide-induced torsades de pointes: a case series. J Emerg Med 2017;53(3):339–44.
60. Wu PE, Juurlink DN. Clinical review: loperamide toxicity. Ann Emerg Med 2017; 70(2):245–52.
61. Chan A, Isbister GK, Kirkpatrick CM, et al. Drug-induced QT prolongation and torsades de pointes: evaluation of a QT nomogram. QJM 2007;100(10):609–15.
62. Moss R, Munt B. Injection drug use and right sided endocarditis. Heart 2003; 89(5):577–81.
63. Silverman M, Slater J, Jandoc R, et al. Hydromorphone and the risk of infective endocarditis among people who inject drugs: a population-based, retrospective cohort study. Lancet Infect Dis 2020;20(4):487–97.
64. Kasper KJ, Manoharan I, Hallam B, et al. A controlled-release oral opioid supports S. aureus survival in injection drug preparation equipment and may increase bacteremia and endocarditis risk. PLoS One 2019;14(8):e0219777.
65. Gray ME, Rogawski McQuade ET, Scheld WM, et al. Rising rates of injection drug use associated infective endocarditis in Virginia with missed opportunities for addiction treatment referral: a retrospective cohort study. BMC Infect Dis 2018; 18(1):532.
66. Schranz AJ, Fleischauer A, Chu VH, et al. Trends in drug use-associated infective endocarditis and heart valve surgery, 2007 to 2017: a study of statewide discharge data. Ann Intern Med 2019;170(1):31–40.
67. Weir MA, Slater J, Jandoc R, et al. The risk of infective endocarditis among people who inject drugs: a retrospective, population-based time series analysis. CMAJ 2019;191(4):E93–9.
68. Nenninger EK, Carwile JL, Ahrens KA, et al. Rural-Urban differences in hospitalizations for opioid use-associated infective endocarditis in the United States, 2003-2016. Open Forum Infect Dis 2020;7(2):ofaa045.
69. Jackson KA, Bohm MK, Brooks JT, et al. Invasive methicillin-resistant Staphylococcus aureus infections among persons who inject drugs - six sites, 2005-2016. MMWR Morb Mortal Wkly Rep 2018;67(22):625–8.
70. Conrad C, Bradley HM, Broz D, et al. Community outbreak of HIV infection linked to injection drug use of oxymorphone–Indiana, 2015. MMWR Morb Mortal Wkly Rep 2015;64(16):443–4.
71. Berg RA, Hemphill R, Abella BS, et al. Part 5: adult basic life support. Circulation 2010;122(18_suppl_3):S685–705.
72. Guy G, Zhang K, Bohm M, et al. Vital signs: changes in opioid prescribing in the United States, 2006–2015. MMWR Morb Mortal Wkly Rep 2017;66:697–704.
73. Colorado Hospital Association, Colorado Chapter of American College of Emergency Physicians, Colorado Consortium for Prescription Drug Abuse Prevention, et al. 2017 Colorado Opioid Safety Pilot Results Report. Greenwood Village (CO):

Colorado Hospital Association; 2018. Available at: https://cha.com/wp-content/uploads/2018/06/CHA-Opioid-Pilot-Results-Report-May-2018.pdf. Accessed June 26, 2020.

74. Colorado Hospital Association. Colorado ALTO Project: Clinician Training Materials. Greenwood Village (CO): Colorado Hospital Association; 2020. Available at: https://cha.com/wp-content/uploads/2018/04/Colorado-ALTO-Project-Clinician-Toolkit.pdf. Accessed June 26, 2020.

75. Colorado Hospital Association. Colorado ALTO Project: Nurse Training Materials. Greenwood Village (CO): Colorado Hospital Association; 2020. Available at: https://cha.com/wp-content/uploads/2018/04/Colorado-ALTO-Project-Nursing-Toolkit.pdf. Accessed June 26, 2020.

76. Berna C, Kulich RJ, Rathmell JP. Tapering long-term opioid therapy in chronic noncancer pain: evidence and recommendations for everyday practice. Mayo Clin Proc 2015;90(6):828–42.

77. Centers for Disease Control and Prevention. Module 6: dosing and titration of opioids: how much, how long, and how and when to stop?. 2017. Available at: https://www.cdc.gov/drugoverdose/training/dosing/. Accessed June 26, 2020.

78. Centers for Disease Control and Prevention. Pocket Guide: Tapering Opioids for Chronic Pain. Atlanta (GA): CDC; 2016. Available at: https://www.cdc.gov/drugoverdose/pdf/clinical_pocket_guide_tapering-a.pdf. Accessed June 26, 2020.

79. Weiner SG, Baker O, Bernson D, et al. One-year mortality of patients after emergency department treatment for nonfatal opioid overdose. Ann Emerg Med 2020; 75(1):13–7.

80. Bernstein SL, D'Onofrio G. Screening, treatment initiation, and referral for substance use disorders. Addict Sci Clin Pract 2017;12(1):18.

81. D'Onofrio G, Chawarski MC, O'Connor PG, et al. Emergency department-initiated buprenorphine for opioid dependence with continuation in primary care: outcomes during and after intervention. J Gen Intern Med 2017;32(6):660–6.

82. Larochelle MR, Bernson D, Land T, et al. Medication for opioid use disorder after nonfatal opioid overdose and association with mortality: a cohort study. Ann Intern Med 2018;169(3):137–45.

83. Herring AA, Perrone J, Nelson LS. Managing opioid withdrawal in the emergency department with buprenorphine. Ann Emerg Med 2019;73(5):481–7.

84. Cisewski DH, Santos C, Koyfman A, et al. Approach to buprenorphine use for opioid withdrawal treatment in the emergency setting. Am J Emerg Med 2019; 37(1):143–50.

85. Kaucher KA, Caruso EH, Sungar G, et al. Evaluation of an emergency department buprenorphine induction and medication-assisted treatment referral program. Am J Emerg Med 2020;38(2):300–4.

86. Edwards FJ, Wicelinski R, Gallagher N, et al. Treating opioid withdrawal with buprenorphine in a community hospital emergency department: an outreach program. Ann Emerg Med 2020;75(1):49–56.

87. Dowell D, Haegerich TM, Chou R. CDC guideline for prescribing opioids for chronic pain–United States, 2016. JAMA 2016;315(15):1624–45.

88. ASTHO Staff. Increasing number of states require naloxone to be co-prescribed with opioids. ASTHO Experts Blog. Arlington (VA): Association of State and Territorial Health Officials; 2019. Available at: https://www.astho.org/StatePublicHealth/Increasing-Number-of-States-Require-Naloxone-Co-Prescribed-with-Opioids/08-15-19/. Accessed June 26, 2020.

89. Gunn AH, Smothers ZPW, Schramm-Sapyta N, et al. The emergency department as an opportunity for naloxone distribution. West J Emerg Med 2018;19(6): 1036–42.
90. Shaw S, Nekouei K, Kaucher K. Integration of pharmacy interns in the discharge counseling of intranasal naloxone rescue kits in the emergency department. Pharmacotherapy 2014;34:E271.
91. Peckham AM, Boggs DL. The overdose education and naloxone distribution program at a VA hospital. Fed Pract 2016;33(11):28–31.
92. Oliva EM, Nevedal A, Lewis ET, et al. Patient perspectives on an opioid overdose education and naloxone distribution program in the U.S. Department of Veterans Affairs. Subst Abus 2016;37(1):118–26.

Comprehensive Cardiac Care
After Cardiac Arrest

Barry Burstein, MD[a], Jacob C. Jentzer, MD[a,b],*

KEYWORDS

- Cardiac arrest • Sudden cardiac death • Resuscitation
- Targeted temperature management • Post–cardiac arrest syndrome
- Postarrest myocardial dysfunction

KEY POINTS

- Cardiac disease causes the majority of cases of cardiac arrest (CA), and coronary artery disease (CAD) is present in more than half of out-of-hospital CA patients who undergo coronary angiography.
- Diagnosing and treating potential cardiac etiologies of CA (including coronary angiography to identify unstable CAD) are primary diagnostic and therapeutic concerns, to prevent recurrent CA or hemodynamic decompensation.
- Postarrest myocardial dysfunction, the systemic inflammatory response, and the hemodynamic effects of targeted temperature management can contribute to the evolving shock phenotype that is common after CA.
- Resuscitation targets should be tailored to the restoration of systemic and neurologic perfusion, recognizing that the injured brain may require a higher blood pressure to maintain adequate cerebral perfusion.

INTRODUCTION

Cardiac arrest (CA) affects more than 500,000 adults in the United States each year; although a majority of patients suffer from out-of-hospital CA (OHCA), more than 200,000 patients suffer from in-hospital CA (IHCA) annually.[1] Cardiovascular disease is a major trigger for CA, as summarized in **Fig. 1**. OHCA and shockable rhythms are associated more often with cardiac etiologies (particularly an acute coronary event); IHCA and non-shockable rhythms more often are noncardiac.[2,3]

Only 12% and 24% of patients survive to hospital discharge after OHCA and IHCA, respectively; hospital mortality in both groups is similar if they survive to intensive care

[a] Division of Pulmonary and Critical Care Medicine, Department of Internal Medicine, Mayo Clinic, 200 First Street Southwest, Rochester, MN 55905, USA; [b] Department of Cardiovascular Medicine, Mayo Clinic, 200 First Street Southwest, Rochester, MN 55905, USA
* Corresponding author. Department of Cardiovascular Medicine, Mayo Clinic, 200 First Street Southwest, Rochester, MN 55905.
E-mail address: jentzer.jacob@mayo.edu

Crit Care Clin 36 (2020) 771–786
https://doi.org/10.1016/j.ccc.2020.07.007
0749-0704/20/© 2020 Elsevier Inc. All rights reserved.
criticalcare.theclinics.com

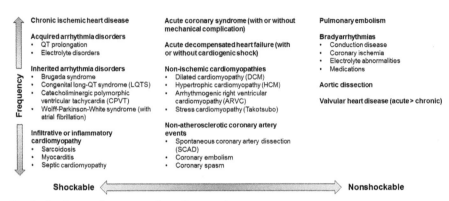

Fig. 1. Cardiovascular causes of cardiac arrest.

unit admission.[4,5] Early deaths (within the first 1–2 days) generally are due to refractory cardiogenic shock (CS), recurrent CA, or multiorgan failure; these causes of death generally are more common in IHCA patients.[5,6] Later deaths typically are associated with anoxic brain injury, which is associated with more than 70% of in-hospital deaths and account for a majority of deaths after OHCA.[7] Optimal cardiovascular care after CA may improve outcomes by providing hemodynamic stabilization to prevent progression of shock, organ failure, and brain injury.

OVERVIEW OF POSTARREST CARDIOVASCULAR CARE

Patients are at extremely high risk of cardiovascular complications in the minutes and hours that follow return of spontaneous circulation (ROSC), with approximately 50% of patients suffering recurrent CA and the majority having circulatory shock.[8,9] Comprehensive cardiovascular care should begin in the emergency department and focus on diagnostic and therapeutic considerations that are likely to improve survival (**Fig. 2**).

	Emergency Department	Critical Care Unit	Ward
Diagnosis	Electrocardiogram Rhythm strip assessment POCUS Focused history Laboratories Neurological assessment	Echocardiography Toxicology screen Troponins	Cardiac MRI Repeat echocardiography
	Coronary angiography		Electrophysiology study
Therapy	Central venous catheter Arterial catheter IV fluids Vasopressors Dual antiplatelet therapy IV heparin Antiarrhythmic agents	Pulmonary artery catheter Inotropic support MCS	CAD and HF optimization
	TTM Coronary revascularization		ICD implantation

Time →

Fig. 2. Overview of diagnostic and therapeutic considerations in postarrest care, by clinical setting. HF, heart failure; IV, intravenous; MRI, magnetic resonance imaging.

The optimal approach should include identification and treatment of the precipitating cause and optimization of tissue and organ perfusion.

DIAGNOSTIC CONSIDERATIONS

The potential etiologies of CA differ between OHCA and IHCA (see **Fig. 1**).[10] Conditions that are amenable to urgent intervention should be identified immediately and treated in order to prevent hemodynamic deterioration or recurrent CA. An electrocardiogram (ECG) should be obtained as soon as possible to identify correctable pathology, such as myocardial ischemia, complete heart block, or hyperkalemia. The ECG also can suggest the presence of pulmonary embolism or cardiac tamponade. The metabolic derangements that characterize the immediate post-ROSC period may mimic or mask typical ECG findings of myocardial ischemia, leading to limited sensitivity and specificity.[11]

Identification of Acute Coronary Syndrome

Acute myocardial ischemia is the leading reversible cause of CA; a majority of patients undergoing coronary angiography after OHCA have underlying coronary artery disease (CAD), making exclusion of unstable CAD a primary goal of initial assessment.[11] Acute coronary syndrome (ACS) is present in at least 50% to 60% of both OHCA and IHCA, especially in the presence of a shockable rhythm.[12,13] CA due to ACS is associated with a more favorable prognosis, likely due to the presence of a treatable etiology.[14]

Nearly all CA patients with ST-segment elevation myocardial infarction (STEMI) have unstable CAD; most CA patients without STEMI have CAD, but unstable CAD is present in only 20% to 35% of these patients.[15–17] Predictors of unstable CAD or acute coronary occlusion (ACO) after OHCA are shown in **Table 1**, and the ACS^2 score can help provide an estimate of the probability of ACO after CA (which should drive a potential benefit of revascularization).[15,18] The diagnostic value of

Table 1		
Predictors of acute coronary occlusion after cardiac arrest		
Evaluation Source	**Established**	**Possible**
Clinical history	Shockable rhythm Chest pain or angina	History of smoking, diabetes mellitus, CAD Heart failure symptoms Brief arrest
ECG	ST-segment elevation	ST-segment depression QRS prolongation
Echocardiography		LV systolic dysfunction Regional wall motion abnormalities
Biomarkers		Elevated cardiac troponin level
ACS^2 score 1. Angina (1 point) 2. Congestive heart failure (1 point) 3. Shockable rhythm (1 point) 4. ST-segment elevations in 2 contiguous leads (2 points)		Higher ACS^2 score (especially ≥2 points) predicts higher likelihood of coronary occlusion.

Adapted from Jentzer JC, Herrmann J, Prasad AP, et al. Utility and Challenges of an Early Invasive Strategy in Patients Resuscitated From Out-of-Hospital Cardiac Arrest. *JACC Cardiovasc Interv.* 2019;12(8):697-708; with permission.

cardiac troponins is limited in the immediate postarrest period, because troponin elevations are present in a vast majority of patients.[19] A very high or rising troponin level is suggestive of ACS, but there is no peak troponin cutoff with high sensitivity and specificity for ACO.[20]

CORONARY ANGIOGRAPHY IN SUSPECTED ACUTE CORONARY SYNDROME

Decisions regarding if and when to perform coronary angiography after CA must take into account the likelihood of ACO as the cause of CA as well as the likelihood of death due to neurologic causes, which would eliminate any potential benefit of revascularization.[15] Consensus guidelines recommend immediate coronary angiography for patients with CA and STEMI, who have a large amount of jeopardized myocardium and the most to gain from revascularization.[21–23] Urgent coronary angiography also should be considered in CA patients without STEMI in the presence of CS or recurrent ventricular arrhythmias (**Fig. 3**).[22–25] The SHOCK trial demonstrated a mortality benefit of early revascularization in patients with ACS and CS; it is uncertain if these findings apply to CA patients with other forms of shock.[26] The CULPRIT-SHOCK study of patients with CS and ACS (including 55% patients with CA) found decreased death and renal injury with culprit vessel revascularization only, compared with multivessel revascularization.[27]

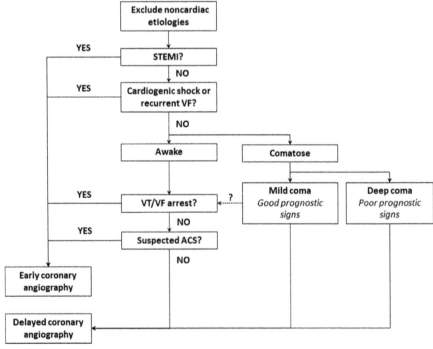

Fig. 3. Suggested approach to patient selection and timing of coronary angiography after cardiac arrest. Early coronary angiography is defined as within 2 hours, and deferred coronary angiography is defined as prior to hospital discharge. (*Adapted from* Jentzer JC, Herrmann J, Prasad AP, et al. Utility and Challenges of an Early Invasive Strategy in Patients Resuscitated From Out-of-Hospital Cardiac Arrest. *JACC Cardiovasc Interv.* 2019;12(8):697-708; with permission.)

Observational studies have demonstrated lower mortality in OHCA patients receiving early coronary angiography, especially revascularization.[28] These non-randomized studies are burdened, however, by selection bias and most have failed to take into account the effects of brain injury on survival after OHCA.[15] Patients with severe brain injury appear not to benefit from early coronary angiography and often die despite receiving optimal cardiac care.[29] The COACT study demonstrated that early coronary angiography does not improve outcomes among hemodynamically stable, comatose CA patients without STEMI compared with delayed coronary angiography after awakening.[16] This suggests that coronary angiography may be deferred initially in comatose OHCA patients without shock or STEMI. All patients in COACT were comatose and a majority of deaths were due to brain injury—these results do not apply to awake patients in whom brain injury is not a concern, and these patients should be strongly considered for early coronary angiography. Markers of severe brain injury have been proposed as potential exclusion criteria for urgent coronary angiography, because they reflect a greater likelihood of noncardiovascular death and lack of benefit from revascularization.[30]

Complications, such as bleeding, vessel injury, and arrhythmias, may occur in approximately 10% of CA patients receiving early coronary angiography and are less frequent in patients receiving delayed coronary angiography.[31] Because of the need for anticoagulant and antiplatelet therapy for percutaneous coronary intervention (PCI), significant bleeding should be excluded prior to proceeding with coronary angiography (including head CT to exclude intracranial bleeding for comatose patients). Patients undergoing early coronary angiography after CA can have potentially harmful delays in reaching temperature goals for targeted temperature management (TTM).[16,32] Coronary angiography and PCI can predispose to contrast-associated acute kidney injury, especially in CA patients undergoing urgent procedures due to periprocedural kidney hypoperfusion.[33]

The authors provide the following recommendations for CA patients achieving ROSC (see **Fig. 3**):

1. Immediate 12-lead ECG with subsequent determination of pretest probability of unstable CAD, severe brain injury, and bleeding risk
2. Urgent coronary angiography should be considered in the patients with the following conditions:
   A. STEMI, including true posterior myocardial infarction
   B. CS without STEMI
   C. Ventricular arrhythmia storm with suspected ACS
   D. Shockable rhythm or suspected ACS in the absence of coma
3. Culprit vessel revascularization only should be prioritized (even in patients with CS), with consideration for staged revascularization after neurologic recovery.
4. Hemodynamically stable comatose patients (including those with suspected ACS) may have coronary angiography deferred until after awakening.

Other Diagnostic Considerations

Point-of-care ultrasound (POCUS) can guide early diagnosis and management by assessing left ventricular (LV) function and/or regional wall motion abnormalities, right heart strain, and pericardial effusion.[34] An invasive hemodynamic assessment, including central venous and arterial catheter placement, is warranted for a majority of patients with CA. For patients with shock after CA, further hemodynamic assessment with a functional hemodynamic monitoring device or pulmonary artery catheter placement with venous oxygen saturation (Svo_2) measurement may be useful.

Formal echocardiography should be performed early in the clinical course to assess for potential causes of CA. A majority of patients who undergo echocardiography after OHCA have reduced LV systolic function, with a median LV ejection fraction (LVEF) of approximately 40%.[35,36] LVEF is quite dynamic after OHCA and generally lower immediately after ROSC.[36] Patients without evidence of CAD warrant nonurgent cardiac magnetic resonance imaging after awakening to exclude occult structural heart disease (especially in patients with preserved LVEF). In cases of CA with a shockable rhythm but without ACS or structural heart disease, specialized testing to exclude inherited arrhythmia syndrome may be considered.[37]

THERAPEUTIC CONSIDERATIONS
Medical Therapy in Acute Coronary Syndrome

It is unknown whether empiric medical therapy for ACS with dual-antiplatelet therapy (DAPT), including aspirin plus a P_2Y_{12} inhibitor (clopidogrel, prasugrel, or ticagrelor) and an anticoagulant (typically, intravenous heparin), is beneficial after CA; most patients in the COACT trial received DAPT and/or heparin.[16] For CA patients with STEMI or suspected ACS undergoing urgent coronary angiography, pretreatment with DAPT and intravenous heparin is reasonable, with DAPT continued after PCI.[21–23] For CA patients receiving initial medical therapy without early coronary angiography, DAPT with or without intravenous heparin can be considered when ACS is suspected and the bleeding risk is low.

Shock After Cardiac Arrest

Hemodynamic instability and vasopressor-dependent shock are common after CA, occurring in 50% to 80% of patients; shock severity and vasopressor requirements are major predictors of adverse outcomes.[38] Shock after CA is driven by the post-CA syndrome, which is triggered by global ischemia and reperfusion.[9] Post-CA syndrome includes postarrest myocardial dysfunction (PAMD) and a systemic inflammatory response syndrome (SIRS) superimposed on the inciting cardiac pathology.[9,39–41] PAMD can manifest as myocardial systolic and/or diastolic dysfunction, contributing to hemodynamic instability and influencing the clinical response to supportive therapies.[9] The pathophysiologic mechanisms that contribute to PAMD and shock after CA are summarized in **Table 2**.

Shock after CA often manifests initially as CS due to PAMD, with an evolving hemodynamic phenotype; vasoplegia and hypovolemia may contribute to the clinical picture, and mixed shock states are common (**Fig. 4**).[38,42,43] Patients often have a honeymoon period of hemodynamic stability immediately after ROSC, and hemodynamic instability may not manifest for several minutes or hours after the initial arrest.[44] Patients initially develop a low-output CS state from PAMD that peaks 6 hours to 8 hours after presentation.[45] Subsequently, the hemodynamic profile often shifts to a progressively more vasodilatory state as SIRS and multiorgan dysfunction develop, often manifesting a mixed shock picture if PAMD persists.[9,45] Vasopressor requirements may persist for greater than 24 hours, correlating with the severity of SIRS and cytokine levels and raising suspicion for the development of sepsis.[9,45,46]

Hemodynamic Targets

Early aggressive resuscitation and hemodynamic stabilization are essential to avoid persistent hypoperfusion that can result in further ischemic organ injury.[47] After CA, the injured brain may demonstrate impaired blood flow autoregulation, which can lead to worsened brain injury due to ongoing brain ischemia.[48] The initial focus of

Table 2
Pathophysiologic processes driving postarrest myocardial dysfunction and shock after cardiac arrest

Ischemia-reperfusion injury	Stress cardiomyopathy
• Cellular sodium/calcium overload	• Catecholamine-induced myocardial toxicity
• Reactive oxygen species excess	• β-Receptor dysfunction
• Intracellular acidosis	• Myocardial apoptosis
SIRS	Underlying cardiac disease
• Nitric oxide–mediated vasodilation	• Cardiomyopathy (ischemic or dilated)
• Microvascular/endothelial dysfunction	• Acute myocardial infarction
• Dysregulated coagulation system	• Demand myocardial ischemia
• Cytokine-mediated myocardial depression	• Myocardial stunning after reperfusion
• Capillary leak	
Metabolic derangements	Iatrogenic factors
• Lactic acidosis	• Myocardial depressants (eg, sedation)
• Electrolyte abnormalities	• Defibrillator shocks
• Adrenal insufficiency	• Cardiovascular effects of hypothermia
• Mitochondrial dysfunction	• Volume overload

Data from Jentzer JC, Chonde MD, Dezfulian C. Myocardial Dysfunction and Shock After Cardiac Arrest. *Biomed Res Int.* 2015;2015:314796.

resuscitation should be on maintenance of adequate mean arterial pressure (MAP) and normalization of clinical perfusion, lactate levels, and urine output. Serum lactate is elevated initially as a result of the no-flow period prior to ROSC, and high lactate levels suggest prolonged hypoperfusion and are associated with worse outcomes.[30,49] Lactate clearance indicates adequate tissue perfusion, and capillary refill time may provide complementary information as a resuscitation endpoint.[50,51] Low central or mixed Svo_2 less than 65% implies inadequate tissue oxygen delivery, and a widened arterial-venous Pco_2 gap likewise may imply ongoing tissue-level hypoperfusion.[52] Early goal-directed hemodynamic optimization strategies have been proposed as part of a care bundle after CA, including TTM and early coronary angiography when appropriate.[53–55]

Neurologic outcomes are worse among CA patients with systolic blood pressure less than 90 mm Hg to 100 mm Hg or an MAP less than 65 mm Hg to 70 mm Hg early after resuscitation.[24,56] Hypotension is a marker of illness severity, and patients with

		Volume Status	
		Wet	**Dry**
Peripheral Circulation	**Cold**	Classic Cardiogenic Shock (↓CI; ↑SVRI; ↑PCWP)	Euvolemic Cardiogenic Shock (↓CI; ↑SVRI; ↔PCWP)
	Warm	Vasodilatory Cardiogenic Shock or Mixed Shock (↓CI; ↓/↔SVRI; ↑PCWP)	Vasodilatory Shock (Not Cardiogenic Shock) (↑CI; ↓SVRI; ↓PCWP)

Fig. 4. Hemodynamic profiles and tailored therapies among patients resuscitated after cardiac arrest. CI, cardiac index; PCWP, pulmonary capillary wedge pressure; SVR, systemic vascular resistance. (Source: American Heart Association. Contemporary Management of Cardiogenic Shock: A Scientific Statement From the American Heart Association. Circulation 2017;136(16):e232-e268.)

hypotension early after CA had greater overall illness severity and neurologic injury at baseline. MAP targets greater than 80 mm Hg have been proposed to improve cerebral blood flow and neurologic outcomes, and an even higher MAP may be required for optimal cerebral perfusion after CA.[48] Randomized trials have not shown improved neurologic outcomes, however, with MAP targets of 85 mm Hg to 100 mm Hg or 80 mm Hg to 100 mm Hg after CA.[55,57,58] The increased vasopressor doses required to maintain higher MAP targets have been associated with an increase in arrhythmias, so the MAP goal must be considered in the context of vasopressor requirements.[59]

The authors suggest that clinicians target a MAP goal of greater than 70 mm Hg and a systolic blood pressure goal of greater than 100 mm Hg after CA. Higher MAP goals greater than 80 mm Hg to 85 mm Hg may be considered for selected patients, including those with preexisting hypertension, assuming this does not require excessive vasopressor doses. Uncontrolled hypertension could be potentially harmful and maintaining MAP less than or equal to 100 mm Hg with short-acting vasodilators may be reasonable.[55]

Fluid Resuscitation, Vasopressors, and Inotropic Support

Capillary leak and relative hypovolemia may develop after CA, resulting in fluid-responsive hypotension.[56] Patients with diastolic dysfunction from PAMD may develop pulmonary edema and respiratory failure with excessive fluid administration.[60] An initial fluid challenge is reasonable for patients who are hypotensive after ROSC, and a bedside assessment of fluid responsiveness may help guide further volume resuscitation (**Fig. 5**).[61] Fluid requirements often increase later in

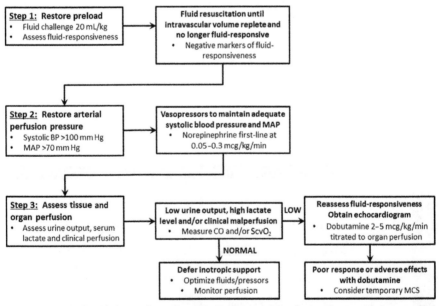

Fig. 5. Suggested early hemodynamic optimization strategy for patients with hypotension or hypoperfusion after ROSC after cardiac arrest. CO, cardiac output; CVP, central venous pressure; Scvo₂, central venous oxygen saturation (normal >70%). BP, blood pressure. (*Adapted from* Jentzer JC, Clements CM, Murphy JG, et al. Recent developments in the management of patients resuscitated from cardiac arrest. *J Crit Care.* 2017;39:97-107; with permission.)

the clinical course as a result of SIRS, vasoplegia, and/or TTM-induced polyuria; development of fluid-responsive hypotension also should raise suspicion for occult bleeding.

If hypotension persists despite adequate volume resuscitation, then vasopressor support should be initiated (see **Fig. 5**). Norepinephrine is a reasonable first option for all forms of shock after CA due to its clinical effectiveness and favorable side-effect profile.[62] A recent study of patients with CS, including many CA patients, showed a lower rate of treatment failure and adverse events (including lactic acidosis) with norepinephrine than epinephrine.[63] If hypotension persists despite adequate fluid resuscitation and high doses of norepinephrine (>0.2–0.3 μg/kg/min), then addition of epinephrine or vasopressin should be considered and a search for secondary etiologies of shock undertaken.[62] Epinephrine may be preferable if heart rate, cardiac output and/or Svo_2 are low, whereas vasopressin may be preferred in the setting of tachyarrhythmias with adequate cardiac output and Svo_2.

Inotropic agents should be considered in patients with low cardiac output (including CS) causing hypoperfusion despite adequate MAP, using the lowest necessary dose.[62] Dobutamine is the preferred inotropic agent in the acute phase, and animal studies have shown favorable responses to low doses of dobutamine in PAMD; a low dose of epinephrine can be used in patients with mixed vasodilatory shock.[64] Caution should be used with any inotropic agent (including catecholamine vasopressors) in patients with ventricular arrhythmias or myocardial ischemia.

Hemodynamic Effects of Targeted Temperature Management

Although beneficial for mitigating brain injury after CA, TTM causes myocardial depression and peripheral vasoconstriction, which can manifest as reduced heart rate, stroke volume, and reduced cardiac output.[65] TTM produces an increase in systemic vascular resistance index, either as a cause or consequence of reduced cardiac output, and the majority of patients undergoing TTM require vasopressor or inotropic support.[66] In the TTM trial, patients had worse hemodynamics and a trend toward worse outcomes at a lower target temperature of 33°C when compared with 36°C, and severe or refractory shock is a potential contraindication to TTM.[24,66,67]

Mechanical Circulatory Support

Temporary mechanical circulatory support (MCS) may be considered for patients with CS who have an inadequate clinical response or adverse effects with vasoactive medications. No temporary MCS device has been shown to improve outcomes among patients with CS in a randomized trial, and patients with CA account for approximately 50% or more of enrolled patients in CS studies.[68] The intra-aortic balloon pump produces modest hemodynamic effects by reducing cardiac afterload while supporting MAP, and failed to reduce mortality in patients with CS after acute myocardial infarction, including approximately 45% CA patients.[69] Newer peripherally inserted ventricular-assisted devices, such as the TandemHeart (LivaNova, London, United Kingdom), Impella (AbioMed, Danvers, Massachusetts), and extracorporeal membrane oxygenation have demonstrated hemodynamic improvements but no increase in survival compared with the intra-aortic balloon pump.[69–71] Failure to improve mortality despite improvements in hemodynamics in these studies may reflect initiation of MCS after establishment of organ failure or irreversible brain injury, at which time it may be too late for hemodynamic support alone to improve outcomes.[72] Although it is possible to predict which patients are likely to die from cardiovascular causes after OHCA, it remains uncertain whether prevention of early cardiovascular death using temporary MCS devices will prevent subsequent death from neurologic causes.[73]

Tachyarrhythmia Management

Ventricular tachycardia (VT) and ventricular fibrillation (VF) are common causes of CA and may recur after ROSC, especially in the immediate post-ROSC period. VT and VF often are driven by myocardial ischemia and LV dysfunction but also occur in inherited or acquired arrhythmia disorders, such as a prolonged QT interval (see **Fig. 1**).[10] Acute myocardial ischemia often triggers polymorphic VT due to enhanced automaticity within the area of ischemic myocardium, whereas monomorphic VT is due most often to myocardial scar and chronic LV dysfunction (with or without an ischemic trigger).[74] Patients with an initial shockable rhythm or subsequent ventricular arrhythmias warrant consideration of coronary angiography to evaluate for myocardial ischemia (see **Fig. 3**).

Antiarrhythmic therapy may be necessary for refractory or recurrent VT/VF, particularly when there is no reversible precipitant. There is no evidence supporting a mortality benefit of prophylactic antiarrhythmic therapy after CA due to VT/VF, and antiarrhythmics generally should be reserved for patients with post-ROSC VT/VF or the need for multiple defibrillations prior to ROSC.[75] Intravenous amiodarone and lidocaine are most commonly used antiarrhythmics for VT/VF; amiodarone appears to have higher efficacy but more adverse effects, such as hypotension and bradycardia.[76] In cases of polymorphic VT due to a prolonged QT interval, lidocaine is preferred over amiodarone because it does not prolong the QT interval further; intravenous magnesium sulfate and correction of hypokalemia are valuable adjuncts.[75] Recurrent VT/VF due to QT prolongation may benefit from pacing to increase the heart rate, which shortens the relative QT interval.[37]

Patients with VT/VF CA not triggered by an ACS should be considered for a secondary-prevention implantable cardioverter-defibrillator (ICD) prior to hospital discharge.[37] When ACS is the trigger for CA, ICD generally is not indicated except when VT/VF occurs beyond 48 hours after the ACS event.[37] Certain patients with potentially reversible causes for CA (other than ACS) still may benefit from ICD therapy due to the presence of an underlying predisposition to recurrent CA.[77] A wearable defibrillator (LifeVest, Zoll, Pittsburgh, Pennsylvania) may be considered for selected patients with VT/VF CA due to ACS, in particular those with reduced LVEF who may be candidates for ICD therapy if LV dysfunction persists after revascularization.[37]

Atrial tachyarrhythmias rarely are the cause of CA without another contributing process but commonly manifest after ROSC. For patients with hemodynamic instability triggered or aggravated by atrial arrhythmias, a rhythm control strategy of electrical cardioversion followed by antiarrhythmic therapy with amiodarone is reasonable.[78] For hemodynamically stable patients, a rate-control strategy targeting a testing heart rate less than 100 beats per minutes is warranted; β-blockers are a reasonable first-line therapy if tolerated, and amiodarone can be used for both pharmacologic rate and rhythm control in patients at low risk of systemic embolism.[78]

SUMMARY

A majority of CA survivors have a cardiovascular trigger for their event, and cardiovascular complications are common after resuscitation from CA. Cardiovascular care after CA should focus on identifying and treating reversible causes of CA and providing prompt hemodynamic stabilization to prevent worsening organ injury. Due to the predominance of noncardiovascular causes of death after CA, it remains uncertain to what extent cardiovascular procedures can reduce overall CA mortality in unselected patients. Hemodynamic optimization and reversal of the triggering etiology, however, should provide patients with the greatest chance of recovery from CA.

DISCLOSURE

The authors have nothing to disclose.

REFERENCES

1. Writing Group M, Mozaffarian D, Benjamin EJ, et al. Heart disease and stroke statistics-2016 update: a report from the American Heart Association. Circulation 2016;133(4):e38–360.
2. Wang HE, Abella BS, Callaway CW. American Heart Association National Registry of Cardiopulmonary Resuscitation I. Risk of cardiopulmonary arrest after acute respiratory compromise in hospitalized patients. Resuscitation 2008;79(2): 234–40.
3. Rajan S, Folke F, Hansen SM, et al. Incidence and survival outcome according to heart rhythm during resuscitation attempt in out-of-hospital cardiac arrest patients with presumed cardiac etiology. Resuscitation 2017;114:157–63.
4. Chan PS, McNally B, Tang F, et al. Recent trends in survival from out-of-hospital cardiac arrest in the United States. Circulation 2014;130(21):1876–82.
5. Australia and New Zealand Cardiac Arrest Outcome and Determinants of ECMO (ANZ-CODE) Investigators. The epidemiology of in-hospital cardiac arrests in Australia: a prospective multicentre observational study. Crit Care Resusc 2019;21(3):180–7.
6. Efendijev I, Folger D, Raj R, et al. Outcomes and healthcare-associated costs one year after intensive care-treated cardiac arrest. Resuscitation 2018;131:128–34.
7. Elmer J, Rittenberger JC, Coppler PJ, et al. Long-term survival benefit from treatment at a specialty center after cardiac arrest. Resuscitation 2016;108:48–53.
8. Kudenchuk PJ, Newell C, White L, et al. Prophylactic lidocaine for post resuscitation care of patients with out-of-hospital ventricular fibrillation cardiac arrest. Resuscitation 2013;84(11):1512–8.
9. Jentzer JC, Chonde MD, Dezfulian C. Myocardial dysfunction and shock after cardiac arrest. Biomed Res Int 2015;2015:314796.
10. Myat A, Song KJ, Rea T. Out-of-hospital cardiac arrest: current concepts. Lancet 2018;391(10124):970–9.
11. Zanuttini D, Armellini I, Nucifora G, et al. Predictive value of electrocardiogram in diagnosing acute coronary artery lesions among patients with out-of-hospital-cardiac-arrest. Resuscitation 2013;84(9):1250–4.
12. Hawkes C, Booth S, Ji C, et al. Epidemiology and outcomes from out-of-hospital cardiac arrests in England. Resuscitation 2017;110:133–40.
13. Wallmuller C, Meron G, Kurkciyan I, et al. Causes of in-hospital cardiac arrest and influence on outcome. Resuscitation 2012;83(10):1206–11.
14. Stecker EC, Teodorescu C, Reinier K, et al. Ischemic heart disease diagnosed before sudden cardiac arrest is independently associated with improved survival. J Am Heart Assoc 2014;3(5):e001160.
15. Jentzer JC, Herrmann J, Prasad A, et al. Utility and challenges of an early invasive strategy in patients resuscitated from out-of-hospital cardiac arrest. JACC Cardiovasc Interv 2019;12(8):697–708.
16. Lemkes JS, Janssens GN, van der Hoeven NW, et al. Coronary angiography after cardiac arrest without ST-segment elevation. N Engl J Med 2019;380(15): 1397–407.
17. Kern KB, Lotun K, Patel N, et al. Outcomes of comatose cardiac arrest survivors with and without ST-segment elevation myocardial infarction: importance of coronary angiography. JACC Cardiovasc Interv 2015;8(8):1031–40.

18. Waldo SW, Chang L, Strom JB, et al. Predicting the presence of an acute coronary lesion among patients resuscitated from cardiac arrest. Circ Cardiovasc Interv 2015;8(10):e002198.

19. Geri G, Mongardon N, Dumas F, et al. Diagnosis performance of high sensitivity troponin assay in out-of-hospital cardiac arrest patients. Int J Cardiol 2013; 169(6):449–54.

20. Dumas F, Manzo-Silberman S, Fichet J, et al. Can early cardiac troponin I measurement help to predict recent coronary occlusion in out-of-hospital cardiac arrest survivors? Crit Care Med 2012;40(6):1777–84.

21. Ibanez B, James S, Agewall S, et al. 2017 ESC Guidelines for the management of acute myocardial infarction in patients presenting with ST-segment elevation: the Task Force for the management of acute myocardial infarction in patients presenting with ST-segment elevation of the European Society of Cardiology (ESC). Eur Heart J 2018;39(2):119–77.

22. O'Gara PT, Kushner FG, Ascheim DD, et al. 2013 ACCF/AHA guideline for the management of ST-elevation myocardial infarction: a report of the American College of Cardiology Foundation/American Heart Association Task Force on practice guidelines. Circulation 2013;127(4):e362–425.

23. Amsterdam EA, Wenger NK, Brindis RG, et al. 2014 AHA/ACC guideline for the management of patients with non-ST-elevation acute coronary syndromes: a report of the American College of Cardiology/American Heart Association Task Force on practice guidelines. J Am Coll Cardiol 2014;64(24):e139–228.

24. Callaway CW, Donnino MW, Fink EL, et al. Part 8: post-Cardiac Arrest Care: 2015 American Heart Association guidelines update for cardiopulmonary resuscitation and emergency cardiovascular care. Circulation 2015;132(18 Suppl 2):S465–82.

25. Yannopoulos D, Bartos JA, Aufderheide TP, et al. The evolving role of the cardiac catheterization laboratory in the management of patients with out-of-hospital cardiac arrest: a scientific statement from the American Heart Association. Circulation 2019;139(12):e530–52.

26. Hochman JS, Sleeper LA, Webb JG, et al. Early revascularization in acute myocardial infarction complicated by cardiogenic shock. SHOCK Investigators. Should We Emergently revascularize Occluded Coronaries for cardiogenic shock. N Engl J Med 1999;341(9):625–34.

27. Thiele H, Akin I, Sandri M, et al. PCI strategies in patients with acute myocardial infarction and cardiogenic shock. N Engl J Med 2017;377(25):2419–32.

28. Barbarawi M, Zayed Y, Kheiri B, et al. Optimal timing of coronary intervention in patients resuscitated from cardiac arrest without ST-segment elevation myocardial infarction (NSTEMI): a systematic review and meta-analysis. Resuscitation 2019;144:137–44.

29. Reynolds JC, Rittenberger JC, Toma C, et al. Post Cardiac Arrest S. Risk-adjusted outcome prediction with initial post-cardiac arrest illness severity: implications for cardiac arrest survivors being considered for early invasive strategy. Resuscitation 2014;85(9):1232–9.

30. Rab T, Kern KB, Tamis-Holland JE, et al. Cardiac arrest: a treatment algorithm for emergent invasive cardiac procedures in the resuscitated comatose patient. J Am Coll Cardiol 2015;66(1):62–73.

31. Jentzer JC, Scutella M, Pike F, et al. Early coronary angiography and percutaneous coronary intervention are associated with improved outcomes after out of hospital cardiac arrest. Resuscitation 2018;123:15–21.

32. Khera R, Humbert A, Leroux B, et al. Hospital variation in the utilization and implementation of targeted temperature management in out-of-hospital cardiac arrest. Circ Cardiovasc Qual Outcomes 2018;11(11):e004829.

33. Lorenzo A, Luciano C, Peter AM, et al. Current risk of contrast-induced acute kidney injury after coronary angiography and intervention: a reappraisal of the literature. Can J Cardiol 2017;33(10):1225–8.

34. Blanco P, Martinez Buendia C. Point-of-care ultrasound in cardiopulmonary resuscitation: a concise review. J Ultrasound 2017;20(3):193–8.

35. Burstein B, Jayaraman D, Husa R. Early left ventricular ejection fraction as a predictor of survival after cardiac arrest. Acute Card Care 2016;18(2):35–9.

36. Jentzer JC, Anavekar NS, Mankad SV, et al. Changes in left ventricular systolic and diastolic function on serial echocardiography after out-of-hospital cardiac arrest. Resuscitation 2018;126:1–6.

37. Al-Khatib SM, Stevenson WG, Ackerman MJ, et al. 2017 AHA/ACC/HRS guideline for management of patients with ventricular arrhythmias and the prevention of sudden cardiac death: Executive summary: a report of the American College of Cardiology/American Heart Association Task Force on clinical practice guidelines and the heart rhythm Society. Heart Rhythm 2018;15(10):e190–252.

38. Neumar RW, Nolan JP, Adrie C, et al. Post-cardiac arrest syndrome: epidemiology, pathophysiology, treatment, and prognostication. A consensus statement from the international Liaison Committee on resuscitation (American Heart Association, Australian and New Zealand Council on resuscitation, European resuscitation Council, Heart and Stroke Foundation of Canada, InterAmerican Heart Foundation, Resuscitation Council of Asia, and the Resuscitation Council of Southern Africa); the American Heart Association emergency cardiovascular care Committee; the Council on cardiovascular Surgery and Anesthesia; the Council on cardiopulmonary, Perioperative, and Critical care; the Council on clinical Cardiology; and the stroke Council. Circulation 2008;118(23):2452–83.

39. Zia A, Kern KB. Management of postcardiac arrest myocardial dysfunction. Curr Opin Crit Care 2011;17(3):241–6.

40. Chalkias A, Xanthos T. Pathophysiology and pathogenesis of post-resuscitation myocardial stunning. Heart Fail Rev 2012;17(1):117–28.

41. Bougouin W, Cariou A. Management of postcardiac arrest myocardial dysfunction. Curr Opin Crit Care 2013;19(3):195–201.

42. Roberts BW, Kilgannon JH, Chansky ME, et al. Multiple organ dysfunction after return of spontaneous circulation in postcardiac arrest syndrome. Crit Care Med 2013;41(6):1492–501.

43. Van Diepen S, Katz JN, Albert NM, et al. Contemporary management of cardiogenic shock: a scientific statement from the American Heart Association. Circulation 2017;136(16):e232–68.

44. Bhate TD, McDonald B, Sekhon MS, et al. Association between blood pressure and outcomes in patients after cardiac arrest: a systematic review. Resuscitation 2015;97:1–6.

45. Laurent I, Monchi M, Chiche JD, et al. Reversible myocardial dysfunction in survivors of out-of-hospital cardiac arrest. J Am Coll Cardiol 2002;40(12):2110–6.

46. Bro-Jeppesen J, Kjaergaard J, Wanscher M, et al. Systemic inflammatory response and potential prognostic implications after out-of-hospital cardiac arrest: a substudy of the target temperature management trial. Crit Care Med 2015;43(6):1223–32.

47. Jentzer JC, van Diepen S, Barsness GW, et al. Cardiogenic shock classification to predict mortality in the cardiac intensive care unit. J Am Coll Cardiol 2019; 74(17):2117–28.

48. Ameloot K, De Deyne C, Ferdinande B, et al. Mean arterial pressure of 65 mm Hg versus 85-100 mm Hg in comatose survivors after cardiac arrest: Rationale and study design of the Neuroprotect post-cardiac arrest trial. Am Heart J 2017; 191:91–8.

49. Lee DH, Cho IS, Lee SH, et al. Correlation between initial serum levels of lactate after return of spontaneous circulation and survival and neurological outcomes in patients who undergo therapeutic hypothermia after cardiac arrest. Resuscitation 2015;88:143–9.

50. Hernandez G, Ospina-Tascon GA, Damiani LP, et al. Effect of a resuscitation strategy targeting peripheral perfusion status vs serum lactate levels on 28-day mortality among patients with septic shock: the ANDROMEDA-SHOCK randomized clinical trial. Jama 2019;321(7):654–64.

51. Lee TR, Kang MJ, Cha WC, et al. Better lactate clearance associated with good neurologic outcome in survivors who treated with therapeutic hypothermia after out-of-hospital cardiac arrest. Crit Care 2013;17(5):R260.

52. Chawla LS, Zia H, Gutierrez G, et al. Lack of equivalence between central and mixed venous oxygen saturation. Chest 2004;126(6):1891–6.

53. Jentzer JC, Clements CM, Wright RS, et al. Improving survival from cardiac arrest: a review of contemporary practice and challenges. Ann Emerg Med 2016; 68(6):678–89.

54. Jentzer JC, Clements CM, Murphy JG, et al. Recent developments in the management of patients resuscitated from cardiac arrest. J Crit Care 2017;39: 97–107.

55. Ameloot K, De Deyne C, Eertmans W, et al. Early goal-directed haemodynamic optimization of cerebral oxygenation in comatose survivors after cardiac arrest: the Neuroprotect post-cardiac arrest trial. Eur Heart J 2019;40(22):1804–14.

56. Nolan JP, Soar J, Cariou A, et al. European resuscitation Council and European Society of intensive care medicine 2015 guidelines for post-resuscitation care. Intensive Care Med 2015;41(12):2039–56.

57. Grand J, Lilja G, Kjaergaard J, et al. Arterial blood pressure during targeted temperature management after out-of-hospital cardiac arrest and association with brain injury and long-term cognitive function. Eur Heart J Acute Cardiovasc Care 2019. https://doi.org/10.1177/2048872619860804. 2048872619860804.

58. Jakkula P, Pettila V, Skrifvars MB, et al. Targeting low-normal or high-normal mean arterial pressure after cardiac arrest and resuscitation: a randomised pilot trial. Intensive Care Med 2018;44(12):2091–101.

59. Asfar P, Meziani F, Hamel JF, et al. High versus low blood-pressure target in patients with septic shock. N Engl J Med 2014;370(17):1583–93.

60. Rhodes A, Evans LE, Alhazzani W, et al. Surviving sepsis campaign: international guidelines for management of sepsis and septic shock: 2016. Crit Care Med 2017;45(3):486–552.

61. Monnet X, Marik PE, Teboul JL. Prediction of fluid responsiveness: an update. Ann Intensive Care 2016;6(1):111.

62. Jentzer JC, Coons JC, Link CB, et al. Pharmacotherapy update on the use of vasopressors and inotropes in the intensive care unit. J Cardiovasc Pharmacol Ther 2015;20(3):249–60.

63. Levy B, Clere-Jehl R, Legras A, et al. Epinephrine versus norepinephrine for cardiogenic shock after acute myocardial infarction. J Am Coll Cardiol 2018; 72(2):173–82.

64. Kern KB, Hilwig RW, Berg RA, et al. Postresuscitation left ventricular systolic and diastolic dysfunction. Treatment with dobutamine. Circulation 1997;95(12): 2610–3.

65. Bro-Jeppesen J, Hassager C, Wanscher M, et al. Targeted temperature management at 33 degrees C versus 36 degrees C and impact on systemic vascular resistance and myocardial function after out-of-hospital cardiac arrest: a substudy of the Target Temperature Management Trial. Circ Cardiovasc Interv 2014;7(5):663–72.

66. Bro-Jeppesen J, Annborn M, Hassager C, et al. Hemodynamics and vasopressor support during targeted temperature management at 33 degrees C versus 36 degrees C after out-of-hospital cardiac arrest: a post hoc study of the target temperature management trial*. Crit Care Med 2015;43(2):318–27.

67. Annborn M, Bro-Jeppesen J, Nielsen N, et al. The association of targeted temperature management at 33 and 36 degrees C with outcome in patients with moderate shock on admission after out-of-hospital cardiac arrest: a post hoc analysis of the Target Temperature Management trial. Intensive Care Med 2014;40(9): 1210–9.

68. Thiele H, Ohman EM, de Waha-Thiele S, et al. Management of cardiogenic shock complicating myocardial infarction: an update 2019. Eur Heart J 2019;40(32): 2671–83.

69. Thiele H, Zeymer U, Neumann F-J, et al. Intraaortic balloon support for myocardial infarction with cardiogenic shock. N Engl J Med 2012;367(14): 1287–96.

70. Ouweneel DM, Eriksen E, Sjauw KD, et al. Percutaneous mechanical circulatory support versus intra-aortic balloon pump in cardiogenic shock after acute myocardial infarction. J Am Coll Cardiol 2017;69(3):278–87.

71. Burkhoff D, Cohen H, Brunckhorst C, et al. TandemHeart Invest G. A randomized multicenter clinical study to evaluate the safety and efficacy of the TandemHeart percutaneous ventricular assist device versus conventional therapy with intra-aortic balloon pumping for treatment of cardiogenic shock. Am Heart J 2006; 152(3):469.e1–8.

72. Ouweneel DM, Engstrom AE, Sjauw KD, et al. Experience from a randomized controlled trial with Impella 2.5 versus IABP in STEMI patients with cardiogenic pre-shock. Lessons learned from the IMPRESS in STEMI trial. Int J Cardiol 2016;202:894–6.

73. Bascom KE, Dziodzio J, Vasaiwala S, et al. Derivation and validation of the CREST model for very early prediction of circulatory etiology death in patients without ST-segment-elevation myocardial infarction after cardiac arrest. Circulation 2018;137(3):273–82.

74. Nijjer SS, Luther V, Lefroy DC. Diagnosis of ventricular tachycardia. Br J Hosp Med (Lond) 2017;78(1):C2–5.

75. Soar J, Donnino MW, Maconochie I, et al. 2018 international consensus on cardiopulmonary resuscitation and emergency cardiovascular care Science with treatment recommendations summary. Resuscitation 2018;133:194–206.

76. Kudenchuk PJ, Brown SP, Daya M, et al. Amiodarone, lidocaine, or placebo in out-of-hospital cardiac arrest. N Engl J Med 2016;374(18):1711–22.

77. Ladejobi A, Pasupula DK, Adhikari S, et al. Implantable defibrillator therapy in cardiac arrest survivors with a reversible cause. Circ Arrhythm Electrophysiol 2018;11(3):e005940.

78. January CT, Wann LS, Alpert JS, et al. 2014 AHA/ACC/HRS guideline for the management of patients with atrial fibrillation: a report of the American College of Cardiology/American Heart Association Task Force on practice guidelines and the heart rhythm Society. J Am Coll Cardiol 2014;64(21):e1–76.

UNITED STATES POSTAL SERVICE ® Statement of Ownership, Management, and Circulation (All Periodicals Publications Except Requester Publications)

1. Publication Title	2. Publication Number	3. Filing Date
CRITICAL CARE CLINICS	000 – 708	9/18/2020

4. Issue Frequency	5. Number of Issues Published Annually	6. Annual Subscription Price
JAN, APR, JUL, OCT	4	$250.00

7. Complete Mailing Address of Known Office of Publication (Not printer) (Street, city, county, state, and ZIP+4®)

ELSEVIER INC.
230 Park Avenue, Suite 800
New York, NY 10169

Contact Person
Malathi Samayan
Telephone (include area code)
91-44-4299-4507

8. Complete Mailing Address of Headquarters or General Business Office of Publisher (Not printer)

ELSEVIER INC.
230 Park Avenue, Suite 800
New York, NY 10169

9. Full Names and Complete Mailing Addresses of Publisher, Editor, and Managing Editor (Do not leave blank)

Publisher (Name and complete mailing address)

DOLORES MELONI, ELSEVIER INC.
1600 JOHN F KENNEDY BLVD, SUITE 1800
PHILADELPHIA, PA 19103-2899

Editor (Name and complete mailing address)

KERRY HOLLAND, ELSEVIER INC.
1600 JOHN F KENNEDY BLVD, SUITE 1800
PHILADELPHIA, PA 19103-2899

Managing Editor (Name and complete mailing address)

PATRICK MANLEY, ELSEVIER INC.
1600 JOHN F KENNEDY BLVD, SUITE 1800
PHILADELPHIA, PA 19103-2899

10. Owner (Do not leave blank. If the publication is owned by a corporation, give the name and address of the corporation immediately followed by the names and addresses of all stockholders owning or holding 1 percent or more of the total amount of stock. If not owned by a corporation, give the names and addresses of the individual owners. If owned by a partnership or other unincorporated firm, give its name and address as well as those of each individual owner. If the publication is published by a nonprofit organization, give its name and address.)

Full Name	Complete Mailing Address
WHOLLY OWNED SUBSIDIARY OF REED/ELSEVIER, US HOLDINGS	1600 JOHN F KENNEDY BLVD, SUITE 1800 PHILADELPHIA, PA 19103-2899

11. Known Bondholders, Mortgagees, and Other Security Holders Owning or Holding 1 Percent or More of Total Amount of Bonds, Mortgages, or Other Securities. If none, check box ▶ ☐ None

Full Name	Complete Mailing Address
N/A	

12. Tax Status (For completion by nonprofit organizations authorized to mail at nonprofit rates) (Check one)
The purpose, function, and nonprofit status of this organization and the exempt status for federal income tax purposes:
☒ Has Not Changed During Preceding 12 Months
☐ Has Changed During Preceding 12 Months (Publisher must submit explanation of change with this statement)

PS Form **3526**, July 2014 [Page 1 of 4 (see instructions page 4)] PSN: 7530-01-000-9931 PRIVACY NOTICE: See our privacy policy on www.usps.com

13. Publication Title		14. Issue Date for Circulation Data Below
CRITICAL CARE CLINICS		JULY 2020

15. Extent and Nature of Circulation		Average No. Copies Each Issue During Preceding 12 Months	No. Copies of Single Issue Published Nearest to Filing Date
a. Total Number of Copies (Net press run)		286	262
b. Paid Circulation (By Mail and Outside the Mail)	(1) Mailed Outside-County Paid Subscriptions Stated on PS Form 3541 (Include paid distribution above nominal rate, advertiser's proof copies, and exchange copies)	171	162
	(2) Mailed In-County Paid Subscriptions Stated on PS Form 3541 (Include paid distribution above nominal rate, advertiser's proof copies, and exchange copies)	0	0
	(3) Paid Distribution Outside the Mails Including Sales Through Dealers and Carriers, Street Vendors, Counter Sales, and Other Paid Distribution Outside USPS®	69	63
	(4) Paid Distribution by Other Classes of Mail Through the USPS (e.g., First-Class Mail®)	0	0
c. Total Paid Distribution (Sum of 15b (1), (2), (3), and (4))	▶	240	225
d. Free or Nominal Rate Distribution (By Mail and Outside the Mail)	(1) Free or Nominal Rate Outside-County Copies included on PS Form 3541	30	21
	(2) Free or Nominal Rate In-County Copies Included on PS Form 3541	0	0
	(3) Free or Nominal Rate Copies Mailed at Other Classes Through the USPS (e.g., First-Class Mail)	0	0
	(4) Free or Nominal Rate Distribution Outside the Mail (Carriers or other means)	30	21
e. Total Free or Nominal Rate Distribution (Sum of 15d (1), (2), (3) and (4))	▶		
f. Total Distribution (Sum of 15c and 15e)	▶	270	246
g. Copies not Distributed (See Instructions to Publishers #4 (page #3))	▶	16	16
h. Total (Sum of 15f and g)	▶	286	262
i. Percent Paid (15c divided by 15f times 100)		88.88%	91.46%

* If you are claiming electronic copies, go to line 16 on page 3. If you are not claiming electronic copies, skip to line 17 on page 3.

16. Electronic Copy Circulation		Average No. Copies Each Issue During Preceding 12 Months	No. Copies of Single Issue Published Nearest to Filing Date
a. Paid Electronic Copies	▶		
b. Total Paid Print Copies (Line 15c) + Paid Electronic Copies (Line 16a)	▶		
c. Total Print Distribution (Line 15f) + Paid Electronic Copies (Line 16a)	▶		
d. Percent Paid (Both Print & Electronic Copies) (16b divided by 16c × 100)	▶		

☒ I certify that 50% of all my distributed copies (electronic and print) are paid above a nominal price.

17. Publication of Statement of Ownership

☒ If the publication is a general publication, publication of this statement is required. Will be printed in the OCTOBER 2020 issue of this publication. ☐ Publication not required.

18. Signature and Title of Editor, Publisher, Business Manager, or Owner		Date
Malathi Samayan — Distribution Controller	*Malathi Samayan*	9/18/2020

I certify that all information furnished on this form is true and complete. I understand that anyone who furnishes false or misleading information on this form or who omits material or information requested on the form may be subject to criminal sanctions (including fines and imprisonment) and/or civil sanctions (including civil penalties).

PS Form **3526**, July 2014 (Page 3 of 4) PRIVACY NOTICE: See our privacy policy on www.usps.com

Moving?

Make sure your subscription moves with you!

To notify us of your new address, find your **Clinics Account Number** (located on your mailing label above your name), and contact customer service at:

Email: journalscustomerservice-usa@elsevier.com

800-654-2452 (subscribers in the U.S. & Canada)
314-447-8871 (subscribers outside of the U.S. & Canada)

Fax number: 314-447-8029

**Elsevier Health Sciences Division
Subscription Customer Service
3251 Riverport Lane
Maryland Heights, MO 63043**

*To ensure uninterrupted delivery of your subscription, please notify us at least 4 weeks in advance of move.